AF686420

# VITAMIN NEWS

VITAMIN PRODUCTS CO. • MILWAUKEE, WISCONSIN

by

Dr. Royal Lee, DDS

INTERNATIONAL FOUNDATION FOR NUTRITION AND HEALTH

Printed in the United States of America

ISBN 0-9713314-1-3

**Published by
the International Foundation
for Nutrition and Health**

3963 Mission Blvd.
San Diego, CA 92109
619-488-8932
www.ifnh.org

# INTRODUCTION TO VITAMIN NEWS

## January 2, 1942

During the past nine years, this periodical has been published for the purpose of relaying to the physician items of technical interest on vitamins. Under this circumstance it has not been possible to arrange the material in a consistent order. A carefully compiled index is supplied to offset this disadvantage.

Since 1930, the Vitamin Products Company has been accumulating clinical information as to the unexpected extent of vitamin deficiency diseases and he have felt a definite moral obligation to pass this information on to such physicians as may be interested.

The vital importance of these facts is exemplified by the situation pictured in our vital statistics which show that more people die from the end results of vitamin deficiency than from all other causes combined, once we admit that heart disease and lowered resistance to infection come in this category.

The biochemical reasons why heart disease and lowered resistance develop as results of vitamin deficiency are only now beginning to be cleared up. This will be observed by a study of the current issue of *Vitamin News*, Pp. 141-142. But, in view of the present recognition of the fact that heart disease and lowered resistance are really an end result of vitamin deficiency, we feel a certain amount of satisfaction in knowing that they were among the first conditions observed to respond to the vitamin C concentrate prepared by the Vitamin Products Company.

V. P. concentrates, we believe, represent the first attempt to make a product of this kind exclusively for the human species in which clinical effectiveness was put above animal feeding tests in determination of their therapeutic or food value. The ultimate elimination of unit measurement of human foodstuffs, based on animal tests, is apparently inevitable in view of the substantiation of our views as to the inadequacy of such a method by the United States Department of Agriculture. (1939 Yearbook, *Food and Life,* Pp. 12, 15, 151.)

Through our work in the vitamin field during the past thirty years we have accumulated an extensive library of well-indexed material on the subject of vitamin and mineral nutrition, which we place at the disposal of physicians or other scientific investigators. Copies of any reference given in *Vitamin News* will be gladly furnished upon request.

## VITAMIN PRODUCTS COMPANY

**MILWAUKEE, WISCONSIN**

*By* **Royal Lee, D.D.S.**

# PREFACE

Knowledge is passed on to following generations through writings of people with visions. Dr. Royal Lee was a person who wanted to share his vision that enabled people to have good health through whole food nutrition.

His knowledge and energy was endless. Dr. Lee learned early on that his life's passion was nutrition. One of his favorite rewards in life was to teach how whole foods with their minerals, vitamins, enzymes and fibers worked together to maintain and to restore health.

He accomplished this by writing and publishing a newsletter called *Vitamin News* on a regular basis for many years. *Vitamin News* has so much knowledge embracing its pages that it will become one of your most honored library pieces.

A federal court mandated, over 40 years ago, that this work and various other writings and research of Dr. Lee's were to be destroyed. These books were to be forgotten. Only through perseverance for the truth did some severely edited copies continue to be printed.

*Vitamin News* slowly disappeared after Dr. Lee's death, eventually ending up on back shelves. They lay there for many years. Until recent times, some issues had been assumed lost.

The Board of Directors of the International Foundation for Nutrition and Health had a vision of its own — to publish, under one cover all of the issues of *Vitamin News*. After nearly four years of research efforts locating the lost material, numbering 22 articles, they edited and consolidated them into this publication. For the first time in nearly 40 years, *Vitamin News* is complete. This statement is relative. *Vitamin News* today is more than complete. The newly compiled version also includes a Table of Contents and full index, items that did not exist prior. Now it is possible to learn nutritional facts, in its original detail, from the greatest intuitionalist of the past century and perhaps centuries to come.

Great men are often years ahead of their time. Dr. Lee, like many other visionaries, often paid a great price. For years, the knowledge that Dr. Lee acquired about soil, plant growth, processing of natural foods and distributing products had been challenged by government agencies, drug companies and others. He fought with vigor and unusual strength for what he believed was truth. Time proved his beliefs to be true and fundamental to health principles.

Dr. Lee also proved to be a great man of his time, not only for his mentorship in the field of nutrition, but as a citizen whose knowledge of electronics helped the United States and it allies win World War II.

I never had the privilege to meet Dr. Lee, but what I did have was a close association with his wife, Mrs. Lee and the many people who worked for him. Mrs. Lee, Herb Moore (a close friend of the Lee family and employee) and I spent hours in conversation of "the good old days" when Dr. Lee was formulating and putting into production his vision and his passion of providing whole food nutrition to maintain health.

Congratulations to the Board of Directors of the International Foundation for Nutrition and Health for providing this publication as a teaching instrument. Dr. Royal Lee would have been proud of your accomplishments.

— Robert J. Peshek, D.D.S.

# ABOUT THIS PUBLICATION

When the International Foundation for Nutrition and Health decided to publish a comprehensive collection of *Vitamin News*, it became evident that there were few, if any, complete versions available. Each publication we ran across had a few pages missing here or a few missing there. That was not good enough for us. Through many phone calls and inquiries, we compiled every issue of the classic, including the full bibliography for the vitamin charts, once thought to be extinct.

In the design of this version, we varied from the original in that we used a consistent type size and font throughout. In our opinion, this will make it easier to read. In addition, we tried to keep all the original indents and design to replicate the pages from decades ago.

In attempting to keep the original feel of the publication, we did little editing of Dr. Lee's words. If you see a redundancy or a slight grammatical error, we included these because they were the original words of the author. Dr. Lee had his own style and we do not consider it our task to change his words. Sanitizing a classic work is not in the interest of anybody.

We hope you enjoy the new, *complete*, *Vitamin News*. We are sure it will always occupy a special space in the reference area of your library. Its information, for the most part, is as relevant today as it was when originally published.

# VITAMIN NEWS – TABLE OF CONTENTS

# VITAMIN NEWS

VITAMIN PRODUCTS CO. • MILWAUKEE, WISCONSIN

// VITAMIN NEWS

VITAMIN PRODUCTS CO. • MILWAUKEE, WISCONSIN

VOL. 1 August 7, 1933 No. 1

This leaflet will be issued twice a month, for the information of our professional friends and customers who desire to hear of the latest developments in the use of vitamin concentrates for the treatment of disease. Such developments have been taking place so rapidly that one not making a special effort to keep abreast of the new announcements will be amazed at their significance.

## VITAMINS and HEART DISEASE

Although "Catalyn" (a food concentrate containing all the necessary vitamins) has been found very effective for the last four years as a remedy for heart weakness and heart disorders in general, it is only within the last year that any of the literature on vitamin subjects has contained any references to this possibility.

Sherman & Smith, *The Vitamins,* page 81, state: "Absence of another vitamin B fraction apparently leads to heart block and a remarkably slow pulse ... "

Dr. D. T. Quigley, in his vitamin chart, (published by the Consolidated Book Publishers, Chicago) under vitamin C, states that a deficiency of this essential results in, among other things, physical weakness, shortness of breath, rapid respiration, rapid heart action and tendency to disease of blood vessels and heart.

Dr. Quigley also states in *Notes on Vitamins and Diets,* page 126 (Consolidated Book Publishers), "Sudden death from heart disease in relatively young or middle-aged persons is caused, in a measure, by blood vessel and heart disease resulting from lack of sufficient foods containing vitamin C."

Valvular involvement arises in many cases from infection. "The organisms may have a special affinity for heart valves and may ... produce organic disease of the heart." (Quigley, page 70.) This susceptibility and low resistance is largely a result of vitamin A deficiency, which is also known as the "anti-infective vitamin."

Vitamin B deficiency is known to produce loss of appetite through its effect of causing a loss of tone of the stomach muscles. This loss of tone also may affect the heart and muscular walls of the arterioles — resulting in heart weakness and edema, respectively. (See Sherman & Smith, page 81.)

That explains the consistent results obtained in dropsy cases with "Catalyn." The accumulation of water in the tissues can result from a great number of factors. The liver, kidneys and heart can be individually and severally to blame. But we are beginning to see that their condition, too, is a consequence of the vitamin deficiency, and the change for the better will begin to occur as soon as the real cause of the situation is corrected.

The real reason that vitamins have not been given their full credit for performing the results we have been able to demonstrate is that the full complement of vitamins have not been commercially available in a sufficiently concentrated form. Vitamins A and D have been over-popularized, and the more important members of the family — "B" and "C" — have been neglected (except by fruit growers' associations, who do not offer concentrations).

It has been noted that more or less disappointing results have attended the use of single vitamin concentrates. This is true of "A" and "D," particularly the "synthetic" D — Viosterol, etc.

The reason for this is: The various vitamins cooperate in producing a given result or in the promotion of a particular function. For instance, as we have mentioned in the beginning of these comments, vitamin A deficiency can induce susceptibility to infection of the heart valves, "B" deficiency can paralyze the nervous control and causes muscular weakness of the heart; and "C" deficiency will cause a shortness of breath, rapid heart action, and rapid respiration.

What physician is not entirely familiar with all these symptoms without knowing the actual causative factors?

Quigley, Page 111, gives us a picture of conditions that is not flattery to our (modern) civilization.

## COMMERCIALISM AND PROPAGANDA IN

## FOOD DISTRIBUTION

> "The most common non-vitamin foods are sugar, white flour, white rice, and macaroni products. These have become common foods, in fact for the average civilized American individual, they constitute from sixty to ninety per cent of the total food intake. These have become common foods because of commercial reason. They can be stored and shipped because of the fact that they are devitalized and devitaminized. They do not furnish a proper food even for insects or germs and so may be handled commercially with considerable ease and profit. The economic situation here involved has forced foods into general use in the civilized world which, if continued, will mean the destruction of those who consume them. A very great number of interlocking organizations connected with the manufacture and distribution of pernicious and unfit food materials has come into existence. They will do everything in their power to continue to sell their goods."

**Edited by Royal Lee**

VITAMIN NEWS

VITAMIN PRODUCTS CO. • MILWAUKEE, WISCONSIN

VOL. 1 August 21, 1933 No. 2

## VITAMINS, CALCIUM METABOLISM and ACIDOSIS

The first commercially important vitamin was vitamin D. Its physiological function is to maintain a normal concentration in the blood of diffusible (serum) calcium. The non-diffusible calcium is probably present in the blood as a component of the blood cells and is obtained from the non-diffusible reserve, which reserve is also the source of supply for all the calcium requirements of the body.

In case of a dietary deficiency of calcium or vitamin D, the serum calcium drops to a low level, the non-diffusible (cell calcium) tending to remain normal.

When vitamin D is supplied without the supplementary dietary calcium, the blood content of non-diffusible calcium will be increased at the expense of the bone reserves.

If there is a deficiency of phosphates in the diet, together with a deficiency of vitamin D, a condition of calcium starvation can be evident, even if there may be ample calcium in the diet. Harris (*Lancet*, May 14, 1933, page 1031) says that more cases of rickets are due to phosphate deficiency than are due to calcium deficiency.

It is well known that the cancellous structures of bones are built up in great detail from the administration of phosphorus. An opposite condition occurs in the aged; the bones become weak and brittle because of the loss of calcium, an end result of phosphate deficiency. Vitamin D in such a case will only aggravate the situation — rob the bone reserves to raise the blood calcium.

There is also a tendency in the adult for the calcium phosphate to become converted in the body into the carbonate — the pathological form — which is insoluble, and can cause considerable trouble. The administration of the phosphoric radical in some form will convert this morbid form of calcium into the useful phosphate, as well as improve the assimilation of other calcium. The lime in drinking water, for instance, being the carbonate, can be of no dietary use unless the phosphoric radical is added, or other alkali phosphates are present in sufficient quantity to afford the opportunity of a chemical interchange. These alkali phosphates are found only in any abundance in wheat bran, which is a food many of us fail to get.

"Bone is a dynamic, not a static, structure. New bone is not formed if either phosphorus (in combination) or calcium is not supplied in sufficient amounts by the blood." (Harris)

All vitamin D can do is to increase the retentivity of the blood serum for calcium. If the diet is rich in this element, the direction of flow of calcium will be from the alimentary organs to the bones. If the diet is deficient in calcium phosphate, the bones will lose this material to the blood.

In the case of growing children (and in pregnancy), there is a great demand upon the non-diffusible calcium reserve. When the serum calcium percentage drops below a certain threshold point, the kidney refuses to excrete any more calcium compounds. Instead, it replaces all calcium in combination, with some other alkali base, ammonium if none other is available. The synthesis of this ammonium is one of the least appreciated of kidney functions. (See *Journal A.M.A*. July 15, 1933.)

We believe that vitamins have an important bearing on this synthesis of ammonium to protect the alkali reserves, and that the cause of acidosis is always kidney failure, and that such failure is a consequence of vitamin deficiency.

Our reason for such a belief is the remarkable and rapid improvement that occurs when "Catalyn" is given to persons having the acidosis complex which usually includes some kidney complications.

Low blood calcium results in nervousness, insomnia, and irritability in the adult. In the child, it causes a quarrelsome disposition, restlessness at night and low-resistance.

We know that phosphorus and calcium are all important constituents of nerve tissues. The results of starving the nervous system of these elements are a hundred times as observable as the results of bone starvation — rickets. And do not forget that unless the phosphoric radical and calcium are amply present in the diet, vitamin D may aggravate the situation by attracting into the blood these mineral elements it should be carrying to the tissues, and that the phosphoric radical is more likely to be needed than calcium, and that the ideal arrangement is to see that all three are present.

**Edited by Royal Lee**

VITAMIN NEWS

VITAMIN PRODUCTS CO. • MILWAUKEE, WISCONSIN

VOL. 1 September 4, 1933 No. 3

# VITAMINS FOR PAIN AND SHOCK

Our definition of "pain" is: The nervous reaction occurring when there is a contact chemically between the nerve endings and cell component materials that normally are retained within cell walls, or some foreign irritant.

These cell components can be released (so as to permit the contact) by:

1. Trauma, or mechanical injury
2. Thermal damage (burns) which can do a better and quicker job in accomplishing the release
3. Electrolytic transfer
4. Cell damage by micro-organisms. (Typical case, malaria, where the infected erythrocytes periodically burst, releasing the toxic products)

These cell components are toxins when released, because of their reaction on the nervous system. The disposal of these toxins causes the depletion of many hormone reserves. (It must be remembered that the chief function of the whole endocrine system is the elimination of toxins.)

Now, when we reflect that the hormones are suspected to be elaborated in the respective endocrine organs by the splitting of vitamin molecules, we begin to see the relation of vitamins to shock and pain.

It also becomes evident as to how a mental impression can (if powerful enough) induce a condition of shock. The impression produces an inhibition of the endocrines and leaves the toxic products that are being constantly produced to do their pernicious work. Shell-shock is a classical example. And the heart failure that results from the shock of bad news which we sometimes see is another case of endocrine inhibition.

We can appreciate the fact that a starved endocrine system can be especially sensitive to the inhibitory effects of mental shocks, while a "well fed" endocrine system can be more or less immune to them.

We can also see why the depression has put so many persons into hospitals and sanitariums. The repeated bombardment of unpleasant and distressing happenings, where a weakness exists because of vitamin deficiency, will induce the development of one or more of a whole category of diseases.

Now, if bad news can kill people, why cannot good news cure them?

It can, in certain selected instances. That is how so many religious cures are really brought about. It explains the bona-fide and authenticated cures that have really taken place through the influence of such agencies.

The endocrine apparatus (as so ably set forth in his monumental work *The Internal Secretions and the Principles of Medicine* by Dr. Charles E. de M. Sajous) is the connecting link between the nervous system and the body functions in general.

It is a frequent observation of experienced clinicians that mental shocks (bad news, etc.) can bring on diabetes, arthritis, heart pathology, increased susceptibility to infection, pernicious anemia, etc., as well as the more common neurasthenic consequences.

Sajous' recommendations as to treatment was the stimulation of glandular function by the use of drugs (strychnine, arsenic, etc.).

Not until the demonstration of the remarkable dependability of vitamins (as "Catalyn") in treating many of these conditions was it realized that this glandular failure was a result of glandular starvation, and should be treated as such.

When we look back over the long years of research by Dr. Sajous and the conclusions that he reached, which are only now becoming the foundation of vitamin therapy, we see what a roundabout way the course of research had to pass before we began to appreciate the importance of those dietary principles that have been and still are so evasive to the chemist — vitamins.

The use of gland extracts and hormone preparations has not been as successful as would be expected for treating these conditions for the reason that it is far more difficult to supply a full complement of the hormones that are elaborated from the vitamins, than it is to supply the relatively few vitamins. By that we mean that it is far more difficult to maintain a balanced endocrine function by giving the gland extracts, and success is possible in far fewer cases, than when the proper supply of all the vitamins is made available.

We might add that in the latter case, nature is permitted to choose the remedy, while in the former, the physician makes the choice.

> "It is becoming increasingly apparent that most, if not all, maladies heretofore attributed to the presence of toxins are, in reality, caused by a deficiency of vitamins."
>
> Dr. D. T. Quigley, M.D., F.A.C.S.

The efficiency of "Catalyn" in eliminating some of the mysterious pains associated with neuritis "rheumatism," menstrual and ovarian disorders, etc. indicates that these are also manifestations of toxic irritation.

In the next *Vitamin News* we will discuss the subject of "Vitamins and Resistance to Infections," in which we will go further into the question of toxins from other sources than damaged cells.

**Edited by Royal Lee**

VITAMIN NEWS

VITAMIN PRODUCTS CO. • MILWAUKEE, WISCONSIN

VOL. 1 September 18, 1933 No. 4

## VITAMINS AND RESISTANCE TO INFECTIONS

The ability of the human body to resist the invasion of its tissues by micro-organisms is dependent upon a number of factors. But probably the best way to ensure the highest degree of resistance for any given individual is to see that his dietary intake of vitamins is amply high.

It is a generally accepted fact that we become susceptible to tuberculosis because of vitamin D deficiency.

It is probable that one cannot contract pneumonia without having a condition of serious vitamin deficiency, usually brought about by the action of some milder infective process that depletes the reserves, such as a severe cold, influenza, etc.

Prof. Barnett Sure, page 187, in his book *The Vitamins in Health and Disease*, in his discussion of the causes of stomach ulcers says:

> "Deficiencies of vitamins A, B and D cause a progressive loss of power of the body surface to control the bacterial life in contact with it."

Stomach ulcers are probably the best instance of a bacterial invasion primarily due to lowered resistance resulting from vitamin deficiency. That is why, even though the ulcers are healed by careful diet, they tend to recur time after time. It is possible that there is present an opsonic deficiency, that interferes with the phagocytic activities which normally control such microbic invasions. And it is highly probable that Erlich's complement and amboceptor are obtained from vitamin molecules, which will explain why vitamins are so necessary to maintain resistance. In fact, it has been suggested that the amboceptor principle is identical with vitamin C.

There is no reasonable doubt but that all these complex molecules — opsonins, hormones, complement, amboceptor, etc. are the "offspring" of vitamin molecules. There are no other dietary sources, and we must recall the primary principle of animal life, that is a process of breaking down of complex organic molecules, with an attendant release of energy. That makes it improbable that these complex molecules are synthesized within the body, although Sherman & Smith relate evidence showing that some vitamins can be synthesized within the bowel by certain vegetable organisms in sufficient amount to eliminate the need for a dietary supply.

The invading organisms in any disease probably produce the far greater part of their effects through the toxins released or created by their activity. It is again, in the disposal of these toxins, that vitamins play an all-important part, as was discussed in the last issue of this leaflet.

Probably one of the most spectacular actions of "Catalyn" is its effectiveness in eliminating toxic products absorbed from burned tissue. It is a lesson to be remembered by anyone observing the mental and physical recovery from the condition of shock that takes place when "Catalyn" is used under these circumstances.

Vitamin A deficiency has the specific effect of rendering the epithelial surfaces vulnerable to bacterial invasion, and infections follow in such locations as eyes, tonsils, sinuses, air passages, lungs and gastro-intestinal tract. To restore the vitamin after the infections have developed is somewhat like locking the stable door after the horse is stolen. For this reason, some investigators who expected great results from the use of vitamin A in concentrated form were disappointed with actual clinical results.

The fact is, to fight the infection after it has gotten into the body requires an ample supply of the rest of the vitamins — mainly B, C and D. "B" to promote catalysis and toxin elimination, "C" to promote phagocytosis, and "D" to maintain the blood calcium which is known to be an important factor in both the resistance to and the elimination of infections.

In *Vitamin News* No. 1, we discussed the relation of vitamins to heart disease. Most persons contracting heart ailments have a history of infection of some kind. Whether pneumonia, rheumatic fever, or some less serious bacterial invasion, the basic reason for the original susceptibility and the ensuing heart disease is vitamin deficiency.

Heart weakness is probably the most specific indication of the deficiency. It disappears as soon as the deficiency is restored. If permitted to exist for long periods, it is natural to assume that there will be degenerative changes, enlargement, coronary sclerosis, etc., as a consequence of the overload on the "machine."

Such a person is more susceptible than normal to infections, colds, and often has a relapse or recurrent attack of pneumonia. The vitamin deficiency sets up the well known vicious circle.

From our experience in observing the results obtained by the use of "Catalyn," we conclude that fifty people out of every hundred have a heart that is being deprived of certain necessary materials because of such deficiency, and that they would be able to work harder, think better and live longer if the deficiency were corrected.

We believe it to be a fact beyond reasonable doubt that the constantly increasing death rate from heart disease is a simple indication of the increasing use of devitalized foods. It is aggravated by the fact that we are finding it less and less necessary to perform manual labor, or to exercise to any degree, and this means a lesser intake of food. We must remember the first principle of dietetics, that our requirement for protein and vitamins is not determined by the amount of work we perform, but the amount of carbohydrate is reflected by the quantity of work.

**Edited by Royal Lee**

# VITAMIN NEWS

**VITAMIN PRODUCTS CO. • MILWAUKEE, WISCONSIN**

**VOL. 1** **October 2, 1933** **No. 5**


## WHY CHILDREN NEED VITAMINS

The child's need for vitamins begins before birth. The morning sickness of pregnancy is nothing more than a warning of vitamin deficiency. After birth, growth and development (physical and mental) are delayed by vitamin deficiency. Susceptibility to the usual children's diseases of rickets, tooth decay, and even a peevish disposition, are due to vitamin deficiency and a consequent incomplete assimilation of calcium and phosphorus, chiefly the latter, as recently demonstrated.

Mellanby has stated that vitamin D is more important than minerals in determining tooth development.

"Dr. Agnew ... stated that his extensive experiments on laboratory animals and humans indicate that phosphorus and vitamin D are the important nutrient elements in the prevention of dental caries. With the laboratory animals, phosphorus assumes a major role, but in humans, vitamin D becomes of great importance." (See *Dental Cosmos,* September 1, 1933, page 919.)

The use of vitamin D preparations alone has been of rather limited benefit, and Viosterol has been shown to be of definite harm in many cases.

We quote again the *Dental Cosmos,* August, 1933, page 780, Marshall: "How illogical then, in fact, how unwarranted, are the efforts of those not sufficiently trained in the medical sciences to attempt therapy by dietary prescription."

Dr. Marshall is absolutely right. To give massive doses of any such potent material is nothing less than reckless. Single vitamin therapy can cause any amount of endocrine unbalance, and the result will differ with each individual. To exclusively make use of single vitamin concentrates requires an insight into the particular requirement of each patient that is practically impossible to attain.

"Catalyn" was developed to make this unnecessary. It is an attempt to supply the entire category of vitamins in the correct proportion, which will successfully treat any deficiency disease if taken in amounts up to four tablets a day. Two per week are considered sufficient to supply the vitamin requirements of the adult or growing child where no accumulated deficiencies exist.

Since vitamins ("C" and "D" in particular) are necessary to the normal assimilation of mineral materials, mineral deficiency in the child is likely to be apparent, where a diet low in vitamins is used. This mineral deficiency in the child is often more apparent than real, because of the limited assimilation of what mineral materials are present, as a consequence of the low vitamin diet.

Candy, all white sugar or its products, and white flour, including its products such as macaroni, spaghetti, etc., should be absolutely barred from the diet of the child. Commercial ice cream is almost as bad. The vitamin and mineral content of these "food" materials is almost nil.

This is not too strong a statement. Dr. Quigley, quoted below, who probably is the best American authority on deficiency diseases, records the same opinion.

All these are energy-producing foods that contain no building materials for the body. The consequences of their toleration are susceptibility to infections, enlarged tonsils, carious teeth, unruly dispositions, stunted growth, rickets, mal-development and very often permanent damage to many of the organs of the body (especially the endocrine glands) that depend upon the vitamin supply for their normal function and development.

Honey, unrefined sugar, and fruits should be the only source of sweets for the child. As a crude comparison, it is just as sensible to put fuel into your automobile and forget the all-important lubricating oil as to permit the diet of the child to consist largely of fuel and no other components. The universal presence of the diseases herein mentioned is ample proof that we have been negligent.

We have been more than negligent. Let us quote Dr. D. T. Quigley, for 17 years instructor in Surgery at Nebraska State Medical School.

> "Officials in medical societies, medical writers, and universities are being subsidized in order to put out propaganda in favor of food conditions as they now are. Some of the officials in medical societies have openly stated that they do not believe in upsetting business. Apparently business for them ranks higher than human life."

The effrontery of the makers of devitalized foods is exemplified by the full page ads in the medical journals attempting to convince the physician of the merits of synthetic glucose (corn syrup) as a food for infants. As examples of artificially, chemically created "foods" totally devoid of vitamins or nutritional mineral materials, such products probably cannot be beat. This looks like pure propaganda, intended to offset the growing suspicion on the part of the consuming public that all is not well with the foods we are being "sold."

The sugar institute has spent large sums advertising in the dental journals, trying to offset the idea always prevalent among dentists, that candy and sugar are bad for teeth. It is true that these foods are not directly injurious to the teeth, but they satisfy the appetite of the child without supplying the vitamins and minerals that should accompany all foods in the correct and sufficient proportion. If they are absent, carious teeth inevitably result. It is nothing short of criminal to satisfy the child's appetite with foods that are obviously incomplete such as Dr. Quigley says form 60 to 90 percent of the total food intake of civilized Americans.

Remember, "Catalyn" is a reliable and quick action remedy for colds, whooping cough, influenza, or any infective disease. It is doubtful whether pneumonia can develop where the vitamin reserve is maintained. The high concentration of "Catalyn" enables you to correct in a few hours the deficiency accumulated over months and years.

**Edited by Royal Lee**

VITAMIN NEWS

VITAMIN PRODUCTS CO. • MILWAUKEE, WISCONSIN

VOL. 1 October 16, 1933 No. 6

## VITAMINOLOGY PLUS ENDOCRINOLOGY

### Equals the long sought Basic Science of Therapeutics

The medical profession has long recognized the fact that there has been no logical or scientific basis on which to study either the causes or treatment of chronic disease.

Prof. Sollman, of the Council of Pharmacy of the American Medical Association, wrote in 1908, "A generation ago therapeutics was an art, promising to develop into a science. At present, it cannot be classed as an art, nor as a science; it can only be classed as a confusion."

Charles E. de M. Sajous wrote in 1909, "Skoda's dictum of several years' standing 'that we can diagnose disease, describe it, and get a grasp of it, but we dare not expect any means to cure it,' has drifted along on the ripples of time, until hardly two years ago the president of a prominent British society, Dr. A. H. Brampton, found it opportune to declare that 'if any daring member has introduced a subject bearing on medical treatment, it has been with an apologetic air and humble mein, well knowing that if his remarks had any reference to the utility of drugs in the treatment of disease they would be subjected to good-humored banter, and received by those sitting in the seat of the scornful with amused incredulity.'"

Sajous introduced Endocrinology as a means of putting the treatment of disease on a more scientific plane. He further says, "When, twenty years ago, I was brought face to face with the mass of heterogeneous material we term the 'Medical Sciences,' and with the yearly crop of contradictory theories upon each disease, mode of treatment, etc., I soon realized that some gigantic flaw alone could account for so great a confusion."

In the attempt to find a rational basis for therapeutical science, Sajous spent his life analyzing the physiology and pathology of the endocrine organs, as set forth in his monumental treatise, *The Internal Secretions and the Principles of Medicine.*

But, tragically enough, Sajous' previous contact with the "medical" science had so colored his judgement that he sought to bring back to functional efficiency the failing endocrine organ that his studies demonstrated was the cause of a particular disease by the stimulative action of drugs — materials foreign to the body.

We now know that the failing endocrine organ was at fault because of *starvation*. We know that the endocrines are only able to perform their necessary functions when a supply of vitamins is available to them.

The atrophy or hypertrophy of the endocrine organs as a result of vitamin deficiency is one of the outstanding consequences noted in animal experiments with vitamin deficient foods. It has been overlooked that these are Primary consequences, and that the balance of the pathological conditions to be seen are chiefly secondary matters that are present because of the endocrine defections.

A ductless gland that is subjected to vitamin starvation will either die or swell up. In diabetes, the cells of the Islets of Langerhans die. In toxic goiter, the thyroid swells, and secretes a morbid active principle. Restoration of the vitamin principles in the case of toxic goiter in almost all cases will restore a normal function, because the parenchymatous tissue is not gone. But in the case of the diabetic, the lost cells are gone forever. Restoring the vitamins necessary will help, because it permits a normal function of those remaining cells, but the situation is precarious, because of the loss of essential tissue.

Lymphoid tissue in particular swells as a result of vitamin deficiency. The lymph gland enlargement that results from infection is an indication of local vitamin deficiency, due to the destruction of leucocytes.

Vitamins are essential to the production of both red and white blood cells. Laboratory reports often show a 50 percent increase of erythrocytes in two weeks, after the administration of "Catalyn" is begun.

The need for the different vitamins in different individuals varies very materially. That is why it is advisable to supply all the vitamins where any deficiency is suspected. Persons with a damaged endocrine, or a degenerated heart, often require heavy supplies to maintain a fair condition of health. The presence of a focal or chronic infection will also necessitate a heavy intake, but with the probability that the condition will then be overcome.

We can here quote again our best authority, Dr. Quigley:

> "A certain amount of vitamin B has come to be associated in the organism with a certain amount of vitamin A. A certain amount of vitamin C undoubtedly functions best in the presence of certain amounts of the other vitamins. Like the products of the glands of internal secretion, there is an inter-relationship of action among vitamins which as yet is not clearly understood." (*Notes on Vitamins and Diets*, Page 121.)

Physiological chemists are faced with the biggest job they have been confronted with yet, in tracing the network of processes of metabolism and regulation involved in the assimilation of vitamins. They have not yet gotten very far up to the present even in the simpler job of explaining what occurs in the assimilation of carbohydrates, the simplest of food materials.

But now that we know what the human body needs, and what the indications are when there is a deficiency, we can wait with more equanimity for an explanation. We can get the benefits to be derived from the use of "Catalyn" without knowing exactly what takes place other than the end result, just as we can enjoy the use of the energy in a chocolate bar without knowing the why or the wherefore.

**Edited by Royal Lee**

# VITAMIN NEWS

VITAMIN PRODUCTS CO. • MILWAUKEE, WISCONSIN

VOL. 1 October 30, 1933 No. 7

## THE COMMON COLD

The common cold is a universal pest. Science has not been able to isolate the microbe causing it, nor produce a specific cure. Some individuals are little affected by an attack, others are very ill. All are susceptible, apparently, to a more or less degree. Children particularly are most susceptible, and those who are made especially ill by cold attacks usually contract any other childhood disease with great ease, and have the most severe cases.

We all recall the children who were "tough," who were poorly dressed, and (in our estimation poorly nourished), who seemed never to be ill. They had good teeth, and pugnacious dispositions.

And we all recall the delicate offspring of the "well-to-do," who were always "catching something," timid of disposition, and whose teeth were so bad as to cause deformities of development.

We know today that VITAMINS spell the difference between these two classes of children. The "poor" child was almost always hungry, ate anything it found of a vegetable or fruit nature immediately in the raw, and got a fair supply of vitamins. The well-to-do child never was hungry, ate only cooked and refined food products, probably never even tasted a raw potato or carrot, was indoors a greater percentage of the time, especially in the fall and spring (to prevent exposure to inclement weather), and deprived of vitamins at every turn.

To quote Dr. Quigley:

> "School children are often found with a nervous condition and anemia, gum infection and decayed teeth, a lack of appetite and constipation, a latent tuberculosis, bow-legs or knock-knees, and eye defects necessitating the wearing of glasses. This means a starvation for vitamin A (eye disease), for vitamin D (tuberculosis and rickets), for vitamin C (mouth scurvy), and vitamin B (constipation, nervousness, lack of appetite and anemia) ... The very great prevalence of these deficiency disorders among school children indicates that unless some radical change is made, the next generation will carry these diseases to a greater degree. It indicates a tendency toward race degeneration." (Notes on *Vitamins & Diet*, Page 98.)

There is little question but that the "flu" epidemic of 1918 was primarily due to vitamin deficiency, brought about by the scarcity of butter, and other high vitamin foods, that were being shipped to Europe while we used substitutes.

Vitamins cannot prevent you from contracting a cold. But if your diet has been low in these essential elements, such a microbic invasion will not be resisted in a normal degree, and you may be quite ill, with a temperature for several days.

The cold attack will leave you in a susceptible condition to contract some other infective diseases — pneumonia, tuberculosis, any of the children's diseases (measles, mumps, whooping cough, etc.) if you are not immune to them because of a previous attack.

This susceptibility is purely due to the further depletion of your vitamin reserves, because of the cold.

Vitamins A, B, C and D are all important in this respect. If a concentrate of these vitamins is taken (such as "Catalyn") at the onset of a cold, it will in most cases be prevented from developing, and will run its course in a very mild form. Several days are required for the body to develop its defensive principles (developing an immunity to specific microbe), and it is during this time that the vitamin supply is important. This immunity only lasts for a few weeks, during which time you cannot catch another cold from this same kind of germ, but of course it is well known that there are several varieties of these.

It will be seen that the use of "Catalyn" will be of utmost benefit in dealing with any infective process. It supplies, as it were, the ammunition for the defensive processes of nature.

The use of vitamin preparations has not, in the past, offered much encouraging evidence of merit as remedies or preventives for colds. The use of viosterol, and preparations of A and D obtained from fish oils has been overdone, as is usual with any new and incomplete scientific discovery. We discover that vitamins are necessary, that their deficiency is the cause of most human pathology, then we immediately overdose ourselves with such vitamin preparations as are available, which in this case affords us disappointing results, and even does harm, (viosterol in overdose is a poison).

We are just beginning to realize that we must make use of all the vitamins in a reasonably normal proportion, to get the results we seek. These vitamins act cooperatively (any table of deficiency consequences shows that most symptoms that develop are present in more than one single vitamin deficiency), and that as with other food materials (proteins, fats and carbohydrates), there is some "balanced" ratio that is best.

"Catalyn" is an attempt to supply this ratio.

In the development and transmission of microbic life in victims of low-resistance, the germs often develop great virulence. This was the case in the 1918 "flu" epidemic. They are then able to produce the disease in others who ordinarily would be resistant.

It appears probable, in view of our four years' experience with "Catalyn," that seventy-five per cent of the physical suffering, as well as most of the economic loss due to the common cold, can be eliminated when this material becomes available to all who need it.

**Edited by Royal Lee**

VITAMIN NEWS

VITAMIN PRODUCTS CO. • MILWAUKEE, WISCONSIN

VOL. 1 November 13, 1933 No. 8

## "A LITTLE KNOWLEDGE IS A DANGEROUS THING"

Various false philosophies of therapeutics have come and gone. Our aboriginal ancestors thought that evil spirits of devils were in possession of the body of the afflicted, and used such terrifying practices as they could devise to frighten them away.

The physician of George Washington's time thought that an excess of blood was the chief cause of many diseases, and tapped the circulatory system for ailments affecting the whole body, and applied leeches for local troubles.

Next came the drug and chemical administering era, which has become by this time pretty well discredited as a means of cure, although useful for providing temporary relief.

There is another class of therapy that has become highly developed as a consequence of the discovery and application of the principles of asepsis — surgery. Surgery, properly used, has saved numberless lives and will continue to do so. But lately, some of the surgically inclined gentlemen have become somewhat over-enthused over certain stunts, such as nerve cutting.

A prominent surgeon has recently announced that he can cure toxic goiter, incipient diabetes, etc., by cutting the nerve supply leading to the thyroid, adrenals, etc.

If your automobile engine idles a little too fast and interferes with the proper shifting of gears, you can cure the condition very successfully by snipping off a few spark plug wires, too. But you never would approach the problem in this way if you were at all familiar with the underlying principles of the mechanism.

Dr. Sajous (referred to in last issue) has pointed out the principles in effect as regards the overactive thyroid and adrenals. He says:

> "The pituitary body governs oxygenation, metabolism, and nutrition in all animals supplied with a thyroid gland and adrenals." (Page 169, 4th Edition, *The Internal Secretions and the Principles of Medicine*.)
>
> "In vertebrates the pituitary body is connected with the thyroparathyroid apparatus, as it is with the adrenals, by direct nerve paths." (Page 171)
>
> "The pituitary body contains the governing center of the thyroparathyroid apparatus and adrenals, and coordinates the secretory activity of these organs." (Page 173)

Sajous also established the fact that the pituitary functions as a "test organ" and reacts to a quantitative or qualitative deficiency of thyroid secretion in the blood stream by stimulating the thyroid into activity.

Suppose a vitamin deficiency, coupled with an iodine deficiency, is responsible for a qualitative impotence of the thyroid secretion. The pituitary stimulus will continue to cause a hyperactivity of the thyroid, and a gland enlargement also can ultimately result. The thyroid secretion that is unable to perform its normal work now poisons the body in general.

Cutting the nerve between the regulating organ and the thyroid will permanently cure the hyperthyroidea, no doubt, so will surgically removing the overworked gland. But the better informed physician will correct the vitamin deficiency and make more heroic measures appear ridiculous.

"Catalyn" is the first specific remedy that can be depended upon to produce immediate results in all uncomplicated cases of toxic goiter. It is effective purely because it contains all the vitamins in such proportions as to as nearly as possible correct the deficiencies resulting from our present-day methods of food preparation.

The iodine deficiency that so far has received the entire blame for goiter conditions is only a contributory factor. It becomes important only when a vitamin deficiency is present. Iodine alone therefore will not cure goiter, but the vitamin treatment does.

These explanations (theories if you please) have not been instrumental in discovering the fact that vitamins cure goiter. That was an accidental occurrence. But they are useful in encouraging others to test the vitamin treatment, because the physician likes to have an understanding of the principles that are behind the treatments he uses. The only proof of a theory is its ability to enable you to predict results. And, the physician who tries "Catalyn" for the first time in a toxic goiter case is due for a pleasant surprise.

Many persons who are underweight or overweight are in that condition as a result of thyroid malfunction. "Catalyn" is useful for both reducing overweight and increasing the underweight by its normalizing action on the thyroid, where this organ is responsible.

It is surprising how many chronic diseases will respond to the following treatment:

> SEE THAT ALL THE ESSENTIAL DIETARY PRINCIPLES ARE AVAILABLE TO THE BODY, IN ABUNDANCE, AND GIVE NATURE AN OPPORTUNITY TO PERFORM ACCORDING TO HER ORIGINAL PLANS.

And, do not forget that after a deficiency disease has developed, often it is too late to do anything without the help of vitamin concentrates, and that "Catalyn" is the only concentrate on the market containing a "balanced ration" of these necessary materials.

**Edited by Royal Lee**

# VITAMIN NEWS

VITAMIN PRODUCTS CO. • MILWAUKEE, WISCONSIN

VOL. 1 November 27, 1933 No. 9

## DENTISTRY AND VITAMINS

Dentists as a class were the first profession to properly appraise and recognize the possible magnitude of the pathological consequences of vitamin deficiency. Today, almost any dentist will agree with the statement that 99 percent of the work he is called upon to do can be considered a direct or indirect result of improper and deficient diet.

Hardly 10 years ago, the dental student was told that there was no proven theory as to the real cause of carious teeth. He was led to think that the lack of coarse foods which mechanically acted to keep the teeth free from bacterial adhesions was the protective factor in those peoples whose diet prevented them from incurring tooth decay. This is the idea behind the false but well advertised slogan that "A clean tooth never decays."

The writer takes some pride in the fact that he was possibly the first to point out the relationship between vitamin deficiency, endocrine depletion, and dental caries, in a paper entitled "Systemic Causes of Dental Caries" read before the senior class at Marquette University in 1923.

Dr. Percy Howe of Boston was cited as to his findings that caries followed children's diseases as a rule, and that those children (among the thousands checked) who had not had these infections had much better teeth. Evidence was presented at that time to show that the vitamin deficiency produced susceptibility to the children's diseases as well as to caries, and the children's diseases reacted to increase the susceptibility to both by a depletion of endocrines that depended upon the dietary intake of vitamins for their nutrition.

All the evidence that has accumulated since that time substantiates the conclusion. Vitamins A, B, C, and D were soon identified as important factors in the situation, B and C in particular, at least as regards to the endocrine situation. The further conclusion was drawn that the only logical method of ensuring protection from all deficiency diseases was to develop a "balanced ration," as it were, of all the necessary vitamins, to supplement the usual denatured diet. "Catalyn" is the commercial result of research done between 1923 and 1929 in the effort to supply such a product.

Clinical tests made with the new product soon demonstrated that it had powers never suspected to be present in a vitamin concentrate. Persons taking it as a pre-natal dental prophylactic, for instance, reported that it eliminated their toxic goiter, heart weakness, etc. Its possibilities as a remedy for the so-called incurable diseases have overshadowed its importance as a dental prophylactic and up to the present, the sale of "Catalyn" has been almost exclusively for these other more urgent purposes.

All these effects were, of course, the direct result of supplying the endocrine organs with the necessary nutrition that had been lacking.

We are now beginning to accept the fact that any case of pyorrhea is nothing more than a relatively mild case of scurvy. It can be treated by the use of germicides, but the basic cause of the infection is the lowered resistance resulting from endocrine starvation.

The virulence of the attacking microbes is as a general rule inversely proportional to the degree of resistance of the victim, meaning that the lower the resistance of the patient, the more likely others are to be infected by germs from that source. It is a well known principle of bacteriology that microbes grown under inhibitive circumstances lose their virulence and vice versa.

When a person with a diseased and infected mouth begins the use of "Catalyn," the pyorrhea begins to clear up, quicker naturally, if other measures supplement it, the job being completed, of course, only if all irritating calculus is removed. Loose teeth will tighten up in an unbelievable manner in 60 to 90 days. There is a definite regeneration of the supporting connective tissues, and receded gums seem to take on a new lease of life. There is a tendency for abscesses to localize with pus formation where there is opportunity for drainage, possibly swelling where there is not. "Catalyn" promotes the formation of red blood cells as well as white; we have laboratory records of cases where the red cell count increased 90 per cent in two weeks, in which there was no response to other remedies.

The dentist needs "Catalyn" for all of his child patients.
For the pregnancy case. (Hyperemesis disappears.)
For the heart case or toxic goiter patient to give them sufficient vitality to stand the ordeal of a "full mouth" extraction.
For all scurvy victims. (Don't laugh, it's the truth.)

And for rickets. "The whole answer to rickets is not to be found in the supplying of vitamin D. There are undoubtedly other factors and these are probably bound up with A, B, and C deficiency and certain mineral deficiencies." (Quigley, *Notes on Vitamins & Diets*.)

We do not expect you to believe these statements without further evidence, but you can supply that evidence yourself if you will give this "balanced ration of vitamins" a test. "Catalyn" has received a wide distribution during the last two years without any advertising other than its merits, and today the major portion of our business is to the medical profession for the treatment of the so-called "incurable" degenerative diseases.

The forces of nature, given the opportunity (by an ample supply of the correct nutritive materials), can do wonders in restoring diseased tissue, and as to functional disorders arising from a vitamin deficiency or a consequent endocrine depletion, the improvement is often actually more than 100 percent.

**Edited by Royal Lee**

VITAMIN NEWS

CATALYN — NATURES SOURCE OF VITALITY — MADE IN U.S.A.

VITAMIN PRODUCTS CO. • MILWAUKEE, WISCONSIN

VOL. 1 December 11, 1933 No. 10

## ARE WE SCIENTIFIC?

The human race gains knowledge at a pathetically slow and tedious pace. And it applies knowledge already gained at a still slower and more pathetic rate.

Just for instance: Alois Senefelder invented the process of lithography, a method of printing that requires no type, just one hundred and forty years ago. He published a complete textbook illustrating and describing his processes in 1818. This leaflet is printed on a machine made no different than his methods suggested except from a plate prepared on a typewriter instead of by hand, that is only this year being made available to the public. In fact, it is the second machine to arrive in this city.

Now just why did it take one hundred and fifteen long years to get this simple device into common use? Very simple; *opposition by the ignorant*, who are exercising that peculiar human trait of condemning anything new that they know nothing about, and who refuse to withhold their opinions until they have had an opportunity to determine the actual facts.

The history of mechanical transportation is another conspicuous example of the inability of man to recognize the marvelous gifts of science when first presented. Steam stagecoaches were built in 1827-30 in London that were remarkably successful. One design, that was used to make regular daily trips of sixty miles over cobble-stone roads, had a top speed of thirty-five miles an hour, carried twenty passengers, and made a total of fifteen thousand miles in about a year. This performance aroused great activity in the construction of such vehicles, but was brought to an end by an act of the Parliament, which, indignant over the explosion of the boiler of one of the machines, killing three people, passed the celebrated law limiting the speed of self-propelled vehicles on public highways to five miles per hour, and which law remained in force until 1898. Now, pneumatic leather tires with rubber inner tubes were patented by a Londoner in 1845, and tested on the horse-drawn buses of that time, which did not need them because of the low speed. It is very evident that we would have had very successful motor vehicles on all the highways of the world before the U.S. Civil War if it had not been for the appalling ignorance of the "learned" majority of Parliament.

And we might mention the fact that it took the French medical societies twenty years to accept the discoveries of Pasteur. And before that, Semmelweiss in Vienna (1846) discovered that if the examining physician in a hospital washed his hands in chlorine-water before each examination, the mortality (from puerperal septicemia) dropped from 11 per cent down to one per cent. Semmelweiss was so ridiculed for his contentions that he finally lost his mind, dying in a lunatic asylum.

Just why is all this? It seems that the average educated (?) man has neither the ability nor the inclination to appraise the merit of anything new.

As Prof. A. E. Wiggam has pointed out, "A research discloses that even a good many men and women trained as scientists have as unscientific attitudes, especially toward social, moral and political questions, as people entirely ignorant of science. A few truly 'scientific citizens' were found who held a strictly unprejudiced attitude of mind toward all questions until they found out sufficient facts on which to base an intelligent judgement. These few scientific citizens are the hope of the world."

Ignorance and education are by no means terms of opposite meaning. There are many educated ignoramuses. Any person is ignorant who ignores facts that he should be concerned with. The person who is naturally ignorant becomes still more so when educated because he sees less reason than before to use his own weak powers of judgement. He is full of ready-made opinions and can find one to cover any situation.

He is in about the same class as Dr. Kettering's "Expert," who "knows all the different ways a thing can't be done." The intelligent person, when confronted by anything new, whether he is educated or not, will reserve his opinion until he has sufficient evidence available from reliable sources to make a decision.

"Catalyn," because of its newness in principle, regardless of its spectacular performance in treating a whole category of heretofore incurable ailments (producing at least some results in 98 per cent of the cases tried, according to physicians' reports), has stirred up a hornet's nest of resentment in certain quarters noted for intolerance. A "Bureau of Investigation" is maintained which has no means of investigating, and which renders swivel-chair opinions without making any effort to determine facts, and which sends out letters to inquirers about "Catalyn," containing such statements as the following:

> "The exploitation of 'Catalyn' is obviously a crude piece of quackery."
>
> "To say that 'heart trouble' is a vitamin-deficiency disease is to make a statement that is meaningless and silly."

To refute the latter statement, we can quote Dr. D. T. Quigley, for many years Professor of Surgery at University of Nebraska College of Medicine:

> "There is sufficient evidence to convince any thinking person that high blood pressure, apoplexy, hardening of the arteries, obesity, stomach and duodenal ulcers, mucous colitis, diabetes, insanity, and cancer and many other chronic conditions often develop on a basis of vitamin deficiency."
>
> "Sudden death from heart disease in relatively young or middle-aged people is caused, in a measure, by blood vessel and heart disease resulting from a lack of sufficient foods containing vitamin C." (Pages 122 and 126 of *Notes on Vitamins and Diets.*)

Do you wonder that Semmelweiss and Pasteur had difficulties in getting their ideas accepted?

**Edited by Royal Lee**

# VITAMIN NEWS

VITAMIN PRODUCTS CO. • MILWAUKEE, WISCONSIN

VOL. 2 January 15, 1934 No. 1

## VITAMIN A

"Vitamin A was discovered by McCollum and Davis in 1915. They found that certain laboratory animals which were deprived of certain foods, such as butter and other animal fats, developed an eye disease and eye infection which eventually led to blindness. They found that an animal which had definitely developed the eye disease might, in cases where the disease had not progressed too far, be cured by restoring the proper food. These food investigations showed that the protective element which they were studying existed in certain fruits, yellow colored vegetables, and the green leaves of vegetables. They found that not only would eye disease develop where this substance was lacking in the diet, but also that certain other parts of the body become diseased, and the character of the disease in these cases was found to be in the nature of an infection. This work proved that food plays a major part in protecting certain parts of the animal body against the more common infections. The animals on the deficiency diets suffered invasion of certain organs and tissues by low grade micro-organisms. The structures in which it was shown that low grade infections had occurred were the eyes, the tonsils, and other lymphatic structures, and the accessory sinuses connected with the nasal cavity (antrums, ethmoid cells, frontal sinuses, mastoids, sphenoids, etc.). In the animals that were killed and examined after such an experimental diet deficiency, abscesses could be demonstrated in the tonsils and sinuses, and in some animals there were also collections of pus in the ear and mastoid cells. The anti-ophthalmic vitamin came eventually to be called vitamin A. (The names vitamin A and B were suggested by McCollum and Kennedy in 1916.) At the present time, vitamin A is considered one of the main elements of protection, in a basic manner, against all infections. It undoubtedly has a very decided effect in protecting against the infections which cause ordinary colds, and which localize in the nasal cavity, the throat, and the respiratory tract." Dr. Quigley, "*Notes on Vitamins and Diets*.

"The body has the power of storing vitamin A to a considerable extent for future needs. An abundant supply of it in early life undoubtedly safeguards the body against later infection as well as provides for present needs. This does not mean, however, that the need of vitamin A is confined to the young. An amount sufficient to support normal growth and health may still be insufficient for the added demands of reproduction and lactation and for resisting the infections more common in early adult life. Long-time feeding experiments conducted on rats have shown increasing benefits throughout succeeding generations in the continued use of liberal amounts of vitamin A." *U.S. Dept. of Agriculture Circular No. 84.*

## VITAMIN A

FUNCTIONS:

(1) Promotes tissue formation.
(2) Increases blood platelets.
(3) Promotes growth and feeling of well-being.
(4) Promotes appetite and digestion.
(5) Prevents infection, notably of eyes, tonsils, sinuses, air passages, lungs and gastro-intestinal tract.

RESULTS OF DEFICIENCY:

(1) Loss of appetite.
(2) Retardation of growth and development.
(3) Physical weakness.
(4) Susceptibility to disease of the eyes (night blindness, corneal ulcers), ears (otitis media), kidneys (renal calculi).
(5) Diseases involving the air passages, lungs, skin, bladder, stomach and colon.
(6) Influences reproduction by failure of ovulation.
(7) Secondary anemia.
(8) Excessive growth of lymphoid tissue.
(9) Dullness or perversion of special senses.

RESULTS OF ABSENCE

(1) Xeropthalmia (eye inflammation and ulcers).
(2) Cessation of growth.
(3) Failure of appetite and digestion.
(4) Formation of pus in ears, sinuses and glands at base of tongue. Pyorrhea.
(5) Prevents conception by failure of ovulation.
(6) Causes phosphatic renal calculi.

## MOST RELIABLE SOURCES:

Whole milk, butter, cheese, egg yolk, some animal organs (mainly in liver oil), green leafy vegetables, yellow corn, yellow sweet potatoes, carrots and other yellow and green vegetables.

Some special effects we have noted from the use of the vitamin A concentrate used in "Catalyn" is the remarkable ability it has of relieving epithelial irritabilities. For instance, stubborn cases of gastro-intestinal irritation (and even ulceration) that failed to respond to other treatments have disappeared as if by magic in a few days after the use of "Catalyn" (or vitamin A concentrate alone) was begun.

Another situation of acute vitamin A deficiency is found in those cases of cystitis where no other offending organism is detected than colon bacillus. A number of such cases on record were all immediately relieved in a few hours' time by the use of this material. There are apparently more people (particularly women) suffering from this condition than we suspect. Cystitis of this kind recurs periodically without any visible reason, at more or less extended intervals, sometimes years apart.

A third situation in which vitamin A is of particular value is in dropsy caused by liver pathology. Here it appears to aid the remaining parenchyma to perform its work. This effect is reasonable, when we recall that the liver is the chief location of vitamin A in the animal, fish liver oils being the main commercial source.

Colds, chronic rhinitis, sinusitis, and psoriasis are more consequences of epithelial irritability that have recently been reported as responsive to our new vitamin A concentrate now available in tablet form, each containing five times the amount of this vitamin in each "Catalyn" tablet, and sold in the same size bottles (36, 120, and 500), and at the same schedule of prices and discounts.

VITAMIN NEWS

VITAMIN PRODUCTS CO. • MILWAUKEE, WISCONSIN

VOL. 2 February 15, 1934 No. 2

# VITAMIN B

The original vitamin B has since been separated into three components — $B_1$ ($B_2$ to some writers) or vitamin G, considered as the anti-pellagra factor, not destroyed by cooking; $B_2$ ($B_3$ to some writers) also known as vitamin F, the growth-promoting factor, not destroyed by cooking; and vitamin B proper, the antineuritic or nerve-nourishing factor, which is destroyed by cooking.

It is this last component that we are now to consider. Besides its action in maintaining nerve tissue, it is also necessary for growth, cooperating with "F" and "G" in this function and probably with other factors as yet not thoroughly investigated.

Vitamin B is of vital importance in cooperation with vitamin C in maintaining normal health of the entire endocrine system. Some observers report atrophy of the organs of internal secretion (in the case of pigeons rendered polyneuritic), while others report increase in size and weight of adrenals, thymus, pancreas, testes, ovaries, spleen, heart, liver, kidneys, stomach, thyroid and brain.

These contradictory findings are easily explained. If an endocrine organ fails to receive the proper nutrition, it is unable to secrete a functionally normal hormone. If the lack of nutrition is severe enough, the result will be atrophy, or death of parenchyma. If the deficiency is less severe, over a longer period, the tendency is for the nervous control (originating in the "test organ" of Sajous, the pituitary) to unduly stimulate the abused endocrine to excessive activity, and an enlarged but morbidly or insufficiently secreting endocrine is the consequence. The pancreas in diabetes is a classic example of the first type of reaction; toxic goiter of the second.

The degeneration of nerve tissue and the paralysis of beriberi are conditions of more severe deficiency of "B," and are not of so great importance to us here in the United States. Pellagra, however, is due to more than vitamin G deficiency alone, the "B" deficiency being responsible, no doubt, for the spinal cord degeneration that precedes the skin lesions and causes them to be bilaterally symmetrical.

Probably the most widespread effect of the universal partial dietary deficiency of "B" is constipation. The action of bran as a remedy for this condition is in no small measure due to the chemical action of the bran particles in irritating the intestinal lining into secretory activity (which latter effect cannot be considered harmless). If you do not believe this, try drinking water in which bran has been soaked as a remedy for that condition.

Loss of muscular tone is another important "B" deficiency consequence. The loss of appetite following "B" deficiency is due to the failure of the empty stomach to contract, because of this condition in the muscular stomach walls, in connection with the established fact that the contraction of the stomach causes the hunger sensation.

This same loss of muscular tone in the heart muscle makes "B" an important factor in many heart cases, as we mentioned in *Vitamin News* No. 1. It is also a factor in the constipation effect, as well as being a common cause of general lassitude and asthenia.

Going back to endocrine considerations, shooting pains in the gonads are frequent symptoms of the deficiency of both "B" and "C." This condition is so common in women that it explains the contention of a prominent surgeon that the major proportion of appendicitis operations on women are traceable to misdiagnosed ovary pains. There is no demonstration of the effectiveness of "Catalyn" more striking than its action in eliminating this symptom.

In fact, "B" is of vital importance to the female sex. In pregnancy the endocrine hyperactivity requires an ample supply of "B" (with its complement "C"), without which goiter, lymphatic and tonsil enlargement, etc. tend to result.

It is the deficiency of "B" and "C" in our civilized diet that is responsible for the difficulties and distress of childbirth that we know is not present among the races of disappearing humanity that eat naturally. Proof of this statement lies in the consistent results obtained where "Catalyn" is used during this period, and as a control for the hyperemesis it is found to be very satisfactory.

Vitamins B and C are vitally necessary for normal lactation, and Dr. Barnett Sure cites the case of an infant that after two weeks' administration of "B" concentrate "Had changed from a thin, pale, spastic, restless, whining infant ... to a happy, rosy-cheeked, smiling baby, whose appetite never seemed to be completely satisfied and whose gain in weight was remarkable."

Cow's milk is notoriously low in vitamin B even when the feed supplied is relatively high in this essential. Therefore, "Catalyn" can be considered the most convenient and certain source of the more difficultly obtainable vitamins A, B, and C for the infant, as well as making the use of cod liver oil, etc. unnecessary though the "D" content, if supplied at the rate of not less than one-half tablet a day.

Although the Vitamin Products Company is now preparing special tablets of some of the individual vitamins to permit the boosting of an obvious single deficiency where there is a necessity to supplement temporarily the administration of "Catalyn," it is not considered desirable to commercially furnish special concentrates of "B" and "C" for the reason that so far no clinical necessity has developed for their specific use in higher concentration than is present in "Catalyn" alone. This is mainly because of the fact that "B" and "C" are so cooperative in action.

Tablets of both "B" and "C" concentrates are available, however, for experimental purposes on special order.

**Edited by Royal Lee**

VITAMIN NEWS

VITAMIN PRODUCTS CO. • MILWAUKEE, WISCONSIN

VOL. 2 March 15, 1934 No. 3

## VITAMIN C

Vitamin C has lately been identified chemically as "ascorbic acid" according to Dr. Szent-Gyorgyi. (*Nature,* London, December 10, 1932, p.888.) (Previously announced as hexuronic acid.)

Vitamin C is one of the most necessary vitamins, and its deficiency results in a wide category of pathologies, the most conspicuous probably being damage resulting from a loss of integrity of intercellular substance in various connective tissues, blood vessel walls, teeth and gums, friability of bones, etc. These are all indications of the loss of strength of the intercellular substance.

Black and blue spots without traumatic cause are due to "C" deficiency causing weakness of blood vessel walls. Vitamin C deficiency is no doubt the major systemic cause of pyorrhea.

Hypertrophy of adrenals with reduced secretion occurs in "C" deficiency. Low blood pressure is the consequence, with fatigability and impaired heart action, tachycardia and shortness of breath.

As vitamin B as well as "C" are known to be necessary to the proper function of the adrenals (see above reference in *Nature*, London), and "B" is also known to be necessary to the nervous control of heart action, it is evident that here we have an explanation of the present-day high mortality from heart disease.

Most heart pathology begins as functional weakness, with enlargement, valvular lesions, and coronary disease as secondary developments. Infection can, of course, play an important part, which may be due to vitamin A deficiency. The valvular trouble in many cases can probably be attributed to enlargement and consequent distortion. The use of vitamin concentrates ("Catalyn") is indicated in all such areas. The improvement is usually definite and progressive. Enlargement and heart weakness are the most responsive to this treatment, coronary disease the least. "Catalyn" is the drugless successor to digitalis.

Vitamin C is also a factor in some anemias.

> "The existence of anemia due to the absence of vitamin C but occurring before frank symptoms of scurvy become manifest has been insisted upon by Weil and Mouriquand who have described the existence of anemia which resisted treatment by iron but which was cured by lemon juice. Recently, Rohmer and Bindschelder investigated a group of 22 anemic infants with a view to determining the existence of 'pre-scorbutic anemia.' In six of these cases the administration of iron did not produce any effect, but when vitamin C was given in addition, a prompt cure resulted." (*Arch. Dis. of Childhood* 8-117-144 April '33)

Vitamin C is cooperative with vitamin D in the calcium metabolism of bone and teeth, possibly in supplying the connective tissue matrix to permit calcification. "Despite a plentiful supply of calcium and phosphorus, little mineralization takes place in susceptible species in the absence of vitamin C." (*Yale Jol. Biol. & Med.* p. 235-244 Jan. 1933)

Peptic and duodenal ulcers have been found to be amenable to treatment with vitamin concentrates (as "Catalyn") according to reports made to us by physicians using it for other ailments in the same patient. This is now explained by the following reference:

"1. Routine necropsies on 1,000 guinea pigs maintained on our stock diet failed to show a single spontaneous peptic ulcer.

2. Of 75 guinea pigs fed on diets deficient on vitamin C, in twenty (or 26%), peptic ulcers developed which were similar in location and in gross and microscopic appearances to those observed in man.

3. Of 80 guinea pigs fed on corresponding basic diets supplemented by vitamin C, in only one did peptic ulcer develop.

4. Diets deficient in vitamins A, B, and D did not cause peptic ulcers if the supply of vitamin C was adequate.

5. Mechanical injury to the mucosa of the duodenum in guinea pigs fed on an adequate diet was followed by rapid and complete healing, while similar injury to guinea pigs fed on a diet deficient in vitamin C resulted in the formation of peptic ulcers.

6. Peptic ulcer in the guinea pig is apparently caused by a partial but prolonged deficiency of vitamin C." (*Arch. of Int. Med.* V. 51 P. 426)

Vitamin C promotes, and is essential to, the production of mucin in the body. Mucin is necessary to the building of connective tissue, and is the gastric protective agent of the mucosa against the digestive agents. The recently discovered effectiveness of gastric mucin (a packing house product) as a remedy for peptic ulcers here is explained. But such therapy does not go to the real cause — vitamin C deficiency — nor prevent associated pathologies due to the same thing.

Probably the best way to get quick results in peptic ulcers is to confine the food intake for two days to orange juice and milk, following this with four "Catalyn" tablets a day for a month or more.

"Partial and prolonged" vitamin deficiencies (or "latent avitaminosis") can now be therefore definitely charged with two of our most common classes of chronic disease — gastro-intestinal ulcers and heart disease. When the human race becomes civilized, it will be made a penal offense to advertise or sell a devitaminized food. The only excuse for such indefensible activities today is ignorance. It is exemplified by the full-page ads in our leading medical journals today touting the use of cheap synthetic glucose — corn syrup — for babies. Babies need above all vitamins and minerals — not energy, which is all that glucose has to offer. Synthetic glucose is not even a safe food for adults, when we realize that the growing incidence of diabetes is nothing more than an indication of too much synthetic and devitaminized carbohydrates.

**Edited by Royal Lee**

# VITAMIN NEWS

VITAMIN PRODUCTS CO. • MILWAUKEE, WISCONSIN

**VOL. 2** **April 16, 1934** **No. 4**

## VITAMIN D

The physiological action of vitamin D is to increase the ability of the blood serum (and lymph) to carry diffusible calcium. This means that dietary calcium is better absorbed, and calcium reserves loosely held in certain tissues (metaphyses of bone) will be absorbed in some degree, while more calcium is thereby made available for tissues having a greater affinity for it. The shafts of the long bones grow under these circumstances at the expense of the metaphyseal calcium.

The kidneys excrete calcium as soon as the serum content rises above a certain threshold point, and the administration of excessive doses of vitamin D can cause nephritis and nephrosis from this overactivity.

The ovaries secrete a hormone that causes (in pregnancy) a great increase of the affinity of the cells in the "storage areas" for calcium, thereby lowering the serum content below the threshold point so that none is eliminated, and the calcium reserves become greatly built up during the first few months, with a temporary increase in the thickness of the bone walls, and a greatly increased need for vitamin D to aid in the absorption, and an increased need for vitamin C to supply the connective tissue matrix for the osseous deposits.

Vitamin C is also highly important to the child in the same connection. It is now recognized that vitamin C rather than vitamin D deficiency is responsible for defective tooth development through the incomplete formation of the connective tissue matrix. It is probable that this connective tissue matrix can only be formed when vitamin C is present, and this is particularly true of teeth. In vitamin C deficiency, this matrix tends to dissolve, with elimination of calcium. This effect is a part of the general degeneration of connective tissue characteristic of scurvy. Pyorrhea and caries will disappear when vitamin C becomes recognized as the specific preventive and remedy for these conditions. (See Sherman-Smith *The Vitamins* pages 161-168). The use of vitamin D has been overrated for these conditions, it being the minor factor. In scurvy, the bones become decalcified, particularly the parts that are the last to undergo ossification, and the joints become swollen and sore.

Oversecretion of the ovarian calcium-depressing hormone is responsible for the nervous, irritable and hysteretic type of woman, because of the nervous irritability occasioned by the low serum calcium. Vitamin therapy is particularly successful in normalizing this type, and the use of "Catalyn" is indicated. Vitamins C, D and F are all factors. This type usually has a prematurely aged appearance, and the effect of vitamin therapy is often an obvious rejuvenation.

There is a vitamin principle present in oatmeal that is antagonistic in action to vitamin D, its effect on serum calcium being somewhat similar to the ovarian hormone in this respect. The use of oatmeal water as a preventive of toxic effects from too much sunlight (such effects being chiefly due to the formation of excessive amounts of vitamin D in the skin with consequent immediate absorption) has long been a practice of persons working in the sun. Like the use of cod liver oil for rickets, long before vitamins were thought of, this practice is now known to have a scientific basis.

Some observers have made the statement that vitamin D caused a reduction in serum calcium. Small doses can do this, by increasing the diffusibility of the serum present in the blood serum, enabling its immediate escape into calcium-starved tissues. Certain of the glands supplying digestive fluids require considerable calcium, and these show one of the first indications of calcium increase when vitamin D is administered. The parotid secretion normally contains three times the calcium of blood serum, and the rise in saliva calcium after vitamin D administration is greater than the rise in serum calcium. It is an established fact that the calcium dissolved out of the tooth enamel surface by fruit acids etc. is replaced from the salivary calcium.

Vitamin D has been charged with causing over-development of osseous structures. But more careful investigations have shown that cases of relative enlargement of diaphyses should be interpreted as caused by the healing of a condition of rickets. Where an ample supply of vitamin D is always available, as in the tropics, the tendency is for bone development to be completed sooner, with consequent reduced stature.

Overdosage of vitamin D is followed by toxic effects, characterized by damage to kidney parenchyma, and pathological calcium deposits in blood vessel walls, liver and kidney. The relation between the toxic dose and the therapeutic dose varies, and is dependent upon the nature of the diet as well as the body requirements for calcium. It has been found that there is no danger of toxic effects during pregnancy and lactation, in animal tests, even with doses that will be very harmful to the animal otherwise. The feeding of oatmeal increases the need for vitamin D in test animals, and brings on rickets more quickly than other foods for the reason before noted. This antagonistic vitamin probably is also beneficial, however, and its use as a food should not be discouraged, rather it should be more used, but with care that vitamin D is not forgotten. It is probable that disease can also result from the deficiency of the oatmeal vitamin, and it is no doubt just as essential to health as vitamin D, which becomes toxic only when there is an absence of such cooperating principles.

To summarize, we can say that vitamin D is an agent that enables the blood serum to pick up calcium, it increases the diffusibility of the serum calcium, increases the absorption of dietary calcium, and increases the amount of calcium available to tissues and organs that must have this element. There are other calcium-regulating principles, however, that control the affinity of these tissues and organs for calcium, upon which the utilization of calcium depends. Unless these are present, the effect of vitamin D is to increase temporarily the serum calcium beyond the renal threshold point until the kidneys restore the normal balance, and this increase may be as much due to absorption from the bone reserves as from dietary sources.

# VITAMIN NEWS

VITAMIN PRODUCTS CO. • MILWAUKEE, WISCONSIN

VOL. 2 May 15, 1934 No. 5

## SUPPLEMENTARY NOTES ON VITAMIN B

Since the publication of *Vitamin News*, February 15, on vitamin B, we have been following up the clinical performance of this vitamin and can offer the information below regarding its uses that deserves immediate attention.

It now appears that vitamin B is an important factor (probably THE important factor) in both diabetes mellitus and pernicious anemia.

Ever since the introduction of "Catalyn" we have received continuous reports of favorable results in diabetes. Until we had enough data to offer a logical explanation and demonstrate what particular vitamin or combination of vitamins was responsible for this action, we hesitated to make definite recommendations for its use for this disease. At the present time, however, we have established these facts:

1. In cases of diabetes associated with low blood pressure, or where there is a history of low blood pressure, vitamin B may be expected to be of definite benefit.

2. In cases where there is a history of high blood pressure, the best treatment is "Catalyn" or vitamin C.

Labbe, Nepveux and Gringoire in *Bull. Acad. de Med. Paris*, 109:689-702, May 23, 1933, make the following statement:

> "In 8 out of 11 cases treated with the B vitamin resulted in an important fall in glycosuria and a notable increase in the hydrocarbon tolerance. In two other cases the vitamin did not modify the glycosuria nor influence the diabetes at all. In the three last cases, however, the diabetes was very serious and had complications, also the vitamin experiment lasted only fifteen days. In the 8 cases favorable to the treatment ... the amelioration was slow and progressive. Increasing the tolerance a very little by a gram a day, the fall in glycosuria averaged 1 gram 70 a day ... When the giving of vitamin B was stopped, the glycosuria reappeared slowly, depending upon how long the vitamin treatment had lasted and to what extent the reserves had been reinforced ... The effect on the general condition from the vitamin B treatment was very favorable. One case put on weight 8 kilo. in 2½ months, another 7 kilo. in 2 months. All, even those whose glycosuria was not diminished, felt greatly benefited from the treatment; they were much stronger and happier ... The dose of 15 grams of vitamin material procured an increased sugar tolerance of from 40 to 50 grams, as much as 32 to 40 units of insulin. This improvement was slow and progressive. Insulin treatment was kept up in the beginning just as if it were the only treatment. In proportion to the increased tolerance of the vitamin treatment, the insulin was diminished or suppressed entirely. The vitamin therapy as given by mouth was much appreciated as a distinct advantage."

We can draw the conclusion, therefore, that if there is any Langerhansian tissue left, the vitamin therapy can be expected to be of benefit through restoration of function of these cells, by a renewed supply of the nutritional elements necessary for the elaboration of the specific hormone. It places diabetes mellitus definitely in the category of a vitamin deficiency disease.

Pernicious anemia also seems to be deserving of the same classification. vitamins B, C, and A are all factors, and should be tested in each case in the order named to determine which is most important. We are completing some work on vitamins E and F to be announced in the next *Vitamin News* that indicates their connection with anemic conditions, also.

The deficiency of vitamins B and C can cause degeneration of the bone marrow, which is admittedly the major etiologic factor in pernicious anemia.

> "Rats stunted by vitamin B deficiency have bone lesions that are identical with those seen in guinea pigs suffering from acute and uncomplicated scurvy. Marrow elements are destroyed and replaced by reticular tissues supporting widely dilated congested blood vessels." (Shipley, McCollum and Simmonds, *J. Biol. Chem.*, 49:399, December 21.)

The use of "Catalyn" for pernicious anemia, plus the supplementary use for a week at a time of the single vitamin concentrates to determine which are important in each individual case (two tablets a day) will often bring out unexpected results. There are so many contributing factors in the causation of pernicious anemia that such procedure is necessary, but these factors probably are all of a deficiency nature. The use of liver extracts, etc. have been effective only because they contained some principle or other that had a bearing in this connection. The limitations of such measures are becoming more and more apparent today, however, and vitamin therapy is unquestionably destined to replace them. It is a far simpler matter to determine what vitamin or group of vitamins are missing, than it is to find out what hormonic principle has been starved out of existence by vitamin deficiency, and attempt to supply such specific hormones.

When the pathological condition has reached the final situation of complete inadequacy or death of the secreting cells, there is no hope of restoration of normal function by vitamin therapy, however, and the continued use of the specific hormone is the only possible alternative. Even in such cases it will be found that the use of the proper vitamins will greatly improve the general physical condition of the patient. Diabetes is the most outstanding example of this set of circumstances. In pernicious anemia, it is probable (to judge from our limited knowledge to date) that vitamin therapy is the best treatment at any stage of the disease.

**Edited by Royal Lee**

CATALYN — NATURES SOURCE OF VITALITY — MADE IN U.S.A.

# VITAMIN NEWS

VITAMIN PRODUCTS CO. • MILWAUKEE, WISCONSIN

CATALYN — NATURES SOURCE OF VITALITY — MADE IN U.S.A.

VOL. 2 June 15, 1934 No. 6

## VITAMINS E AND F

Vitamin E was first established as a fat-soluble principle that was necessary to prevent atrophy of certain gonad structures in both male and female, resulting in sterility. The damage is more permanent in the male, while relatively curable by restoration of the vitamin in the female.

Vitamin A is just as essential to prevent sterility as the vitamin E, but "E" has been termed the anti-sterility vitamin because that characteristic led to its discovery, which, being relatively recent, accounts for the lack of information in the literature regarding its other important attributes.

Clinically, our vitamin E concentrate has been found valuable in the treatment of sterility of both sexes. Probably the most common indication of vitamin E deficiency is disappearance of the sex instinct, or its failure to appear at all, the former situation being more common in the male sex; the latter in the female.

It should be understood that the vitamin E is not a sex stimulant. In treating a condition of deficiency the effect on this function is merely that of a tendency to renew normality.

In our experience, mysterious pains, suspected to be of neuritic or arthritic origin, in persons beyond middle age, have been one indication frequently encountered that can be successfully treated with vitamin E concentrate, particularly those cases complaining of severe pains that were not variable in location, and seemed to be originating from a small center of activity.

Vitamin E cooperates with vitamin A, not only in preventing sterility, but in the other functions of vitamin A — the maintenance of normal epithelial metabolism. It is a useful aid in correcting conditions like eczema, urticaria and dermatitis.

Vitamin E from different cereal sources has been found by us as well as other investigators to have quite different characteristics. This we consider to be due to the varying proportions of two distinct vitamins.

We have taken the liberty of designating the new one vitamin "F" ("F" being otherwise an orphan in the vitamin alphabet since the accepted change in the previous "F" back to "B"). We consider this "F" to be identical with Mirvish's calcium depressor found in oatmeal. It is also present in considerable amounts in rye, but there appears to be little in wheat. It is biochemically an antidote for vitamin D, as it causes a reduction in serum calcium. The use of oatmeal water by farmers and others as a beverage while at work in the hot sun is scientifically justified by this discovery. Sunstroke can be considered as largely a condition of vitamin D toxicosis, and vitamin F the preventive.

Both vitamins F and E are fat-soluble nominally, being found in the oil or fat component of the cereal, but they are also soluble in considerable degree in water. The vitamin E present enormously stimulates the propagation of the yeast and other micro-organisms in an aqueous extract of wheat germ while the same extract with the oil removed is fairly stable.

The "F" seems to be more water-soluble than the "E," and the report once made that vitamin E was of value in anemia is, no doubt, due to the presence of "F." We have found our "F" concentrate particularly valuable as an aid in anemias, and it creates a healthy, slightly tanned color of the skin, that is hardly compatible with anemic conditions, in a surprisingly short time. This, no doubt, is part of the vitamin D antagonizing action.

Vitamin F probably acts on the blood calcium by first converting the non-diffusible into the diffusible, thereby permitting its escape into the tissues, ultimately arriving within the cells causing their distension and opposing tissue edema. This effect improves the function of glandular organs, and tones up all tissues, noticeable particularly in the skin. It is a growth factor; in the young probably feeds the thymus, in particular; in the adult, the spleen and gonads — these are the calcium depressors.

Because it causes the appropriation of calcium by the soft tissues and muscles, while the action of vitamin D is to cause appropriation by bone growth, it will in the absence of vitamin D aggravate and help to bring on rickets. Where both vitamins are present, a normal balance permits a proper supply of this necessary calcium to both classes of tissues.

Vitamin F, then, is valuable for:

1. Anemic conditions (of deficiency origin).
2. As a remedy in edematous conditions (is effective in those cases where other measures fail).
3. For cosmetic effect — improves the skin color, and "deflated" tissues are restored.

Neither our vitamin E concentrate tablets nor the "F" concentrate tablets are free from the other vitamins. Rather, they are made from sources in which one vitamin predominates, and the accompanying complementary vitamin is permitted to remain. Therefore, the concentrate should be selected for a particular case with the more outstanding necessity in mind and it can be taken for granted that results desired from the other vitamin will be accomplished by the use of the one concentrate.

There is a possibility that vitamin F will be found useful in the treatment of arthritis — for the only reason that vitamin D aggravates that disease, and "F" is the antagonist of "D." We have already mentioned that our vitamin E (with its accompanying "F") is useful in treating arthritic pains. We will have more information to offer on this subject in the near future.

**Edited by Royal Lee**

VITAMIN NEWS

VITAMIN PRODUCTS CO. • MILWAUKEE, WISCONSIN

VOL. 2 July 15, 1934 No. 7

## VITAMIN G

In the early investigations of vitamin B, the antineuritic vitamin, it was soon found that it contained a separate factor that was necessary to growth, that was more resistant to heat than the B, and occurred associated with B in varying proportions, being relatively high in yeast and low in corn. Different animal species were found to have varying requirements for the two components, pigeons being relatively immune to deficiency of the growth factor, while rats were susceptible to a deficiency of either.

The growth factor became separately designated as vitamin G, and it is now known that a deficiency of this principle is a factor in the causation of secondary anemia, pellagra, cataracts of the eye, and various forms of dermatitis.

In pellagra, Mellanby has stated that vitamin A deficiency (caused by use of white corn as the principle food) is the cause of spinal cord degeneration, and the associated deficiency of G causes the skin lesions in areas affected by the cord deficiency. This theory explains the "symmetrical" appearance of the skin lesions. It also indicates the impossibility of a complete cure, in view of the cord degeneration.

As to its relation to anemic conditions, where there may be so many contributory factors, vitamin G has been found to be of great benefit in certain types that fail to respond properly to other treatments. It can be safely stated that anemia can specifically result from vitamin G deficiency, but that vitamin G is not necessarily beneficial in any case of low erythrocyte count. vitamin C is also known to be an important factor and so are E and F. Vitamin G is likely to be found of value in secondary anemias while the others are more valuable in pernicious anemia.

Sherman-Smith say of vitamin G:

> "Vitamin G is evidently a substance of coordinate importance with the longer known vitamins as an essential factor in normal nutrition and deprivation or serious shortage of this substance results in wide-spread injury to the body. Conversely, the liberal feeding of this substance may be expected to play a significant part in inducing a better-than-average nutritive condition."

Vitamin G deficiency has been demonstrated to be a specific cause of cataract of the eye in test animals.

We quote the *Journal of Nutrition*, January 1934, pages 97-106:

> "Of 72 rats receiving diet 625 (deficient in G), 70 developed cataracts between the 40th and 87th day ... diagnosed by gross observation with the naked eye."

Cataract is here suggested as a more reliable and constant indication of G deficiency than the dermatitis heretofore considered specific, as its appearance is more consistent and unmistakable.

"Catalyn," because of its vitamin content, has been demonstrated to be a valuable remedy for cataract. The cataract is known to be a deposit of calcium carbonate, and to aid in its resolution "V-P Phosphade" is very useful in supplying the phosphorus radical to make the conversion to calcium phosphate. Because there are always many other less conspicuous deposits of calcium carbonate in the body tissues the "Catalyn" and "V-P Phosphade" must be taken for several months as a rule before the cataracts are affected. When the rest of the deposits are dissolved, however, the cataracts disappear with relative suddenness.

The reference given above is only six months old. "Catalyn" with "V-P Phosphade" has been successfully used for cataract for three years.

It will be here noted that vitamins A, C, D, F and G (probably also E) are concerned with some phase of calcium metabolism. A, causing by its absence kidney stones, C, being responsible among other things for the proper health of bone and teeth, D, ditto, but of less importance, F, being an agent that increases the diffusibility of calcium, making it available to the muscle and nerve functions, while G deficiency results in morbid soft tissue deposits of calcium. Only vitamin B is omitted from this category, probably because of our present ignorance, as its antineuritic effect is no doubt wrapped up in a calcium reaction.

Some day the sciences of vitamin therapy and endocrinology will be established as secondary to the study of the biochemical reactions of the alkali metal salts, with calcium as the major factor. The problems of old age itself are matters of calcium metabolism, in all probability, and most of the symptoms of senility are due to direct changes in calcium metabolism because of hormonic and vitamin deficiencies.

Why is vitamin G deficiency more productive of its specific reaction in old age? Because the vitamins act as nutritive agents for the endocrines and as age progresses, the endocrine organs become less efficient. More of the nutritional materials may be required to maintain the function.

This hypothesis applies to vitamins B, C and E as well. In children, vitamins A and D are required in relatively higher amounts, somewhat less in later years.

**Edited by Royal Lee**

# VITAMIN NEWS

VITAMIN PRODUCTS CO. • MILWAUKEE, WISCONSIN

VOL. 2 September 15, 1934 No. 8

## NERVOUS INSOMNIA

Nervous insomnia, like many other conditions directly due to avitaminosis, has been considered a result of the "high speed" of modern civilization. It is quite true that overwork, worry, mental stress, etc., aggravate the ailment. But the real cause is lowered resistance to such stresses, lowered stamina, increased nervous irritability because of deficient nutrition.

The metabolism of calcium and magnesium must be normal to ensure a properly functioning nervous system. Not to speak of the possibility of dietary deficiency of these two mineral elements, their assimilation and use can normally occur only in the presence of vitamins, all of which (with the possible exception of B) are concerned. Vitamin A deficiency is known to be the cause of kidney stones. Vitamins C and D are the best known factors in bone and tooth development. Vitamins E and F are necessary to convert the blood calcium (and probably magnesium) into a form that is useful to muscles and nerves; (we are beginning to find that arthritis in most of its forms is due to E and F deficiency), and G deficiency causes cataract of the eye as the most pronounced consequence of the precipitation of calcium occurring in the soft tissue.

Extreme irritability of the nervous system occurs if there is a deficiency in the blood of calcium or magnesium. Children with low blood calcium are unmanageable, restless at night, and have a "chip on the shoulder" disposition. Animals deprived of dietary magnesium will die in a convulsive fit on the slightest disturbance.

Did you ever see a hungry baby go peacefully to sleep? Nor will an adult go peacefully to sleep if he is starving himself with respect to vitamins.

"Catalyn" is the first physiological remedy offered for insomnia. There is probably no other effect produced by this vitamin product that is so easily demonstrated. Unlike drugs, its effects are purely constructive, and the amount required becomes less and less.

The correct dosage must be tested for each individual; one to three tablets upon retiring being the usual range to begin with. Because of its physiological action, an overdose can not induce excessive sleep, but will, on the other hand, cause wakefulness by its well known effect of eliminating fatigue.

Another effect of "Catalyn" is to clarify and normalize brain function. It is a commonly observed fact that school children on "Catalyn" treatment for some other purpose, soon receive much better marks in their school subjects, especially those who have had difficulty keeping up.

Dr. H. M. Johnson in his researches on sleep found that periodic changes of position were made.

> "The typical sleeper's period of rest between changes of position varies with his age. In infancy, he rests only five minutes at a time; the period lengthens to about fifteen minutes at maturity, then drops back gradually to seven or eight minutes with old age. Manual laborers rest for longer periods than brain workers; women rest 30 per cent longer than men." (*Fortune Magazine*, September, 1934.)

In our bulletin on our product, "V-P Phosphade," (a source of dietary phosphorus as $-PO_3$ and magnesium) we mention the fact that phosphate deficiency (caused mainly by the use of white flour products) brings about a tendency for deposition of calcium as carbonate in the soft tissues, and that this change is responsible for increased restlessness at night as well as "writer's cramp," "accelerator foot," etc.

Dr. Glenville Giddings found in a series of sleep experiments on children that during an epidemic he could predict the onset of disease several days in advance by the increased mobility of the child patient during sleep. Too, he found that while fever itself had no appreciable effect on childrens' motility, antipyretics made them restless indeed. (*Fortune*, same article.)

These facts all fit together with what we have said regarding deficiency conditions.

Normal body function is a situation of delicate balance, particularly hormonic balance and osmotic balance. Supply the complete nutritional picture, and the forces of nature will accomplish the rest. It is really surprising how far-reaching are the results of a few "Catalyn" tablets and a few doses of "V-P Phosphade" in cases where there are indications of calcium deposits. These are not irreparable damages.

The degree of recovery, for instance, is quite remarkable in some cases of arteriosclerosis, subjected to this treatment. The use of vitamin concentrates was the missing link necessary to the success of the long-known decalcifying agents. In fact, the normal diet should contain sufficient of both the decalcifying agents (phosphates in whole wheat) and the vitamins to prevent such pathology. But when the pathology is found we need quick action, calling for concentrated forms of each essential.

**Edited by Royal Lee**

VITAMIN NEWS

VITAMIN PRODUCTS CO. • MILWAUKEE, WISCONSIN

VOL. 2 October 15, 1934 No. 9

## MORE ON THE METABOLISM OF CALCIUM

All the vitamins, with the single possible exception of vitamin B, are known to be directly concerned with calcium metabolism. To illustrate, vitamin A deficiency is definitely proved to be the major cause of kidney stones; vitamin C is necessary to normal development of teeth and bone tissue (in scurvy the bones become decalcified); vitamin D is necessary to bring about the alimentary absorption of calcium; vitamin E (and its partner F) are essential in carrying calcium to the nervous and muscular tissues; while in vitamin G, deficiency cataracts of the eye develop (deposits of calcium carbonate).

It has been stated before in *Vitamin News* that calcium metabolism and the physiology of vitamin assimilation were practically synonymous, just as the chemistry of carbon compounds is to organic chemistry.

A study of hormones brings out similar facts. There are hormonic principles in the sex glands, spleen and suprarenal cortex, that depress the serum calcium; parathyroid hormone raises serum calcium, as also does adrenalin. The posterior pituitary pressor principle is a calcium control, as its hypersecretion causes deposition of calcium in the blood vessel walls.

Vitamin B enters the picture, too, but indirectly. Its deficiency causes an insufficient secretion of the gonad-stimulating principle, with a consequent reduction in the gonad-calcium depressor. The gonad-calcium depressor probably depends for its existence on the vitamin E and F intake which are known to reduce blood calcium by increasing the diffusibility of the serum calcium and causing its appropriation by nerve and muscle tissue.

Calcium is an important element in the function of the muscle cell. Muscular soreness is soon apparent as a consequence of any severe muscular activity where there is a deficiency of available calcium.

And the pains of neuritis and arthritis in all probability are due to the same deficiency of a certain kind of diffusible calcium. The diffusible blood calcium is known to be of at least two kinds — one passes to the negative pole and one to the positive in electrolysis.

Therefore, theoretically, we can have at least six calcium-control hormones — a depressor of the non-diffusible, of the negative diffusible and of the positive diffusible; also a stimulator of each.

As an offhand guess, I would say that the stimulator of the non-diffusible is posterior pituitary; stimulator of the diffusible are parathyroid and adrenalin. And we have three depressors left to balance the situation — suprarenal cortex, gonad and spleen.

Vitamin F, the fat-soluble growth principle found associated with E, and acting to oppose the action of vitamin D in maintaining calcium balance in the blood, appears to be the specific antidote for D poisoning. It is apparently present in cod-liver oil and this would account for the great difference in toxicity of cod-liver oil D as compared to irradiated ergosterol.

It is quite probable that the presence of F is as essential to the assimilation of calcium as D — the D is necessary to the alimentary absorption into the blood and the F is necessary to prepare the blood calcium for use by the tissues. The fact is significant that pregnant animals are immune to D toxicosis. Possibly the animal in this circumstance even synthesizes F, as the human infant does to obtain its necessary supply of vitamin C during the first months of its existence as has been recently demonstrated by Rohmar, Bezzonoff and Sanders. Personally, I am sure that the disorders of calcium metabolism of older people — loss of bone calcium, arthritic and neuritic tendencies, and even eye disorders — loss of accommodation of iris and lens as well as cataracts — are due to a lack of vitamins A, E, F and G and their inefficient assimilation in the small amounts ordinarily received.

The aggravation of rickets by the F in oatmeal is because F ensures a calcium supply to nerve and muscle at the expense of bone. Too much D can cause a too high blood serum calcium content, unless an ample F and E supply are present to insure its conversion into forms useful to the soft tissues. An enzyme — phosphatase — is the local stimulator of bone ossification, and after adult age is reached the phosphatase content of bone tissue is automatically lowered, reducing the bone demand for calcium, and increasing the danger of D toxicosis — another name for high serum calcium, which can cause hypertension, arteriosclerosis, etc., even while the muscular and nervous tissues are sadly needing calcium because of the dietary deficiency of vitamins A, B, C, E, F and G.

Both vitamin A and E deficiency cause damage to the semeniferous epithelium where the gonad hormone is secreted. Quite possibly, each contributes an atomic group to the gonad hormone molecule that is so necessary to normal calcium metabolism.

Abnormalities in calcium metabolism because of various factors bring on premature old age (we have noted the fact before that the natives who live in the South American tropics become weakened and aged at thirty years, and usually die before thirty-five. The African native, being coal-black, escaped these consequences.).

Calcium unbalance results in osmotic unbalance, with cell shriveling and a "dried up" appearance on one hand, and cell distension and obesity on the other. The deficiency of all causing the second situation as a rule, with too much D (along with a deficiency of the rest) being instrumental in helping to bring about the first. The people in the southwestern United States are particularly conspicuous as to skin degenerations (deep wrinkles and a weatherbeaten appearance) as compared to the people of the North and East, because of the formation of vitamin D in their skins from the relatively greater exposure to sunlight.

**Edited by Royal Lee**

# VITAMIN NEWS

VITAMIN PRODUCTS CO. • MILWAUKEE, WISCONSIN

VOL. 2 November 15, 1934 No. 10

## VITAMIN F and CALCIUM METABOLISM

Recently, there have been quite a few reports on the successful treatment of kidney stones by the use of vitamin A or special diets high in A. It has been known for some time, of course, that test animals deprived of vitamin A developed renal calculi.

Reports have also been made of the benefit to eye conditions, that were due to disorders of calcium metabolism, obtained from the use of vitamin A and carotene (which can be converted into vitamin A by metabolic changes after ingestion). Even cataract has been successfully treated with vitamin A.

It is becoming apparent from the experiences of those using vitamin A for these purposes that other factors were involved that affected the outcome of the treatment. Often initial results were obtained that were very encouraging but with a later cessation of improvement.

That is a very commonly observed phenomenon in attempting to treat deficiency diseases. If the pathology in question is (as is usually the case) a consequence of a number of associated deficiencies, the replacement of a part of the group will produce some improvement, but the recovery will, of necessity, have to stop before normality is reached.

As stated in the last issue of *Vitamin News*, all the vitamins, with the possible exception of B, are involved in calcium metabolism. That is why the use of "Catalyn" has been observed to be effective in so many of the diseases in which calcium metabolism is involved.

But the value of vitamin E or F to supplement "Catalyn" in the treatment of kidney stones, cataract, and other eye conditions has been becoming more and more apparent of late. In fact, we are almost ready to assume that most of the eye pathologies which have always been considered an inevitable penalty of oncoming years, are rather due to endocrine aging that can be largely offset by an added intake of the proper vitamins, and that most of this aging is premature, due to the same nutritional deficiency.

The eye tissues begin to show a functional change because of calcium deposits probably before there is evidence of them elsewhere. The determinations of Hesse (1929) of the calcium content of blood-vessel walls probably will correspond in the main with the calcium content of eye tissues — 0.16% at two years, 0.38% at thirty-four years and 1.97% at fifty-six years. A 500% increase between the ages of thirty-four and fifty-six.

While in test animals vitamin G deficiency invariably causes cataract of the eye, in human clinical experience the use of this single vitamin is not so specifically useful to dissolve the cataract as vitamins A, C and F, and it appears that F is particularly valuable as an aid in hastening the process. The use of vitamin F concentrate has also been noted in most of the test cases to improve the ability of the eye lens to accommodate to various focal distances, and has thereby necessitated the refitting of glasses. It has caused the disappearance of photosensitiveness, and this, of course, is merely improved ability of the iris to respond to light stimulus.

Possibly all these are improved muscular functions.

Vitamin F has also produced quite rapid improvement in a few cases of prostate enlargement that failed to respond to the administration of "Catalyn."

And the F seems to be a salutary stimulus to the liver and improves in some cases the bowel elimination, possibly through the agency of the liver effect.

And, so far, those stubborn cases of hypertension that refuse to respond to "Catalyn," have fallen before vitamin F treatment. These were, no doubt, due to the arterial wall impermeability and incipient hardening due to the well-known calcium accumulations as per Hesse's analyses.

The administration of viosterol has been demonstrated to cause hypertrophy of the medial (muscular) layer of the arterioles and marked hypertension, in a few weeks, under moderate doses. F, as the physiological antagonist of vitamin D, may be the long-sought specific against arteriosclerosis. So far, all indications are pointing that way.

Our recommendation is one or two tablets of vitamin F (and two or three "Catalyn" tablets) a day for any of the cases where it is desired to test its effects.

Where "Catalyn" has been used for a period of time and it may not be considered necessary to continue its use, the F, of course, may be given alone. Over two tablets a day should be considered a waste of material for a long continued treatment, as it appears that the F principle does not require heavy dosage.

We feel that F is worthy of trial in cases of arthritis, neuritis, hypertension, enlarged prostate, photosensitiveness, all cases of the old and feeble, and in vitamin D toxicosis.

**Edited by Royal Lee**

# VITAMIN NEWS

VITAMIN PRODUCTS CO. • MILWAUKEE, WISCONSIN

VOL. 2 December 15, 1934 No. 11

## THE CHRISTMAS SPIRIT

Christmas is the time we think of others — the children in particular. As our contribution, we shall here offer what advice we are able, to those who are in a position to make use of it, regarding the dietary precautions to ensure the best gift of all; good health and a sound physique.

The writer, in 1923, had occasion to investigate the causes of rickets, now known to be due to vitamin D and C deficiency. The disease was known to appear chiefly in very poor or quite well-to-do families. The explanation became apparent that the very poor child failed to get enough food to receive the necessary vitamins for development, while the child in the wealthy family received only highly refined and sterilized foods, whereas in the middle class family, the children had an opportunity to supplement their diets with raw foods, vegetables, etc. obtained during the preparations of the meals, to which the child in the wealthy family failed to have access.

The wider use of fresh vegetable salads, etc. has altered the picture today over what it was a number of years ago.

Probably the greatest offender in causing vitamin deficiency in children is the use of candy and sugar products. All candy and sugar products are devitalized and supply fuel only, to produce energy, and have no other food constituents. The child needs materials for construction — minerals, proteins, and vitamins — and if they are supplied candy and sweets, their appetites are satisfied without supplying the necessary building materials. To make a crude simile, it would be just as foolish to try to build an automobile with gasoline as structural material.

White flour products are just as damnable, as child food. Test animals die from mineral and vitamin deficiency in three or four weeks if fed on white flour alone, while maintaining health indefinitely on whole wheat.

Fresh whole wheat flour (obtainable in health food stores in all large cities) for making muffins, pancakes, etc. supplies this cereal in its most palatable form. The bread supply should be only whole wheat or rye.

The white flour milling companies have made frantic efforts to side-track the growing consciousness on the part of the public that white flour is bad. (The bleaching processes that are necessary to ensure keeping qualities have been proved to leave certain nitrates in the flour the cumulative effect of which may make the flour actually poisonous.) The makers of devitalized foods (sugar, corn syrup, white flour, etc.) attempt to ingratiate themselves with the medical and dental organizations by spending large sums in advertising in the journals. "Corn Syrup for Infant Feeding — it is so well tolerated" is a favorite advertising slogan in such propaganda. A solution of agar or gelatine would be well tolerated too — if food values were of no merit.

As a matter of fact, it is an unwise thing to select any item of diet for a child on the principle that it contains carbohydrates. The list of foods necessary to supply minerals and vitamins will inevitably supply a sufficiency of the energy source as an included and unavoidable component. The difficulty, it is clear, is not to get carbohydrates but to avoid its excess in forms that do not contain the other essentials.

Honey and raw unrefined sugar (obtainable at health food stores) in limited amounts, can be used to satisfy the craving for sweets, if it is present. It usually is not in the child properly supplied with natural foods. It is of interest in this connection that the Negro child of the south, obtaining its sweets from the chewing of sugar cane, always has perfect teeth — the cane sap contains its quota of minerals and vitamins.

Milk, being a food complete in itself, is to be highly recommended, but no irradiated milk, as the irradiation process kills the vitamin A. Pasteurization destroys the vitamin C, and the difficulty of obtaining unpasteurized milk with a reasonably low bacteria count greatly reduces its usefulness in the diet.

Milk contains no excess of vitamins or minerals that will compensate for the use of other devitalized foods, as is often claimed.

Plant leaves are the only foods that contain an excess of mineral salts and vitamins A and C that can be so used. But their incidence in the usual diet is so low that this effect never or seldom occurs. The green leaves — turnip greens, lettuce, spinach — are best in vitamin content. The calcium and mineral content depends largely on the degree of deficiency existing in the soil on which they were grown.

Meats, of cold-storage origin, are worthless sources of vitamins, and are not fit for the child's diet. Fresh meats, fish and fowl, are in another class, and are valuable sources of growth-promoting vitamins (A & G).

The use of fresh vegetable juices (carrot, celery, cabbage, etc.) are a wonderful aid in supplying increased vitamins and minerals. The juice from a pound of carrots, for example, contains most of the food values of the carrot — but is far more palatable and more easily imbibed than an equal quantity of the raw vegetable. (Juice extractors for the vegetables are now available. We refer you again to the health food store.) Fruit juices are in the same class, but are not as valuable as sources of minerals as the vegetables. Carrot juice is high in vitamins A and B whereas orange juice is looked upon as a good source of C.

The first reaction observed from a diet high in candy and white flour is the typical lack of appetite due to A, B and C deficiency. The child so afflicted is difficult to handle for that reason — they refuse the foods they should have. That is where our vitamin concentrates are particularly useful. The use of two "Catalyn" tablets with one vitamin A tablet a day brings back that lost appetite in a very short time.

And please do not forget — that in children's febrile diseases, the temperature can be quickly controlled with "Catalyn."

**Edited by Royal Lee**

## ABSTRACTS ON THE EFFECT OF PASTEURIZATION ON THE NUTRITIONAL VALUE OF MILK

### INHERENT CHARACTERISTICS OF MILK DISTURBED BY PASTEURIZATION

" ... Pasteurization was also found to affect the hematogenic and growth-promoting properties of the special milk (raw milk from specially fed cows whose milk did not produce nutritional anemia — whereas commercially pasteurized milk did) ... "

Krauss, W. E., Erb. J. H. and Washburn, R. G. Studies on the Nutritive Value of Milk II. The effect of Pasteurization on Some of the Nutritive Properties of Milk, *Ohio Agricultural Experiment Station Bulletin* 518, page 11, January, 1933.

*The Lancet*, page 1142, May 8, 1937 states that resistance to tuberculosis increased in children fed raw milk instead of pasteurized, to the point that in five years only one case of pulmonary TB had developed, whereas in the previous five years, when children had been given pasteurized milk, 14 cases of pulmonary TB had developed.

"Human or cow milk added to an equal volume of agar did not support the growth or allowed only slight growth of B. diphtheriae, Staph. aureus, B. coli, B. prodigious, B. pyocyaneus, B. anthracis, streptococci, and unidentified wild yeast. The factors in human milk inhibiting bacterial growth ('inhibins') were inactivated by heating at 56 degrees C (pasteurization temperatures — 60 degrees — 70 degrees C.) for thirty minutes by standing twelve to twenty-four days at 5 degrees C., but not by repeated freezing and thawing. The 'inhibins' in cow's milk were not inactivated by heating at 80 degrees C. for seven minutes but were destroyed by heating at 85 degrees C. for seven minutes. Attempts have not been made to identify the natural antiseptics."

Dold, H., Wizaman, E., and Kleiner C., Z. Hyt Inf., Antiseptic in Milk. *The Drug and Cosmetic Industry,* 43,1:109, July, 1938

"Milk, an animal product, is the essential food of all infant mammals. Mammals are so classified in the scale of living things because of the common characteristic of the female nursing her young. The infant mammal is accordingly carnivorous in his natural habits irrespective of whether the adult of the species is herbivorous or carnivorous.

"If the adults on a carnivorous diet show conditions of deficiency on cooked meat, is it not reasonable to suppose that growing infants on entirely cooked carnivorous diets will do likewise? Many experimenters, such as Catel, Dutcher, Wilson, and others, have shown such to be the case in animals fed on pasteurized milk.

"Can human infants be born of mothers who are deficient, and yet attain a fair degree of skeletal development if given a proper raw milk supply? The three infants in Figure 4 were born of mothers known to be hypothyroid. Prior to the birth of the infants shown, all three mothers had given birth to children within three years. Each of the previous children was asthmatic, showed infantile rickets, and possessed poor skeletal development. The first child shown in Figure 4 was breast fed from birth, with the mother living under excellent health-promoting conditions. The second child was on powdered milk for four weeks, and on raw certified milk after that without cod-liver oil or orange juice. Both the first and the second child began supplemental feedings when they were about five months old and were very healthy babies. The third baby was always sickly and had been on formulae since birth. These formulae included powdered milk, pasteurized milk, boiled milk, boiled certified milk and canned milk. She had suffered from severe gastric distress during her entire infancy and when eight months old she developed asthma. She is very small though her parents are of larger build than the parents of the other two children.

"The strictest bacteriological standards for milk must always be maintained. The feeding of cattle should receive greater attention. It should be determined experimentally, if possible, whether health and resistance are undermined by pasteurization. If so, on our attempt to protect the child from milk-borne infections, we may be denying his heritage of good health by removing from his milk vitamins, hormones, and enzymes that control mineral assimilation and promote body development and general resistance to disease. Is it also possible that these same elements are as important to the adult invalid who needs milk as to the infant?

"Let us have closer cooperation between raw-milk producers and public-health officials so that the growth-producing factors of raw milk can be studied. We cannot afford to pasteurize milk if it is found that pasteurization diminishes the potency of the growth-promoting factors that determine the skeletal development of our children. We cannot afford to lessen the resistance of our children to respiratory infection, asthma, bronchitis and the common cold when factors preventing them are present in greater amounts in properly produced clean raw milk than in pasteurized milk."

Pottenger, F. M., Jr., Clinical and Experimental Evidence of Growth Factors in Raw Milk, *Certified Milk*, January, 1937

"Some have questioned whether pasteurized milk is really involved in the production of scurvy. The fact, however, that when one gives a group of infants this food for a period of about six months, instances of scurvy occur, and that a cure is brought about when raw milk is substituted, taken in conjunction with the fact that if we feed the same number of infants on raw milk, cases of scurvy will not develop — these results seem sufficient to warrant the deduction that pasteurized milk is a causative factor. The experience in Berlin, noted by Neumann (Neumann, II., *Deutsch. Klin.*, 7:341, 1904) and others, is most illuminating and convincing in this connection. In 1901 a large dairy in the city established a pasteurizing plant in which all milk was raised to a temperature of about 60 degrees C. After an interval of some months, infantile scurvy was reported from various sources throughout the city. Neumann writes about the situation as follows:

> 'Whereas Heubner, Cassel and myself had seen only thirty-two cases of scurvy from 1896 to 1900, the number of cases suddenly rose from the year 1901, so that the same observers — not to mention a great many others — treated eighty-three cases in 1901 and 1902.'

An investigation was made as to the cause, and the pasteurization was discontinued. The result was that the number of cases decreased just as suddenly as they had increased ... "

Hess, A. F., Infantile Scurvy. V. A. Study of Its Pathogenesis, *Am. J. Dis. Child.*, November, 1917

"Although pasteurized milk is to be recommended on account of the security which it affords against infection, we should realize that it is an incomplete food. Unless an antiscorbutic, such as orange juice ... or potato water is added, infants will develop scurvy on this diet. This form of scurvy takes some months to develop and may be termed subacute. It must be considered not only the most common form of this disorder, but the one which passes most often unrecognized. In order to guard against it, infants fed exclusively on a diet of pasteurized milk should be given antiscorbutics far earlier than is at present the custom, even as early as at the end of the first month of life."

Hess, A. F., Infantile Scurvy, III. Its Influence on Growth (Length and Weight). *Am. Jl. Dis. Child.*, August,1916

"One of the most striking clinical phenomenon of infantile scurvy is the marked susceptibility to infection which it entails — the frequent attacks of 'grippe,' the widespread occurrence of nasal diphtheria, the furunculosis of the skin, the danger of pneumonia in advanced cases ... "

Hess, A. F., Infantile Scurvy. V. A. Study of Its Pathogenesis, *Am. J. Dis. Child.*, November, 1917

" ... Recently, Minot and his colleagues came to the conclusion that adult scurvy can be precipitated by infectious processes; in other words, that latent scurvy can by this means be changed to manifest scurvy. In general, therefore, investigations in the laboratory as well as clinical observations are in agreement in stressing the interrelationship of scurvy and bacterial infection."

Hess, A. F. Recent Advances in Knowledge of Scurvy and the Antiscorbutic Vitamin, *J.A.M.A.*, April 23, 1932

This illustrates the futility of pasteurization of milk to prevent infection from diseases the cows may sometimes have, such as undulant fever. The infant is then made subject to the common infectious diseases, and deaths from these common diseases are not attributed, as they should be, to the defective nature of the milk.

## EFFECTS OF PASTEURIZATION OF MILK ON TOOTH HEALTH

*Lancet*, page 1142, May 8, 1937 says that in children the teeth are less likely to decay on diet supplemented with raw milk than with pasteurized milk.

"Dr. Evelyn Sprawson of the London Hospital has recently stated that in certain institutions children who were brought up on raw milk (as opposed to pasteurized milk) had perfect teeth and no decay. Whether this was due actually to the milk being unheated, or possibly some other quite different and so far unrecognized cause, we cannot yet say; but we may be sure of one thing, that the result is so striking and unusual that it will undoubtedly be made the subject of further inquiry."

Harris, L. J., *Vitamins in Theory and Practice*, page 224, Cambridge University Press, 1935.

## EFFECTS OF PASTEURIZATION OF MILK ON GROWTH

... Fisher and Bartlett "point out by statistical treatment that the response in height to raw milk was significantly greater than that to pasteurized milk. Their interpretation of the data led to the assertion that the pasteurized milk was only 66 per cent as effective as the raw milk in the case of boys and 91.1 per cent as effective in the case of girls in inducing increases in weight, and 50 per cent as effective in boys and 70 per cent in girls in bringing about height increases."

Krauss, W. E., Erb, J. H. and Washburn, R. G., Studies on the Nutritive Value of Milk. II. The Effect of Pasteurization on Some of the Nutritive Properties of Milk, *Ohio Agricultural Experiment Station Bulletin 518*, page 7, January, 1933.

" ... Daniels and Loughlin observed that young rats fed long heat-treated milks, evaporated, condensed and pasteurized by the 'hold' method failed to grow normally, but if the precipitated calcium salts were incorporated into the various milk, growth was normal ... "

Daniels, A. L., and Loughlin, R., *Journal of Biological Chemistry,* 44,381, 1920 as abstracted by Holmes and Pigott, Factors That Influence the Antirachitic Value of Milk in Infant Feeding, Oil & Soap, 12.9:202-207, Sept., 1935

## CALCIUM AVAILABILITY IN PASTEURIZED MILK

"Kramer, Latzke and Shaw (Kramer, Martha M., Latzke, F., and Shaw, M. M., A Comparison of Raw, Pasteurized, Evaporated and Dried Milks as Sources of Calcium and Phosphorus for the Human Subject, *Journal of Biological Chemistry*, 79:283-295, 1928) obtained less favorable calcium balances in adults with pasteurized milk than with 'fresh milk' and made the further observations that milk from cows kept in the barn for five months gave less favorable calcium balances than did 'fresh milk' (herd milk from a college dairy)."

Krauss, W. E., Erb. J. H., and Washburn, R. G. Studies on the Nutritive Value of Milk, II. The Effect of Pasteurization on Some of the Nutritive Properties of Milk, *Ohio Agricultural Experiment Station, Bulletin 518*, page 8, January, 1933.

In the *Lancet*, page 1142, May 8, 1937 it is shown that chilblains are practically eliminated (result of higher calcium values of raw milk or improved assimilation of calcium) when raw milk rather than pasteurized milk is used in the diet of children.

## PASTEURIZATION DESTROYS VITAMIN A

" ... According to S. Schmidt-Nielsen and Schmidt-Nielsen (*Kgl. Norske Videnskab. Selsk. Forhandl.*, 1:126-128, abstracted in Biological Abstracts, 4:94, 1930), when milk pasteurized at 63 degrees C. (145 degrees F.) was fed to mature rats, early death or diminished vitality resulted in the offspring. This was attributed to the destruction of vitamin A."

Krauss, W. E., Erb. J. H. and Washburn, R. G., Studies on the Nutritive Value of Milk, II. The Effect of Pasteurization on Some of the Nutritive Properties of Milk, *Ohio Agricultural Experiment Station, Bulletin 518*, page 9, January, 1933.

## PASTEURIZATION DESTROYS VITAMIN B COMPLEX

"Pasteurization of milk destroys about 38% of the B complex according to Dutcher and his associates ... "

Lewis, L. R., The Relation of the Vitamins to Obstetrics, *American Journal of Obstetrics and Gynecology*, 29,5:759, May, 1935.

"Mattick and Golding (Relative Value of Raw and Heated Milk in Nutrition, *Lancet*, 220:662-667) reported some preliminary experiments which indicated that pasteurization destroys some of the dietic value of milk, including partial destruction of vitamin $B_1$. These same workers found the raw milk to be considerably superior to sterilized milk in nutritive value."

Krauss, W. E. Erb, J. H. and Washburn. R. G. Studies on the Nutritive Value of Milk, II. The Effect of Pasteurization on Some of the Nutritive Properties of Milk, *Ohio Agricultural Experiment Station, Bulletin 518,* page 9, January, 1933.

" ... On the 7.5 cc. level two rats on raw milk developed mild polyneuritis toward the end of the trial; whereas three rats on pasteurized milk developed polyneuritis early, which became severe as the trial drew to a close. On the 10.0 cc. level none of the rats on raw milk developed polyneuritis, but three on pasteurized milk were severely afflicted."

Ibid, page 23.

"Using standard methods for determining vitamins A, B, G and D, it was found that pasteurization destroyed at least 25% of the vitamin B in the original raw milk."

Ibid, page 30.

## PASTEURIZATION DESTROYS VITAMIN C

" ... The pasteurization of milk has been found to destroy 20 to 50 percent (of the Vitamin C), the fraction that has undergone reversible oxidation ... "

Bastedo, W. A., *Materia, Medica, Pharmacology, Therapeutics and Prescription Writing*, Fourth Edition, Reset, page 78, W. B. Saunders Co., Philadelphia, 1938.

"Current objection to pasteurization is mainly on the ground of vitamin destruction. vitamins A (fat-soluble) and B (water-soluble), both abundant in milk, are quite resistant to heat, but the antiscorbutic vitamin C is weakened or destroyed by pasteurizing temperatures. Infants fed exclusively on a diet of pasteurized milk will develop scurvy. Fortunately, the addition to the diet of readily accessible antiscorbutics such as orange juice or tomato juice is tolerated by infants much earlier than used to be supposed, even in the first month of life. The reasonable procedure, therefore, appears to be to use pasteurized milk to insure protection against disease germs of various kinds and to supply the vitamin deficiency through other foods. The success in infant feeding based on this principle is evidenced especially in the amazing reduction in infant mortality in summer months."

Jordan, E. O., *A Textbook of General Bacteriology,* Twelfth Edition, Revised, page 691, W. B. Saunders Co., 1938

"Within the past few years, an increasing number of patients affected with heavy scurvy have been brought to the Oregon Children's Hospital. As the prophylactic amount of vitamin C (15 mg. daily) is contained in 300 cc. of breast milk, scurvy is rarely found in breast-fed babies.

"The vitamin C of cow's milk is largely destroyed by pasteurization or evaporation."

Overstreet, R. M., *Northwest Medicine*, June, 1938, as abstracted by Clinical Medicine and Surgery, The Increase of Scurvy, 42, 12:598, December, 1938.

"Samples of raw, certified, certified Guernsey and certified vitamin D milks were collected at the different dairies throughout the city of Madison. These milks on the average are only a little below the fresh milks as recorded in Table I, indicating that commercial raw and certified milks as delivered to the consumer lose only a small amount of their antiscorbutic potency. Likewise, samples of commercial pasteurized milks were collected and analyzed. On an average they contained only about one-half as much ascorbic acid as fresh raw milks and significantly less ascorbic acid than the commercial unpasteurized milks.

"It was found that commercial raw milks contained an antiscorbutic potency which was only slightly less than fresh raw milks and that pasteurized milks on the average contained only one-half the latter potency. Mineral modification and homogenization apparently have a destructive effect on ascorbic acid."

Woessner, Warren W., Elvehjem, C. A., and Schuette, Henry A., The Determination of Ascorbic Acid in Commercial Milks, *Journal of Nutrition*, 18,6:619-626, December, 1939.

# NOTES

VITAMIN NEWS

VITAMIN PRODUCTS CO. • MILWAUKEE, WISCONSIN

VOL. 3 January 15, 1935 No. 1

## THE PRESENT STATUS OF VITAMIN A

A year ago in *Vitamin News* we discussed the known effects of vitamin A deficiency, its sources, and some of the therapeutic uses of the concentrate.

The experience of the year as regards our tablet of vitamin A concentrate indicates that it may be found useful in treating the following conditions:

1. Lack of appetite in undernourished children. (One tablet a day, with one "Catalyn" tablet.)

2. Lowered resistance of the epithelium to bacterial invasion and epithelial irritability. This includes such otherwise diverse conditions as susceptibility to colds, gastritis, cystitis, and nephritis. It is possible that there may be other factors causing these diseases, but when vitamin A deficiency is present they tend to persist and are not as amenable to the heretofore conventional therapeutic measures. Albuminuria without apparent cause, especially in children is often controllable with one tablet a day of vitamin A. Acute cystitis is often immediately controlled, so are certain types of gastritis.

3. Constipation. Certain individuals have found that an occasional vitamin A tablet maintains a normal bowel function. As yet we have no theory to offer, except that vitamin A is known to be essential to liver function. vitamins B, C and F are known to sometimes have this effect also.

4. Dropsy, where there is present liver dysfunction. The fact must be recalled also that vitamin A is essential to kidney function as well as of the liver, and its value in this situation may be attributable to the beneficial action on each organ.

5. Renal calculi. Stones or gravel in the kidney or bladder can be considered a definite result of vitamin A deficiency. The accompanying susceptibility to infection because of the same deficiency is a serious matter. The calculi tend to become abscessed, and the only rational treatment (besides surgical removal) is a high vitamin diet and vitamin concentrates. Two tablets each of vitamin A and "Catalyn" produce definite results. Many persons with renal calculi have a mottled ruddy complexion — sometimes a "whisky nose" — which begins to clear up in a few days under the above treatment. The actual dissolution of the calculi, however, is a slow matter. They become sharper (star shaped) as they dissolve, and may cause trouble at any time. The value of vitamin A to allay the irritability of the urinary system is here most apparent.

Vitamin A is formed in the body from carotene, the coloring material in butter, yellow vegetables and cereals. It is also obtained from eggs, liver, carrots and the green leafy vegetables.

Carotene in a purified form has been widely sold as vitamin A. This should not be considered as an effective source of this vitamin. It is our opinion that most persons who have a deficiency of vitamin A have for some reason lost their ability to convert the carotene into the vitamin. McCollum has stated that in certain countries where the diet was confined to vegetables high in carotene (squash as an example), some persons (presumably those who had lost the conversion power) became yellow in color, simulating jaundice, differing only in that the whites of the eyes were not affected.

Sherman and Smith, in *The Vitamins,* say that an alcoholic extract of carrot was known to protect rats from xerophthalmia where pure carotene prepared from carrot was without effect. (Page 244). This indicates that some rats also can fail to be able to make the conversion.

It is our prediction that some other dietary factor as yet unidentified will be found to be necessary for this conversion. Meanwhile, we offer our concentrate of vitamin A to those who are sufficiently critical to expect a definite clinical result in each case where its use is indicated.

We believe that a serious mistake has been made in the acceptance by the U.S. Pharmacopeia of carotene as a unitary standard of vitamin A. It is a premature decision to accept carotene as a measure of what the as yet unknown vitamin will accomplish. It is a justification of our attitude of record to refrain from making the attempt to offer our customers a unit specification of vitamin content that fails to take into account clinical performance, but is based on some other unrelated means of standardization.

We prefer to stake our reputation on our care in the selection of raw materials, and on our care in so processing these materials as to insure a potent final product. We have as yet to receive a complaint from any physician that he failed to get results in a case that according to his experience should have responded. No pharmaceutical product should be purchased without taking into account the reputation of the manufacturer, and in the history of all food products no better standard has been developed.

**Edited by Royal Lee**

CATALYN — NATURES SOURCE OF VITALITY — MADE IN U.S.A.

# VITAMIN NEWS

VITAMIN PRODUCTS CO. • MILWAUKEE, WISCONSIN

VOL. 3 February 15, 1935 No. 2

## FURTHER COMMENTS ON VITAMIN A

The *A. M. A. Journal* of December 29, 1934 carried an article by Drs. Shibley and Spies, calling attention to their work in which it was found that vitamin A failed to produce the expected results as a protective agent against colds, in particular, and was not as valuable a prophylactic against other infections as it had been considered by other investigators.

This report needs analysis before acceptance. The specific action of vitamin A that relates to infections is its ability to ensure an epithelial integrity that will prevent the mechanical entrance of germs. Colds and influenza are believed to be caused by a filterable virus so the ability of vitamin A to protect against the entrance to these infective agents may be of little or no value in those particular infectious diseases.

Vitamin A deficiency in test animals, however, is particularly effective in reducing the resistance to pus germs — with resulting infections of sinuses, tonsils, mastoid, etc. Here we have visible microorganisms to deal with, and not a filterable virus that can penetrate openings too small to admit germs that can be seen in the microscope.

The resistance of the organism to a filterable virus is not dependent at all upon the first line of defense — the epithelium — nor is it dependent upon the second line of defense — the phagocytes, but upon the third line of defense — the rapid development of immunity. As Sajous has stated, we depend upon vitamin intake for the defensive agents that are needed to produce specific immunity, and it is the experience of every physician who has used our product, "Catalyn," that it ordinarily causes immunity to be developed at a far more rapid rate than normally is possible. Vitamins B and C are chiefly instrumental in this effect. Sajous even went so far as to state that in his opinion vitamin C and Erlich's complement were identical. It is, therefore, evident that immunity may be impossible without vitamin C, and without "C," the third line of defense is non-existent.

As it has been demonstrated that the number (and probably the activity as well) of the phagocytes is limited by vitamin deficiency, we begin to realize the all-important part vitamins play in protecting us from microbic attack. The integrity of each of the three lines of defense is dependent upon an adequate vitamin supply.

We consider the findings of Drs. Shibley and Spies also illustrative of the fallacy of using vitamin concentrates standardized by animal tests in clinical research. The real and only way to test a vitamin that is supposed to prevent colds is to use it to treat colds in human subjects. According to their method of testing, the products used by Drs. Shibley and Spies did not contain therapeutically useful amounts of vitamin A. That would be our conclusion, rather than that vitamin A were not of benefit for the diseases under consideration, for there is too overwhelming a volume of evidence supporting the affirmative side of that question.

We are also inclined to accept this explanation for the failure of these investigators to find their vitamin A concentrates of benefit, because of the consistent failure of the product to protect against respiratory infections in children, or in reducing the incidence of otitis media and scarlet fever.

It is more than probable that a widespread reduction in the supply of vitamin A such as occurred during the World War (mainly because of butter substitute) was the basic reason for the influenza epidemic that spread over the entire civilized world. The paucity of other high vitamin foods and the attendant low intake of all vitamins, no doubt, was an aggravating factor. Infective agents are known as a general rule to increase in virulence in proportion to the lack of opposition by the normal defensive factors of the subjects affected. A person with low resistance may develop a severe attack of influenza, for instance, and thereby infect another subject who normally would resist the disease and fail to contract it from a person suffering from a less virulent form. That is how epidemics get under way.

The severity of the cold and influenza epidemics noticed in some of our large cities recently has caused some observers to suggest that possibly the general irradiation of milk may be responsible, because of the attendant destruction of vitamin A. There is no doubt but that the practice of irradiating foods indiscriminately has become more or less a commercial racket, and further investigation of the real facts is imperatively necessary.

**Edited by Royal Lee**

NATURE'S SOURCE OF VITALITY CATALYN MADE IN U.S.A.

# VITAMIN NEWS

NATURE'S SOURCE OF VITALITY CATALYN MADE IN U.S.A.

VITAMIN PRODUCTS CO. • MILWAUKEE, WISCONSIN

VOL. 3 March 15, 1935 No. 3

## VITAMIN B NOTES TO DATE

A year ago, in these pages, attention was called to the fact that a deficiency of vitamin B resulted in such reactions as enlargement and undoubted malfunction of a list of organs including adrenals, thyroid, thymus, pancreas, gonads, spleen, heart, liver, kidneys, stomach and brain.

The effect on the pancreas was further discussed in the May 15th issue, showing that a deficiency of vitamin B can cause diabetes mellitus and that an improvement usually follows the use of concentrates of that vitamin.

The enlargement of spleen, stomach and heart because of B deficiency is explainable on the grounds of muscular dystrophy, known to be a specific consequence of B deficiency. It is that muscular weakness of the stomach walls that causes the lack of appetite in the B-deficient child. The spleen has recently been demonstrated to be (before senile atrophy) a muscular organ acting as a reservoir for blood, so that a loss of muscle tone in that organ can act to cause its enlargement as well as a loss of vascular and tissue tone that is dependent upon such an "elastic" reservoir, not to speak of the loss of vascular tone due to the direct action of the deficiency on the muscular layer of the vessel walls.

The intestinal walls also lose their contractile power in B deficiency with resultant constipation and stagnation. The flow of digestive juices is inhibited. (Pernicious anemia can be brought on mainly because of degeneration of the blood-forming tissues in the bone marrow.) In vitamin B deficiency in rats, "Marrow elements are destroyed and replaced by reticular tissue supporting widely dilated congested blood vessels." (Shipley, McCollum and Simmonds, *Journal of Biological Chemistry*, 49, 399.)

There is some mutual action between vitamin B and vitamin E. Too much B (yeast extract) has been demonstrated to be a cause of sterility in rats. Too much E (spinach extract) has been known to cause anemia. Probably these two vitamins each require the complementary presence of the other in metabolism, and overdosage of one without the other can thereby cause an acute deficiency of the missing principle.

We have had reports of cases in which our B concentrate caused such vascular contraction as to produce coldness of extremities and contraction of the pupils. Normal persons have no such reaction, and in all probability it is due to deficiency of some cooperative principle, possibly E.

Hyperthyroidea causes an excessive requirement for vitamin B (Cowgill). Possibly this is because of the pancreatic demand, in that more oxidation of carbohydrate requires an increased pancreatic secretion, which we have seen is dependent upon the B intake. At any rate, it is well established that the B requirement is parallel with the metabolic rate.

The dietary habits of recent times, in which we ingest large amounts of carbohydrates — white flour and refined sugar — without the vitamin B necessary to the normal assimilation of the carbohydrates, has without reasonable question been the basic cause of the constantly increasing incidence of diabetes mellitus in all civilized countries.

White flour and refined sugar, lacking vitamin B and the minerals they once contained, cannot be considered fit foods either for the adult or the child. The sale and use of such foods is excusable, if at all, only on the grounds of ignorance. The crime is particularly inexcusable because of the irreparable nature of the pathology produced. Dental caries, maldevelopment of bone — 80% of rickets is due to the phosphate deficiency (occurring because of our failure to include in the diet the outer portions of cereals) according to a London laboratory report — low resistance to infective disease (that causes often a permanent endocrine disorder), stunting and delay of growth, heart pathology starting as muscular weakness, arteriosclerosis and other pathologies due to the excessive accumulation of calcium carbonate in the tissues (otherwise prevented by the phosphates lost in flour milling), to say nothing of the diseases directly due to disorders and malfunction of any one of the list of organs given at the beginning of this paper, that could occupy volumes, were we to go into detail.

The facts are becoming so obvious that it is incredible that there should be such an apathetic attitude shown by the general public toward the situation. New laws are urgently needed for the protection of all against the minority who find it necessary because of competitive conditions to denature food products — not exactly for profit, but because if they do not, they will soon be bankrupt. A higher price is necessary to cover losses due to the greater perishability, and unless we have uniform laws requiring all to maintain the same standard, the business will go to those who denature, bleach and refine their products to prevent loss and quote a lower price.

The low price certainly fails to benefit the consumer who pays ten or a hundred times the amount saved for medical services, and has his life shortened fifteen or twenty years besides.

**Edited by Royal Lee**

VITAMIN NEWS
VITAMIN PRODUCTS CO. • MILWAUKEE, WISCONSIN

VOL. 3 April 15, 1935 No. 4

## MORE INFORMATION ON VITAMIN C

A year ago last month we summarized the consequences of vitamin C deficiency somewhat as follows:

1. Scurvy symptoms of more or less degree (skin hemorrhages due to weakened capillaries, pyorrhea, loose teeth, decalcification of bones, susceptibility to dental caries).

2. Impaired adrenal (and thyroid) function, with consequent cardiac and vascular disease.

3. Anemia due to impaired iron metabolism.

4. Stomach and duodenal ulcers. (Vitamin C being essential to the normal secretion of gastric mucin.)

Today we are beginning to see a little light as to the bio-chemical reactions that are back of these symptoms.

Sollmann, *Pharmacology,* p. 367 says that a preponderance of potassium ions causes the parasympathetic nerves to be more sensitive to stimulus, while a preponderance of calcium ions increases the sensitiveness of the sympathetic nerves.

In vitamin C deficiency, we have a reduction in calcium ions, altering the calcium potassium ratio. It is possible that the result is hypersensitiveness of the parasympathetics because of the increase in relative potassium. The drug atropine, a parasympathetic paralyzer, is known to be specifically a remedy for gastric ulcer, and its action as such is no doubt due to the reduction of a parasympathetic stimulus, causing among other things an abnormal secretion of gastric juice with its excessive acid.

It has been said on good authority that the action of vitamin A is to maintain the function of the sympathetic nerves, and that of vitamin C to maintain the autonomic (in Howell's terminology, the parasympathetic). According to this, vitamin A is a diffuser and distributor to nervous tissues of potassium. We know that vitamin C is a diffuser and distributor of calcium to the tissues from the blood.

That explains how vitamin C deficiency, through a reduction of calcium ions, can deaden the sympathetic (vasodilator) stimulus to the arteriole musculature, which is normally necessary to maintain dilation, and, thereby, interfere with the blood supply to certain organs or extremities, such as occurs for instance in certain forms of arthritis.

Acetylcholine is a new drug that renews circulation in such situations, and is known as a parasympathetic (and sympathetic) stimulant, opposing atropine in effect. vitamin C, however, is the physiologic dilator of the arterioles, and there is no better example of the superiority of the therapeutic use of vitamins over drugs (if one were needed) than this, for here we have two drugs of opposite biologic reaction (one a parasympathetic paralyzer, the other a parasympathetic stimulator) that may both be indicated for the same basic disorder — vitamin C deficiency.

It is in the later years of life that the consequences of vitamin C deficiency become most apparent. It is undoubtedly a factor in the cause of cataract of the eye. H. K. Muller in *Nature* (London), Aug. 19, 1933 p. 280 says: "Experiments on the significance of the aqueous humor in the lens' metabolism ... have shown that the power of the aqueous humor of cattle and of the rabbit to reduce methylene blue does not depend on the presence of an enzyme, but essentially upon a reducing substance ... which can be titrated with iodine (vitamin C). The vitamin C of the aqueous humor stands in, close to metabolism of the lens. It is traceable ... only in minimal amounts in the aqueous humor of the rabbit's eye after the lens has been removed ... The lens, either secretes vitamin C into the aqueous humor or it reduces some component of the aqueous humor already present. The vitamin C of the aqueous humor must be brought into relationship with the genesis of cataract. Within four hours after oral administration of naphthalene in doses sufficient to cause cataract, the capacity of the aqueous humor to reduce iodine disappears." (Showing disappearance of the vitamin C.)

Probably all the vitamins concerned in calcium metabolism are factors in the treatment of cataract. (That includes all the vitamins with the possible exception of B.) As each case of each patient presents a different combination of relative deficiencies, with the common added complication of more or less degeneration of the endocrines which are the medium of action for vitamins, it is difficult to make a blanket recommendation of treatment. Nevertheless, to date, the majority of cases under treatment have reported favorable results, the time necessary to dissolve the opacities varying from four to fourteen months. The basic dosage is four "Catalyn" tablets a day and two doses of "V-P Phosphade" reduced to three "Catalyn" tablets where one or two special vitamin tablets daily may be considered necessary because of individual circumstances.

**Edited by Royal Lee**

# VITAMIN NEWS

VITAMIN PRODUCTS CO. • MILWAUKEE, WISCONSIN

VOL. 3 May 15, 1935 No. 5

## VITAMIN D

Since offering our observations on vitamin D in *Vitamin News* of April, 1934, quite a number of new facts have appeared.

The use of the synthetic vitamin D (irradiated ergosterol, etc.) has been shown to be highly inferior to vitamin D from natural sources. Even the natural vitamin varies as much as 15 to 1 in its potency for different species when taken from different sources (See *Country Gentleman*, April 1935, page 108). The statement is made that vitamin D from tuna fish, in equal amounts as regards effect on the rat, is but 1/15th as effective to produce the vitamin D effect when given to the chick. Dr. Steenbock (*Journal of Biological Chemistry*, July 1932, pages 249-264) states that irradiated ergosterol must be given in quantities of 40 to 120 times the equivalent amount of cod liver oil vitamin D (calculated in rat units) to produce the same degree of bone calcification. He further concluded that ergosterol and yeast, when irradiated, are inefficient sources for vitamin D for the chicken, which was the animal experimented upon.

No doubt we can prepare to accept a new law of vitamin therapy that a vitamin effect can be produced in different species by entirely different chemical principles.

Steenbock has stated his opinion that the antirachitic substance in cod liver oil and viosterol are different chemically (*Journal of Biological Chemistry*, 97:249).

The use of cod liver oils rich in vitamin A with added viosterol has not been found particularly better than the cod liver oil alone, thus exploding the idea that the use of vitamin A with viosterol would afford results comparable with the cod liver oil (*American Journal of Diseases of Children*, Vol. 46, page 250).

The synthetic vitamin is very much more toxic than the natural product, as one can infer from the statement above, where 40 to 120 times are necessary to get the same result — the toxicity then being evidently 40 to 120 times that of the natural vitamin.

In the *Archives of Internal Medicine*, September 1932, page 433, Dr. Spies states that severe and persistent damage can be produced to such vital organs as the aorta, lungs and kidneys by repeated administration of toxic doses of viosterol.

Several cases of persistent hematuria and albuminuria in children have come to the writer's attention where the only possible relevant circumstance that could be found in the case history was a long continued heavy dosage of viosterol. (The use of "Catalyn" and our vitamin A tablets was instrumental in clearing up the condition in each case. The hematuria case has required the continued administration of the A tablets, however, to prevent recurrence.)

It is particularly unfortunate that the rat was selected as the test animal for vitamin D. It must be recalled that the rat is one of the few species that is able to manufacture its own supply of vitamin C (by the action of its specialized intestinal flora), and it is possibly because of this circumstance that it can use the synthetic vitamin so successfully.

Vitamin C is an important co-operative factor in the assimilation of calcium. C deficiency is known to be accompanied by a decalcification of bone, and the action of D is purely that of increasing the affinity of the blood for that element. It is probable that vitamin C causes the diffusion of the blood calcium to the bones and teeth, as distinguished from the supply to the nerve and muscle tissue, accomplished by another principle. (We believe by our vitamin F.)

Vitamin D, therefore, can only increase the blood calcium, and other factors must be present to insure its distribution. Too much D without its cooperating factors can cause a reversal of the flow of calcium to the tissues needing it, and we believe that this is what takes place in senility, osteomalacia, scurvy, etc. It has definitely been shown that the toxic action of D is due entirely to a too high blood calcium.

It has also been shown that in pregnancy toxicosis from the administration of D is practically impossible because of the mobilization at this time of the hormonic promoters of calcium diffusion that are necessary for this physiological emergency, to store in the bones all ingested calcium against the fetal requirements. The renal threshold for calcium automatically rises to prevent loss of the element, and the renal ammonia synthesizing function is called upon to supply a substitute alkali base to take the place of the Ca molecule in salts eliminated.

The albuminuria of pregnancy is due to the deficiency of vitamins (A and C in particular) in the kidney. The abnormal renal demand for these vitamins is also the basic cause of the hyperemesis. "Catalyn" supplies these vitamins in the proper form, and 3 or 4 tablets a day are recommended. Any physician who observes the course of a pregnancy where the vitamin supply is sufficient will never forget the difference between physiological and pathological childbirth.

**Edited by Royal Lee**

VITAMIN NEWS
VITAMIN PRODUCTS CO. • MILWAUKEE, WISCONSIN

VOL. 3 June 15, 1935 No. 6

## EVOLUTION OF VITAMIN THERAPY

The writer has received comments numerous times from physicians receiving this leaflet to the following effect — "I have been reading *Vitamin News* for some time and find it very interesting. It all sounds reasonable, but do those theories stand the acid test?" (Needless to say, these comments come from those who have not yet prescribed our products.)

First, permit me to say that before the statement is made in these pages that any particular disease responds to treatment with vitamin concentrates, clinical results substantiating that statement must be in our hands, showing quite consistent performance of the concentrate in question for the purpose stated. These facts are discovered many times through the use of the concentrates for treating a patient for some other condition, and finding that more was accomplished than was expected. This is the cue for making tests on other uncomplicated cases with often surprising results. Almost every physician using vitamins for therapeutic purposes has occasion to discover new — to him, at least — forms of disease that can be reliably treated by vitamin concentrates.

When we have accumulated sufficient evidence to be sure of consistent performance of the product for the purpose, often after checking the possibility of geographical differences in the etiology of the disease in question, we begin to include the new disease in our literature. That is the process by which we have accumulated the imposing, not to say staggering, list of diseases that can be expected to respond to vitamin therapy.

We have been severely criticised for making those claims, but the criticiser is always the inexperienced person who is not familiar with the results that we are accomplishing. A test of vitamin therapy on a heart or dropsy case, a prostate case, a hyperthyroid or two — the more desperate the better — and the criticiser becomes a friend and a booster. The only reason our business has increased 1000 per cent in three years is because those results speak for themselves. We have had physicians tell us that they could see improvement in an hour after the administration of one "Catalyn" tablet in children's diseases in acute stages. The reaction is so consistent as to be almost infallible. Why?

It is a known fact that most great discoveries are made first and explained afterwards. We are beginning to see some light as to how vitamins work in such cases. In the *Proc. Soc. Exp. Bio. & Med.*, April 1935, page 1157, the statement is made, "Vitamin C under certain conditions increased the resistance of guinea pigs to injections of a standardized diphtheria toxin" (when injected with the toxin).

Also, Ibid, page 1089, "Yavorsky, Almaden and King examined human tissues from autopsy for their vitamin C content and noted that generalized infections were more common among those having a low vitamin C content. Worringer and Sala reported scurvy in infants following diphtheria and pertussis." These are merely laboratory confirmations of clinical findings made constantly by users of our products in the last five years. A child suffering from vitamin deficiency will not show much of an indication of this situation until it succumbs to an attack of whooping cough, diphtheria, etc. But then, its chances of recovery may, and often do, depend upon the vitamin reserves it may possess. The use of therapeutic measures other than vitamin concentrates certainly is not to be condemned, but the real cause of the susceptibility and low resistance is that deficiency, and its correction is one of the imperative duties of the physician.

One of the most outstanding effects of vitamin therapy is improvement in heart function. Readers of our literature who have written to the Bureau of Investigation of the American Medical Association asking if there were any truth in the claim that vitamins were of value in heart conditions were replied to with a form letter stating that "it is ridiculous to assume that there is any connection between vitamins and heart trouble." But of late such references are appearing in the scientific literature as the following from *Jour. Bio. Chem.*, page 197 (Japanese): "It may be concluded therefore that the function of heart muscle is severely injured by polished rice feeding owing to the deficiency of hydrogenase activity as well as oxidizable substances." And the Japanese investigators have caused and cured heart enlargement in test animals by withdrawing and replacing vitamin B in the diet." (Reported in the *Tohuku Jour. Exp. Med.*, 1935.)

> "The triad, 'gas, belching, and fullness after meals,' heard by the surgeon as well as the internist is ascribed in the absence of an organic pyloric cause, to delayed emptying time resulting from atonic gastric musculature. Other symptoms accompanying these include constipation, nausea, regurgitation and headache. A physical sign of importance is a successive gastric splash with which there is frequently found a palpable cecum and iliac colon. X-ray and laboratory examination reveal evidence of ptosis, hypo and achlorhydria, splastic colon with stasis, subnutritional states and mild hypothyroidism. Chronicity and resistance to treatment is typical. Accompanying gall bladder disease is quite rare.
>
> "It is believed that these cases are the result of a deficiency of the B antineuritic factor of vitamin B. This deficiency is attributed to the downward trend in the use of meat and cereal with the corresponding increase in the use of sugar. Most cereals now used are degerminated and white bread is of questionable vitamin B content. A series of 75 cases constituted the clinical study of this report. In commenting on the fact that 50 per cent of the patients had had appendectomy performed, attention was directed to the effect of vitamin B deficiency on the integrity of lymphoid tissue.
>
> "Excellent results followed the administration of vitamin B. However, since sufficiently bulky foods could not be consumed because of limited digestive capacity, it was necessary to administer vitamin B in a concentrated form of wheat germ." (*American Journal of Digestive Diseases and Nutrition* for February, 1936, Volume 2, No. 12, pages 764 and 766. Abstract of Article by Fitts, John B.)

**Edited by Royal Lee**

VITAMIN NEWS

VITAMIN PRODUCTS CO. • MILWAUKEE, WISCONSIN

VOL. 3 July 15, 1935 No. 7

## VITAMIN E

In our discussion of vitamin E a year ago in these pages, it was pointed out that the action of vitamin E (besides its more commonly known function of preventing sterility) was the promotion of mineral metabolism, in particular the promotion of the diffusibility of calcium and magnesium. This action of increasing the diffusibility of mineral salts enables such altered salts to pass through the vascular walls and thereby causes a loss of minerals to the blood. The alkali salts in question had been attached to protein molecules, the entire molecule being too large to pass through the vessel wall.

Other vitamins (A, C and F) apparently do somewhat the same thing. The form which the alkali salt assumes in becoming diffusible, and the particular alkali elements of their proportionate relation in respect to each of these vitamins are matters still under investigation.

It is probable that the mineral supply to different organs is controlled by different vitamins, and the organs or tissues, no doubt, select the form of molecule specifically useful by some process of biochemical affinity. The fact we need to emphasize is that unless the vitamins are present to properly prepare these elements, the nutrition of some tissues or organs will inevitably be impaired.

At the last convention of the American Medical Association, a Canadian investigator announced that vitamin E has been found to have a prophylactic value in the prevention of cancer. This announcement is especially interesting in view of the fact that, as stated in these pages last year, this vitamin promoted the supply of magnesium to the tissues (as well as that of calcium) and also in view of the fact that certain foreign investigators had established an apparent relationship between magnesium deficiency and cancer. This began from a study of the geographical distribution of cancer, there being exceptionally few cases in the Nile valley, one of the few fertile agricultural regions in the world where there is an abundant supply of magnesium in the soil. This was followed by tests of magnesium salts as remedies for cancer with partial success.

We have always held that deficiency of minerals from a metabolic standpoint was more often due to the inability to assimilate because of vitamin deficiency than because of actual dietary lack. Not that such dietary shortage does not frequently occur, but that in the great majority of cases it is vitamin deficiency that makes that shortage apparent. A good illustration is the case of iodine deficiency in goiter, where the primary cause is vitamin B and C deficiency, necessitating a higher intake of iodine to prevent trouble, the use of B and C concentrates being a far more satisfactory remedy than iodine after the condition has developed.

No doubt the use of vitamin E will become a valuable aid in the control of cancer. However, the cure of cancer may not be as simple as the treatment of other deficiency diseases, because of the fact that there are often so many associated degenerative complications involving irreparable organic changes.

Interesting in this connection is our statement of last year (*Vitamin News*, Vol. 2, No. 6) that the common neuritic and arthritic pains of older persons were usually greatly helped by our vitamin E concentrate. The diffusive action on calcium and magnesium would explain that, too, these elements being essential to nerve function.

Recently, we have made available to our customers a new preparation of vitamin E — wheat germ oil, in capsule form. We do not consider this product as economical as our tablets of vitamin E when considered as a source of that vitamin, but it has another important pharmaceutical effect — that of a vermifuge for children — that will be appreciated by the physician.

The accompanying reference is offered with the statement that clinical reports to us on our wheat germ oil capsules ("Cerol") have fully substantiated the findings.

**Edited by Royal Lee**

VITAMIN NEWS

VITAMIN PRODUCTS CO. • MILWAUKEE, WISCONSIN

**VOL. 3** **August 15, 1935** **No. 8**

## VITAMIN F

### (A growth-promoting vitamin of our own designation)

As announced last June in *Vitamin News*, our vitamin F is a calcium-diffusing principle that causes the distribution of blood calcium to the muscular system, and probably to other tissues.

It is found in cereals (first in oatmeal by Mirvish), especially rye (rye owes to its F its known property of causing muscle rather than fat development in growing animals), and, no doubt, in wheat germ to some extent. (See Blumberg, *Journal of Biological Chemistry*, page 277, January 1935). The latter article offers evidence that there is present in wheat germ oil a factor besides vitamin E, which is necessary to growth, that we consider identical with our vitamin F.

The term "Vitamin F" has been an orphan in the vitamin family since $B_2$ was changed from F to G. Therefore, we appropriated it with possibly too little regard for the formalities when we applied it to our new calcium metabolizer — especially in view of the fact that it was being applied at about the same time to the unsaturated fatty acid (linoleic acid) that has already been found to be a necessary dietary constituent. (This is the vitamin F referred to besides the growth vitamin in the Blumberg article above.)

However, it is not exactly in line with the past practices of terminology to put fatty acids in the vitamin category. The term "vitamin" has been reserved to describe something required in far more infinitesimal amounts, because of its catalytic rather than nutritional effect, and which had to have some name during the years of investigation necessary to determine its chemical nature. So in all probability linoleic acid will not be officially accepted by this title.

Clinically speaking, the main use so far developed for our vitamin F concentrate is in the treatment of stubborn prostate cases that fail to respond properly to "Catalyn." (Maybe one out of ten of those receiving "Catalyn" will get added benefit from one vitamin F tablet a day in addition.)

It has been found to have an effect on the eye musculature, too, in that if the person taking the one F tablet a day is wearing spectacles, he may find in a couple of weeks that he will need to be refitted with weaker lenses.

This fact, together with the known action of F as a diffuser of calcium, suggested that it might be valuable in cataract, but experience has not encouraged us in that respect. The use of "Catalyn" and a certain amount of "V-P Phosphade" has been the most successful combination to date, with vitamin A and C concentrates offering the best promise as supplements where indications pointed toward their specific deficiency.

The indiscriminate use of F is not to be encouraged. It has the opposite action of vitamin D on the blood calcium (it is a good remedy for persons susceptible to sunstroke, as noted last June in these pages), and is, therefore, capable of causing radical effects in heavy dosage. This reduction in blood calcium is due to the increased diffusibility of the calcium when " is present. (These remarks may apply to magnesium, too, both as to D and F.) If the alimentary supply of calcium is deficient — as is usually the case — vitamin F can bring about an oversupply to muscular tissues at the expense of the requirements of other classes of cells that more directly depend on the blood calcium. Vitamins A and C are known to accomplish some of their effects (maybe all) through their influence on the alkali ion supply to the sympathetic and parasympathetic nervous systems. (See *Vitamin News*, April, 1935.) There is no doubt but that F also is a factor in the whole alkali ion balance, but we are as yet not prepared to offer an acceptable complete hypothesis. It is not impossible that C and F act in synergetic cooperation.

The use of F because of its calcium-diffusing power, was at once suggested for arthritis. The clinical reports have been very contradictory. In some cases, the arthritic pains were quickly controlled. (They often are aggravated in the first stage of "Catalyn" treatment.) In other cases (hypertrophic arthritis), where the ankylosed joints had begun to break apart through "Catalyn" treatment, the use of F caused a freezing again. The latter result is reasonable in that F is a distributor of calcium to the tissues, and in hypertrophic arthritis there is already too much. In atrophic arthritis, the results seem to have been beneficial, as would be expected.

The role of the thyroid as the physiological eliminator of calcium seems to have been overlooked. It is known that the most consistent result from the administration of thyroxin is the quantitative elimination of calcium. The metabolic rate should be determined in any serious case involving hypercalcemia. It is well to recall also that the administration of vitamins (as "Catalyn") while being the first physiological remedy for hyperthyroidea, will also prevent toxic effects from the administration of thyroid in subjects that otherwise cannot tolerate any dosage (this being due to the paucity of vitamins in the diet — as well as to nervous strain and overwork — that exhausts the vitamin reserves).

The thyro-adreno-pituitary group requires vitamins A, B, C and D for nutrition. To include gonad and prostate, we must include vitamins E and F. Unbalance in the functional relationships of these endocrines is most likely to occur in middle age, when the endocrine activity normally slows, because a parallel rate of regression of the different glands is not maintained. The most common disturbing factor is endocrine starvation — or vitamin deficiency. The hormone output of the thyro-adreno-pituitary group is apparently controlled from a common center through the sympathetic innervation, and this stimulus often causes an overactivity of one member when another fails to respond. Vascular hypertension results if the adrenals are overactive from this cause; hyperthyroidea, if it is the thyroid. That is why the surgical remedy of cutting the nerve supply to the overactive gland has been a demonstrably effective remedy. Such heroic measures are seldom necessary if the dormant endocrine is revived by vitamin therapy — "Catalyn." It produces results in almost all of the hyperthyroid cases and about 80 per cent of the hypertensive.

**Edited by Royal Lee**

VITAMIN NEWS

VITAMIN PRODUCTS CO. • MILWAUKEE, WISCONSIN

VOL. 3 September 15, 1935 No. 9

# VITAMIN AND MINERAL METABOLISM IN HEART DISEASE

Heart pathology can be of three classess — nervous control is impaired; muscle tissue may be weak; hypertrophied, later degenerated or starved because of coronary disease; or infection or hypertrophy of muscle may have impaired valvular function.

Vitamin concentrates (in the form of "Catalyn") will accomplish a great deal for the weak or enlarged heart or for the patient with tachycardia.

The speeding up of the heart is the normal reaction to a deficiency of certain essential nutritional elements in the blood. Oxygen deficiency is the commonly recognized stimulus, but it is becoming apparent that other deficiencies can also cause the specific nervous stimulation that causes an increase of pulse rate. Three things are necessary to muscular activity — oxygen, sugar and the oxidizing ferment (the catalyst) that promotes the oxidation of the fuel, without which the "combustion" with the consequent release of energy cannot take place. Vitamin C is necessary to ensure a supply of the catalyst. (Sajous considered the oxidizing ferment as originating from C and similar chemically.) Therefore, it is not difficult to see why augmentation of vitamins can slow the heart. The muscular tissue is able to get its required amount of necessary supplies with a normal velocity of the "conveyor system" — the blood stream.

Vitamin B deficiency, on the other hand, causes a slowing of the heart, probably because of the direct action of the deficiency on the nervous system. Therefore, a deficiency of both B and C vitamins can obviously be a serious matter for the heart. The heart muscle itself then suffers because of the insufficient supply of essential nutrition, which without the B deficiency would be compensated for by an increased blood velocity.

Valve trouble overloads the muscle tissue and "Catalyn" is of great value here in maintaining or restoring compensation. Often, the regurgitation decreases so markedly meanwhile as to lead one to suspect that the myocardial hypertrophy that is thereby reduced was acting to aggravate the valve trouble by the mechanical distortion of the valve structures.

In heart disease characterized by fibrillation, less specific benefit can be expected. A certain amount of improvement will occur, but there has been degeneration and atrophy of nerve tissue that cannot be repaired.

In coronary occlusion, usually accompanied by angina pectoris, an improvement in the quality of the heart nutrition can be productive of considerable improvement in the heart performance. "V-P Phosphade" should be used for the first month or two for treatment, as it does two important things:

1. It lowers the blood viscosity, thereby improving the circulation produced by a given amount of heart power.

2. It dissolves the calcium carbonate responsible for the calcification of the coronary arteries that is usually the primary cause of the condition. (The coronary arteries have been found calcified when no other arteries in the body showed this pathology.)

Where there is a general arteriosclerosis, of course, the "V-P Phosphade" is also an essential part of the treatment. The dietary source of the phosphate radical is from the phytin component of cereals, mainly in wheat bran or brown rice. Phytin is chemically a combination of inosite and phosphoric acid with variable amounts of calcium and magnesium. In assimilation it is split by an enzyme (present in the small intestine and also in the blood) into inosite and phosphoric acid. The phosphoric acid of course immediately combines with the sodium carbonate or bicarbonate present to form sodium phosphate. This phosphate, however, differs in activity from the ordinary kind in that it is more loosely combined and can take place in new reactions more readily — such as, for instance, the double decomposition reaction with calcium carbonate.

As most of the phosphorus ingested is in the form of phytin, we must consider that element as an acid mineral as contrasted with the basic (or alkali) minerals as found in the green leaf vegetables. These alkali minerals require vitamins as a class for their assimilation, and a deficiency of either the basic minerals or the vitamins can cause almost the same general deficiency symptoms. In fact, where there is a failure to obtain results from vitamin therapy, it is usually because of a deficiency of these basic minerals.

These organic minerals (from green leaf vegetables) are now available in tablet form as "V-P" Organic Mineral Tablets. One of the most conspicuous effects of these tablets is their cooperative action with vitamin B in improving the function and sensitivity of the sympathetic nervous system. This causes an improved bowel function, especially because of the specific action in correcting the condition known as "lazy colon."

"V-P" Organic Mineral Tablets are a concentrate of the unaltered colloidal minerals in green leafy vegetables, made without heat. By the removal of unnecessary bulk, the possible dosage is increased to a point where one or two tablets a day produces immediate and definite results.

**Edited by Royal Lee**

// VITAMIN NEWS

VITAMIN PRODUCTS CO. • MILWAUKEE, WISCONSIN

VOL. 3 October 15, 1935 No. 10

For the past two years we have enjoyed the privilege of compiling in these pages information and notes relating to the use of vitamin concentrates for therapeutic purposes. In this issue, we are departing from that policy to submit a few actual case reports as received by us from the physician. They will convey an idea of what can be expected from the use of really effective vitamin concentrates. Any of our distributors can offer many similar reports from local sources.

"Mr. B. Age 67. Weight 204 pounds.

SEPTEMBER 18, 1934. Symptoms: Bright's disease with dropsy, cardiac asthma, insomnia, circulation poor, urination difficult, no appetite, bowels constipated, sleeps only at intervals in reclining chair. Under constant medical care for ten months. Heart attacks frequent. Abdominal distention, legs swollen to twice normal size. On pressure, tissue is unyielding, hard as wood to the touch. Three-inch running sore on right leg.

SEPTEMBER 20. Weight 204 pounds. Urine shows 5% albumin. Began taking three "Catalyn" a day with one F concentrate, 1 teaspoonful "V-P Phosphade."

SEPTEMBER 24. Weight 199 pounds. Kidney action improved. No heart attack since starting treatment.

OCTOBER 17. Weight 174 pounds. Urine shows 1% albumin. Patient now able to sleep in bed with comfort. Bowels normal. Breathing while not normal, is much improved.

NOVEMBER 23. Weight 154 pounds. Albumin 1%. Breathing normal. Heart action normal. Ulcerated leg completely healed. Abdomen normal size. Legs normal. Ankles and feet still slightly swollen. Urinating two quarts daily.

JANUARY 5, 1935. Weight 151 pounds. 1% albumin. Ankles still slightly swollen. Patient is now active and able to walk and exercise in moderation without fatigue.

JANUARY 28. Began taking two "Catalyn" a day with two A concentrate and two E concentrate on alternate days.

FEBRUARY 26. Patient normal. Urine albumin-free. All physical symptoms disappeared.

MAY 10. Patient in normal health. No return of former symptoms. Walks 20 blocks per day. Feels fine. Looks good. Maintains weight at 151 pounds."

(SIGNED) Dr. M.D.W.

"A baby, 19 days old. Eczema from head to foot. I gave it one-half tablet "Catalyn" each day, and in only ten days it was clear.

Woman, 33 years old. Migraine for 20 years. I have treated her for three years, and I have never been able to give her any relief 'til I started her on "Catalyn."

I have six patients with high blood pressure; every one responded to "Catalyn."

A woman, 75 years old. Acute nephritis, temperature 105; a great deal of pus and albumin. Cleared up in three weeks' time with "Catalyn."

Woman, 35 years old. Low blood pressure. Systolic 80, Diastolic 54. I had treated this case for three years with no improvement. After taking "Catalyn" for four months, Systolic 100; Diastolic 70. Improvement in every way.

I have not had one case that didn't show improvement, that took 'Catalyn.'"

(Signed) Dr. C. B.

"In the case studied there has been a chronic infection of practically all of the sinuses, as shown by X-ray. Frequent occlusion or collapse of the eustachean tubes with a temporary loss or diminution of the ability to hear. Unable at times to breathe freely. Pus continually draining, offensive odor, and of a bright yellow color. Absorption of pus produced an anemia, headaches daily, and loss of appetite.

Treatment: Operation was resorted to with no improvement other than obtained by removal of some polypoid growth which with the enlarged turbinates were at times rendering it impossible to breathe freely. Diet and blood tonics were instituted and after weeks of careful diet, was somewhat overcome. Infra-red lamps relieved headaches for only a short time. Vitamin concentrates in the form of "Catalyn" tablets were then started, which produced a marked improvement within ten days' time. The first noticeable change was a lessening of the pus discharge with a change in its character, as from a bright yellow color it assumed a cream color and cheesy, flaky appearance. The headaches gradually disappeared and the appetite which had been affected by the unavoidable swallowing of the pus, improved. "Catalyn" was discontinued for a time and there was a slow return of the old symptoms. After a time, "Catalyn" treatment was resumed and in a short time symptoms began to subside. It is believed that if the "Catalyn" had been continued without interruption, there would have been a complete cessation of all the symptoms."

(SIGNED) Dr. E. A. J.

# VITAMIN NEWS

VITAMIN PRODUCTS CO. • MILWAUKEE, WISCONSIN

VOL. 3 November 15, 1935 No. 11

## MUSCLE PHYSIOLOGY AND VITAMINS

Probably the most outstanding feature of the physiological action of vitamins is the effect upon muscle metabolism and function.

Vitamin B is known to be necessary to maintain the normal tone of involuntary muscle. Vitamin C is known to be necessary to promote the chemical reactions that release the energy in muscle contraction — to act as the spark does in the automobile engine. Vitamin D is necessary to ensure the assimilation from the alimentary system of the calcium so necessary to muscular activity — without which toxic wastes accumulate, and we feel that soreness of muscles which is a result of unaccustomed overwork. But vitamin F is quite necessary to ensure the diffusion of that calcium into the muscular tissues from the blood, the function of the D being limited to getting that conveyor system — the blood stream — loaded up.

It is important that we be familiar with the controlling factors in muscle physiology, as normal muscle function is the foundation of life itself, and in fact, we might say that the difference between plant and animal life is based upon the evolution of the muscle cell and its attendant metabolism.

Asthenia, fatigability, or common laziness — are all traceable to disturbances in muscular metabolism. If the situation becomes bad enough to involve the heart muscle, which is no doubt the hardest worked muscle in the body, we call it heart disease. Often, the heart begins to break down before the general physical condition indicates that the rest of the muscular system is affected. That is usually due to disease of the coronary artery, causing an interference with the blood supply to the heart muscle. The best procedure, of course, is rest, plenty of vitamins and time to permit the development of collateral circulation. Cases have been known where an autopsy in an individual that had died of other causes and who had been doing manual labor up to his death, showed that a long-standing total occlusion of the coronary artery existed, collateral vessels carrying all the blood supply. The prognosis of such cases, therefore, is not necessarily discouraging. The most helpful thing to do is to improve the quality of the blood supply to the heart to compensate for the lack of quantity, which will also increase in time.

The heart is a throttle-governed engine. The throttle action is through the nervous control that acts on the muscular layer of the coronary artery. A shock — especially that of mental origin, bad news, etc. — can cause a constriction of the coronary that may last for weeks. Meanwhile, especially if the subject has been a victim of malnutrition, permanent damage can occur to the heart muscle. Even death can be a consequence of such a reaction. The term "broken heart" is no mere figure of speech. Every physician of much experience has seen such a shock precipitate myocardial disease.

The success of the "lie detector" depends upon this throttle control of the heart, in that the mental stimulus of fear causes a release of power to the heart, with a temporary rise of pulse rate and a parallel rise in blood pressure. This mental control is supplemented by hormonic control, a pancreas hormone being known to dilate the coronary selectively and has been isolated for use as a remedy in coronary occlusion and angina pectoris. (Known as "Kallikrein" in Germany and as "Padutin" (trade name) in this country; used only as a hypodermic remedy.)

There is a distinct difference in the physiology and the metabolism as well between the striped and smooth muscle. The difference is based upon a law of physics — the law of conservation of energy. Energy is required to produce motion, according to this law, but not to maintain a pull. The smooth or involuntary muscle in general maintains a pull rather then performing work. It is called upon to perform work at times, but its main office is the maintenance of "muscle tone." The striped or voluntary muscle on the other hand is able only to create a pull by the expenditure of energy. To offer a mechanical analogy, a spring can exert a pull, but to make use of the pull as a source of power will result in the discovery that the spring can not generate power but only deliver back what was put into it when it was stretched.

It is probable that the unstriped muscle maintains its pull without the expenditure of energy, but is able to establish its own tonicity without outside help by its momentary ability to expend energy. Were this not true, nature would have made a big mistake in basic design, in requiring a constant expenditure of energy where a "spring" would serve. In smooth muscle then we probably have a unique device that can act as a "spring" or "motor" as may be required. The striped muscle is probably able to act only in the capacity of motor, but more efficiently because it does this exclusively.

This difference in nature is indicated in the difference in metabolism, by comparing the two types of muscle physiology.

Striped muscle produces creatin which it requires in its metabolic reactions, and smooth muscle does not, and is probably the distinguishing feature that indicates the difference between the power-producing striped muscle cell and the tonus-producing smooth cell.

The smooth muscle tonus requires a nerve stimulus for its maintenance. Vitamin B deficiency destroys this, so that such deficiency can be a major factor in the cause of hemorrhoids, varicose veins, destruction of parenchymatous elements of the bone marrow (resulting in pernicious anemia), intestinal atony and lessened peristalsis reduction in pulse rate due to vascular dilation, enlargement and degeneration of various glandular organs, especially pancreas, to mention a few functional and organic changes that can be traceable to this form of starvation.

Did you ever stop and ask yourself just how you would know if YOU were not getting a sufficient amount of vitamins in your food? The first indication would necessarily have to be either simple asthenia, low resistance to infection, or some symptoms of chronic functional or organic disease. In fact, it is impossible to study foods and their methods of preparation without admiring the adaptability of the human machine to the miserably small proportions of essential vitamins and minerals in the average diet.

Let us not forget that wholesome food can only be perishable food — not the devitalized, sterilized and denatured product upon which neither insects, molds nor microbes can exist — and neither can we, but most of us try to, to our own discomfiture.

**Edited by Royal Lee**

# VITAMIN NEWS

VITAMIN PRODUCTS CO. • MILWAUKEE, WISCONSIN

VOL. 3 December 15, 1935 No. 12


## THE METABOLISM OF FAT

Fats in digestion are reduced to fatty acids. Fatty acids are converted (after desaturation) in the liver to glycogen (by the aid of a pancreatic principle or the organic compound betaine) and thereby become fuel for the production of heat and muscular energy.

The betaine is probably supplied normally by the pancreas, because in experiments with animals, removal of the pancreas will not result fatally if insulin and betaine are given. Without the insulin, blood sugar rises; without betaine, liver fat rises and blood sugar drops. The liver fat will increase from a normal 3% to 35% under these circumstances.

In diabetes, it is common for the blood fat to rise unduly, as well as the liver fat. If we assume that the end-product of fat is blood sugar (glycogen), and that the consumption of glycogen is hindered by the shortage of insulin, we realize how and why the fat content of blood and liver can rise. It rises merely because the demand has decreased and the supply has not.

This increase in blood and liver fat can cause serious symptoms alone. It is an accepted fact that diabetic coma is a direct result of the high blood fat rather than high blood sugar (Joslin, *New Eng. Med. Jol.* v.209, p.525). The blood fat may rise from a normal 1 or 2% to 25%. Such a situation is possibly a case of inability to convert fat to sugar rather than wholly a case of inability to metabolize sugar (insulin deficiency).

No doubt, one factor causing a slowing of the conversion of fat to sugar in the liver is the already high blood sugar in the diabetic, but let us not forget that the pancreas is also the source of the betaine that is necessary for this job.

Another very significant fact is that betaine is associated in food materials with vitamin B, being found in wheat bran to the extent of .35%. Another source of betaine is lecithin, from which it is supposedly formed by oxidation of its choline component. If this is a reliable source, there should be less danger of a deficiency, as eggs are well loaded with lecithin. Otherwise, cereals — unrefined — are also good sources, as lecithin is present in the germ. A vegetarian diet, with refined cereals, could very possibly be deficient also in lecithin, however.

The above hypothesis explains why the diabetically inclined person is usually overweight. He does not convert the normal amount of fat into sugar, therefore stores it up in the tissues. The main reason that he does not make the conversion is because his blood sugar does not disappear at the normal rate (because of insulin deficiency).

But many persons are fat because of reasons other than insulin deficiency. Might it not be possible that betaine deficiency is the reason in some cases? Or a pancreatic disorder that prevents the proper secretion of the betaine factor?

It is quite possible that the average non-diabetic obesity case (excluding from consideration the hypothyroid) can be oversupplied with fat because of an inability to convert fat to sugar. We know that certain hormonic controls have a bearing on the situation, and the center of such control is in all probability located in the pituitary gland, both anterior and posterior hormones being factors. The anterior pituitary "thyrotropic" hormone apparently promotes thyroid activity, while it has long been known that a posterior pituitary principle was instrumental in reducing intestinal alimentary absorption as much as 50%.

A posterior pituitary hormone (pitressin) also contracts the coronary artery. Last month was mentioned the fact that this artery was dilated by a pancreatic hormone, and we can see that this "heart throttle" control is a balance between these two influences — besides the control of the nervous system.

To further complicate the picture, it is known that a duodenal hormone apparently must be present in the blood stream to release both the pitressin of the pituitary and the "padutin" of the pancreas. Disease of the duodenum (ulcers, etc.) is common. Therefore there can be obesity (or other disease) because of a shortage either of a duodenal hormone, or pancreatic hormone (we have three now, the "padutin," the betaine carrier, and insulin), all of which probably need the duodenal stimulus, or of the pitressin, without which intestinal absorption can double and the heart throttle open wide.

It is known that overdosage of pitressin can cause fatty degeneration of the liver. This also occurs if the betaine principle (from the pancreas) is lacking. Pitressin is known to promote glycogen production by the liver so the fatty degeneration it causes may be a secondary consequence of an exhaustion of the betaine supply of the pancreas, which is necessary to convert fats to glycogen. The secretion of pitressin gradually decreases with age, no doubt an automatic compensative measure to maintain hormonic balance.

To meddle with the normal hormonic balances is a dangerous thing to do unless the patient is in critical need of help. In time, there is no doubt but that the use of hormones, especially for the older patient, will become indispensable, but pending the time when our knowledge is more complete and a full complement of the necessary hormones can be obtained (to say nothing of the difficulties of administration), the use of vitamin concentrates to insure an ample nutrition to the endocrines is a sane policy to pursue. Correct nutrition must precede more difficult therapeutic measures, or we will find ourselves treating symptoms rather than causes.

**Edited by Royal Lee**

CATALYN NATURES SOURCE OF VITALITY MADE IN U.S.A.

# VITAMIN NEWS

CATALYN NATURES SOURCE OF VITALITY MADE IN U.S.A.

VITAMIN PRODUCTS CO. • MILWAUKEE, WISCONSIN

**January 15, 1936** **VOL. 4**

## ALPHABETICAL TABLE OF RECOMMENDATIONS OF VARIOUS "V-P" CONCENTRATES USEFUL IN THE TREATMENT OF DISEASE

The recommendations here given are not to be considered final or beyond improvement by the physician who has obtained some experience of his own in connection with the use of "Catalyn," "V-P Phosphade," and "V-P Concentrates." They are rather suggestions for those whose experience is limited. On the other hand, they do represent the consensus of opinion of the users of our products with whom we have been able to maintain contact.

There is also to be considered the difference in the patient and his vitamin requirements because of geographic location, differences in sunlight, differences in mineral content of drinking water and food locally produced, as well as differences in climatic conditions. These factors alone will considerably alter the picture of vitamin requirements, both in health and disease, for different parts of the country.

The dosage specified is for adults and children over twelve years of age. Younger children should receive less at the discretion of the physician.

The time of administration is not important except in connection with the effect upon the appetite and upon the assimilation of food. In general, vitamin concentrates given twenty to thirty minutes before meals tend to reduce the appetite, and often cause an automatic weight reduction in the patient (mainly true of "Catalyn"). If the concentrates are taken with or after meals, the tendency is for the efficiency of assimilation to be enhanced, with a resulting probability of weight increase. This effect is valuable in convalescence and anemia, etc.

These recommendations are intended to apply only to the deficiency angle of the disease discussed. Other factors of importance from a therapeutic viewpoint are, of course, left to the discretion of the physician, and often are of equal or greater moment than the deficiency angle.

It is a common mistake for the enthusiast in any specialized therapeutic field to become over-encouraged as to the merits of his methods simply because he can see results in such a high percentage of the cases he treats. That only means, however, that he has favorably influenced ONE of the many possible factors responsible for the pathological situation. The deficiency factor is of extreme importance, and in most of the diseases here listed, is the major factor.

At the same time, the use of vitamin concentrates is compatible with almost any other type of remedial measure, with the exception of the use of certain drugs, particularly digitalis. "Catalyn" (mainly due to its content of B and C) restores a normal intolerance and increases the stimulative reaction to digitalis. Where digitalis is being given, the dosage of "Catalyn" should begin gradually (not over one tablet per day) until it is determined whether the digitalis action is being accentuated. In the case of addiction to narcotics, the effect of "Catalyn" is to aid greatly in alleviating the distress in "tapering off." It is probable that most drugs act and produce their desirable effects by mobilizing the vitamin reserves. That is why the "day of reckoning" is inevitable — we are ultimately faced with an overdrawn account.

Please note also List of Reactions that can occur when "V-P" Concentrates are used.

**ACIDOSIS:**

From a vitamin deficiency viewpoint, one cause of acidosis is the impairment of the kidney function of ammonia synthesis, which is necessary for the retention of the alkali reserves by substituting ammonia for the alkali metals in salts eliminated in urinary solution. Vitamin A at the rate of three tablets per day is effective in restoring this function.

Albuminuria is an indication of such vitamin deficiency, particularly the acidosis and albuminuria of pregnancy. To retain calcium for the needs of the fetus, the synthesis of ammonia is imperatively essential.

**ACNE:**

Three tablets per day of "Catalyn."

**ALCOHOLISM:**

*Chronic:* Four tablets of "Catalyn" per day often kills the pathological craving for alcohol.

**ANEMIA:**

*Pernicious:* Two "Catalyn" tablets and two vitamin B tablets daily (one of each after lunch and dinner) to three of each daily after one week if definite improvement is not evident. The dosage of vitamin B may be pushed to six tablets per day if it is desired to speed up the improvement, but is ordinarily not necessary.

Where a case of pernicious anemia is known to have been unresponsive to treatment with liver extract, it may be found advisable to increase the "Catalyn" rather than the vitamin B. These cases usually improve steadily under vitamin treatment, as the failure to get results with the liver extract is usually due to the cumulative vitamin deficiency present.

*Secondary:* In most secondary anemias, "Catalyn" alone is sufficient in dosage up to four tablets per day (one tablet after each meal and one at bedtime). If any kidney disease is present, as is often the case, two or three tablets daily of vitamin A are of great help. Where an infection has been a factor, the addition of vitamin C (two tablets per day) is advisable for the first two weeks along with the "Catalyn."

**ANGINA PECTORIS:**

Two "Catalyn" and two vitamin E tablets daily, increasing to three of each per day after two weeks if improvement is not definite. One teaspoonful daily of "V-P Phosphade" (taken as directed on bottle) is quite essential.

**ARTERIOSCLEROSIS:**

Same schedule as for angina pectoris except that the dosage of "V-P Phosphade" may often be stepped up to two or three doses per day to advantage if well tolerated. vitamin A should also be given up to three tablets daily if there is any kidney pathology.

We recommend the "V-P Phosphade" in connection with the vitamin concentrates because it supplies the phosphate radical necessary to aid in the elimination of the pathological calcium carbonate in the tissues that may be partially responsible for the condition

(See High Blood Pressure)

**ARTHRITIS:**

*Atrophic (Chronic Infective Arthritis, Arthritis Deformans, Rheumatoid Arthritis):* Two "Catalyn" tablets and two vitamin C tablets daily, increasing to three of each after two weeks if improvement is not definite. One teaspoonful daily of "V-P Phosphade" (taken as directed on the bottle) is quite essential; more if well-tolerated.

Arthritis in some cases, at least, being aggravated by exposure to cold, which automatically reduces the phagocytic activity (promoted by "Catalyn"), indicates that such activity is a factor of importance in the treatment or prevention of the disease.

In atrophic arthritis, there is a degeneration of bone, in fact a collapse of the bone tissue, due to the loss of the calcified elements in the affected areas.

Sometimes the symptoms are aggravated for the first few days with later continued improvement. This action is due entirely, we believe, to the promotion of phagocytic activity.

*Hypertrophic:* Exercise caution here. The minimum dosage of one "Catalyn" tablet, one-half teaspoonful of "V-P Phosphade" in a six-ounce glass of water and one "V-P" Organic Mineral tablet given daily for one week, then increasing the "Catalyn" to two tablets daily and the "V-P Phosphade" to one teaspoonful. Increase weekly until four "Catalyn" tablets, one teaspoonful of "V-P Phosphade" and one "V-P" Organic Mineral tablet are being taken daily.

*Note: Should the reaction be too great on increasing the dosage, return to the minimum and continue there until patient can tolerate the increased dosage.*

**ASTHENIA:**

Ninety per cent of asthenic cases will respond to vitamin therapy — "Catalyn" alone should ordinarily be given a trial first. If there is no improvement in one to two weeks, when three tablets are used, vitamin A and B concentrates should be tried, three tablets per day (one week test of each). If there are no results, try one tablet daily of vitamin D or F for a week's test.

The use of the wrong concentrates may aggravate the asthenia, as we are dealing with an unbalanced condition, and some of the vitamins oppose one another in action. If the test shows that the asthenia is being aggravated, drop the dosage used and use one vitamin for the rest of the week, before continuing with the next test.

**ASTHMA:**

Two tablets daily each of "Catalyn," vitamin A and vitamin C are usually effective in controlling asthma, the greatest promise of favorable results being in the young patient. It is advisable to start with half of this dosage, increasing to the full amount after the first week.

**BACKWARD CHILDREN:**

One "Catalyn" tablet daily for children less than 7 years of age. Two "Catalyn" tablets daily for children from 7 to 10 years of age. Three "Catalyn" tablets daily for children from 10 to 18 years of age.

Applies both to physical and mental backwardness. An improvement in school work is a frequent source of comment in these cases.

**BERIBERI:**

Incipient beriberi is often a complication, especially in cardiac diseases. Bloating (dropsy) and anemia are indications of the need for vitamin B.

(See Heart Disorders)

VITAMIN NEWS

VITAMIN PRODUCTS CO. • MILWAUKEE, WISCONSIN

February 15, 1936 VOL. 4

## ALPHABETICAL TABLE OF RECOMMENDATIONS OF VARIOUS "V-P" CONCENTRATES USEFUL IN THE TREATMENT OF DISEASE – Continued

**BOILS:**

*Acute:* One vitamin A tablet and one "Catalyn" tablet taken hourly should show pronounced results within 48 hours.

*Chronic tendency to:* Two tablets each daily of vitamins A, C and E are usually effective in correcting the susceptibility to boils. Often, vitamin A alone does the job. Each of these vitamins is known to increase the calcium supply to the tissue fluids.

**BURNS:**

Two "Catalyn" tablets per hour during the first six hours; then four "Catalyn" tablets per day during the course of the healing. It is a great aid in preventing and combating the toxicosis and shock.

**CALCULUS: *Renal* (See Kidney Dieseases). Therapeutic Food Manual.**

**CARIES:**

*Dental, Susceptibility to:* Two or three vitamin C tablets daily for the adults; in children, one tablet per day.

**CATARACT:**

Cataracts have been eliminated by the administration of vitamin concentrates, but the effect is not certain, and different vitamins appear to be responsible in different cases, "Catalyn" having caused the disappearance of cataracts in many cases where it had been administered for other purposes.

The failure to respond to the use of vitamins is, no doubt, because irreparable damage has occurred to some of the endocrine organs. We have a parallel situation in diabetes mellitus in which vitamin B is very useful, provided the pancreatic insulin-secreting cells have not been totally destroyed.

The parathyroids, thyroid, spleen, gonads and pituitary are among the endocrines that influence calcium metabolism. The ultimate solution of the cataract problem lies, no doubt, in replacing some one or more of the specific hormones that are lacking because of endocrine disability, which disability is, no doubt, due mainly to vitamin starvation.

Experimental dosage for cataract: One teaspoonful of "V-P Phosphade" first thing in the morning in a full glass of water, one vitamin A and one "Catalyn" tablet at breakfast, one "Catalyn" tablet and one "V-P" Organic Mineral tablet at lunch (noon), one "Catalyn" and one vitamin G tablet at dinner (evening).

**CATARRH: (See Rhinitis, Chronic).**

**CHLOROSIS: (Same schedule as for Secondary Anemia).**

**CHOREA (St. Vitus Dance):**

One "Catalyn" tablet and one vitamin C tablet daily, increasing to two tablets of each after one week. One-half teaspoon of "V-P Phosphade" daily in one-half glass of water is very helpful in getting more speedy results. Improvement is more definite in children than in adults.

**COLDS AND INFLUENZA:**

Two "Catalyn" tablets, one vitamin A tablet and one "V-P" Organic Mineral tablet per hour is recommended during acute period (for 4 to 8 hours usually), until the temperature is down, or under control.

Where the expected results are not obtained in treating colds by this schedule (it is 90% effective), there probably is a severe deficiency of the inorganic alkali minerals. Calcium lactate or any of the proprietary inorganic alkalizers are here indicated and are often required to get the best results in connection with the vitamin concentrates.

**CONSTIPATION:**

None of the vitamins can be considered a direct remedy for constipation, but where the liver is at fault, four vitamin A tablets daily are often very effective. This form of constipation (exhausted liver) is one that defies any other treatment. Vitamin B is very beneficial where peristalsis is impaired, one tablet each meal being taken until normality is restored. Where a "lazy colon" is responsible, two tablets daily of the Organic Mineral tablets, one with each of the two largest meals, often restores a normal colonic reflex. In fact, an overdosage of the "V-P" Organic Mineral tablets may result in abnormally frequent bowel movement, but with little or no other effect on the bowel function.

**CYSTITIS:**

*Acute:* Two tablets of vitamin A per hour during the first six hours; then four tablets per day with two "Catalyn" tablets daily, for two or three weeks.

*Chronic:* One vitamin A tablet and one tablet of "Catalyn" one-half hour before each meal if the patient is overweight, and one-half hour after meals if underweight.

**DIABETES MELLITUS:**

One "Catalyn" and one vitamin B tablet at each meal (increased to two tablets of vitamin B at each meal after the first week, if the case is severe.

All diabetics are able to note more or less improvement in general health under "Catalyn" treatment, much of the effect probably being due to other factors than any specific aid to the pancreas.

If patient is on Insulin, it may be advisable to decrease the Insulin dosage about 10 percent weekly during the vitamin treatment.

(See also comment under Acidosis, which shows the importance of vitamin A in diabetes, in combating the tendency to acidosis present in this condition.)

**DROPSY:**

Four "Catalyn" tablets per day (one each meal and one at bedtime). The only cases of dropsy that do not recover on this schedule are those in which the heart, liver or kidney degeneration has reached a point where the removal of the cause is no longer a factor in controlling the condition. If response after ten days on this schedule is not satisfactory, add two vitamin A and two vitamin E tablets daily.

There is no more spectacular result to be demonstrated in vitamin therapy than the treatment of the average case of cardiac decomposition with kidney involvement, resulting in dropsy, in the immediate response of both kidneys and heart to vitamins A, B and C ("Catalyn"). The elimination of the excess water by way of the kidneys in five to seven days is the story in seven out of ten cases. It is an object lesson that is only comparable to the action of vitamins in treating the disorders of pregnancy (See comments under Acidosis).

**ECZEMA:**

One vitamin E tablet at each meal.

**EYE DISORDERS:**

*Accommodation, Defects of:* vitamin F, one tablet per day, has been found very effective in improving both lens and iris accommodation. A change in spectacle lenses is often necessary after a few weeks' treatment.

*Irritability of Eyes:* Vitamin A, three tablets per day, has proved to be very effective in the control of chronic irritability and inflammation of the eyes. Usually accompanied by kidney symptoms of vitamin A deficiency (albuminuria, cystitis).

**GASTRITIS:**

One tablet of "Catalyn" and one vitamin A tablet one-half hour before each meal if the patient is overweight, or taken one-half hour after each meal if the patient is underweight.

**GOITER: (See Thyroid Dysfunction)**

**HEART DISORDERS:**

*Angina Pectoris:* Two "Catalyn" and two vitamin E tablets daily, increasing to three of each per day after two weeks if improvement is not definite. One teaspoonful daily of "V-P Phosphade" (taken as directed on the bottle) is quite essential.

*Coronary Occlusion:* Same schedule as for Angina Pectoris.

In view of the fact that the best authorities consider that coronary occlusion, even though complete, may not be fatal if there is time for the collateral circulation to develop, the value of vitamin concentrates in improving the quality of the blood supply to the heart muscle is obvious. Sometimes the additional use of one or two vitamin C tablets per day with the above schedule is of noticeable benefit. It is, we believe, the vitamin E which controls the pains in these cases.

*Heart Enlargement:* Four "Catalyn" tablets per day. It is advisable to start with two tablets per day at first to see that it causes no untoward reaction in case the patient has been taking digitalis, as "Catalyn" restores normal sensitiveness to that drug.

*Rapid or Erratic Pulse:* (patients under 40 years of age): One tablet of "Catalyn" per day for the first week, increasing one a day each week until four a day are being taken, which dose is continued for the duration of the treatment. If the patient is overweight, the tablets should be taken one-half hour before meals; if the patient is underweight, one-half hour after meals.

*Rapid or Erratic Pulse:* (patients over 40 years of age): Same treatment as above with the addition of one teaspoonful of "V-P Phosphade" daily, taken as directed on the bottle.

**HYPERTENSION:**

One tablet of "Catalyn" with two or three (minimum) doses of "V-P Phosphade" per day for the first week, two tablets per day of "Catalyn" for the second week, three tablets per day for the third week and four tablets per day after the fourth week. In this way, the "V-P Phosphade" is given an opportunity to partially remove the cause of the high blood pressure before the full dosage of "Catalyn" is reached, as were a patient suffering from myocardial disease, the improvement in heart function could possibly cause an increase in blood pressure in the beginning of the treatment, the high blood pressure being due, in this case, to obstruction of flow with the heart attempting to maintain flow in spite of this obstruction.

If the "V-P Phosphade" is not well tolerated (if it causes gastric irritation) reduce dosage and give two "V-P" Organic Mineral tablets and two vitamin A tablets, daily, with it.

# VITAMIN NEWS

VITAMIN PRODUCTS CO. • MILWAUKEE, WISCONSIN

March 15, 1936 VOL. 4

## ALPHABETICAL TABLE OF RECOMMENDATIONS OF VARIOUS "V-P" CONCENTRATES USEFUL IN THE TREATMENT OF DISEASE – Continued

**HYPOTENSION:**

One "Catalyn" tablet at each meal and one at bedtime. There is probably no other effective remedy for hypotension. There is a fair response in most cases.

**INFECTIONS:**

The effect of "Catalyn" on any chronic focal infection is to aid in combating it through an increase in phagocytic activity, provided there is any avenue of drainage. Where there is no drainage, stimulation of the phagocytic activity will cause a congestion and pressure in the infected area, causing pain, Nature's reaction to forced drainage, which must occur before the infection can be cleared up.

Dosage: One "Catalyn" tablet at each meal.

*Acute:* Four "Catalyn" tablets as an initial dose, followed by one tablet per hour until the infection is under control, as indicated by temperature, etc. Where pyogenic organisms are responsible, a great increase in pus discharge will be observed, due to the enhancement of phagocytosis.

**INFLUENZA (See Colds):**

**INSOMNIA:**

One to three "Catalyn" tablets taken just before retiring. In insomnia, the small dosage should be tried, increasing nightly until four tablets are being taken. If no results are manifest, vitamins can be ruled out. But most cases get relief and there are soon many other physical evidences of improvement apparent as well.

The treatment should be continued at a medium dosage after the insomnia has disappeared, for thirty to sixty days to build up the patient, as otherwise a recurrence can be expected soon.

**KIDNEY DISEASE:**

*Albuminuria:* (especially the albuminuria of Pregnancy): Four vitamin A tablets per day. (See Acidosis for further comments.)

*Bright's Disease:* Four vitamin A tablets daily.

*Calculi:* One "Catalyn" tablet and one vitamin A tablet at each meal and at bedtime.

*Nephritis:* Four vitamin A tablets daily.

**LOW VITALITY:**

One tablet of "Catalyn" daily for the first week, increasing one tablet a day each week until four a day are being taken, which dose is continued for the duration of the treatment. If the patient is overweight, tablets should be taken one-half hour before meals; if underweight, one-half hour after meals.

**LYMPHATIC GLAND ENLARGEMENT:**

This condition is usually a consequence of lowered resistance and infection as a result. Four "Catalyn" tablets daily for thirty to sixty days.

**MENOPAUSE:**

*Endocrine, Unbalance of:* Same schedule as for Menstrual Dysfunction.

**MENSTRUAL DYSFUNCTION:**

One "Cerol" capsule daily and one tablet of "Catalyn" one-half hour before each meal if the patient is overweight; one tablet one-half hour after each meal if the patient is underweight. Amenorrhea is particularly responsive to this treatment.

The abdominal pains attendant to menstrual dysfunction are caused by congestion of the ovary with consequent painful tension on the ovarian capsule (often mistaken in acute stages for appendicitis) and are usually relieved promptly with "Catalyn."

Gland swelling in general is a vitamin deficiency reaction, notable in ovaries, prostate, thyroid.

**MIGRAINE:**

One "Catalyn" tablet per day often is of great benefit in migraine headaches. Some cases fail to respond. Those that do respond, show almost immediate improvement (the next periodic attack is reduced in severity or does not appear).

If "Catalyn" is not effective, one "Cerol" capsule per say sometimes produces results.

**NERVOUS CONDITIONS:**

One "Catalyn" tablet before each meal if patient is overweight. One tablet of "Catalyn" one-half hour after each meal if the patient is underweight. To either schedule add one-half teaspoonful of "V-P Phosphade," taken as directed on the bottle, per day.

**NEURASTHENIA:**

Two "Catalyn" tablets and one "V-P" Organic Mineral tablet per day. Double this in ten days if definite improvement is not under way.

**NEURITIS:**

Neuritic pains can usually be controlled by the use of vitamin E tablets, three or four per day. If the cause is known to be an infection, three "Catalyn" tablets a day for thirty days should be given to aid in its elimination.

**OBESITY:**

We hesitate to recommend "Catalyn" or vitamin voncentrates for reducing purposes, because so much depends upon the cooperation of the patient.

The direction in our dosage charts is to give "Catalyn" one-half hour before meals in obesity because under such circumstances it often tends to reduce the appetite and thereby lower the food intake. If taken after meals, the assimilation is improved, and the patient will tend to gain weight.

In the case of a patient on a strict reducing diet, it will be found that two or three "Catalyn" tablets daily will prevent weakness and insure against the usual consequence of dieting — lowered resistance.

**PELLAGRA:**

The pellagra victim is usually, if not always, suffering from a multiple vitamin deficiency, and our recommendation is three "Catalyn" tablets and three vitamin G tablets daily.

These may be best taken one tablet of each after each meal. Quite satisfactory results can be expected in the treatment of pellagra with this schedule. Any symptoms of deficiency of other vitamins, particularly vitamins A, B and C, should be watched for and treated, if necessary, with two or three tablets of the proper concentrate daily.

**PNEUMONIA:**

One "Catalyn" tablet every one-half hour until the temperature is under control, which is usually accomplished within eight to twelve hours, with obvious improvements in two hours.

**PREGNANCY:**

*Disorders of:* Two or three "Catalyn" tablets and one "Cerol" capsule (along with one or two vitamin A tablets per day if albuminuria is present). (See Acidosis.)

The hyperemesis of pregnancy is usually easily controlled with "Catalyn," three tablets daily. This should be continued through the lactation period. One "Cerol" capsule daily or one tablet of vitamin E is also advisable. (See "Cerol" literature.)

The use of "Catalyn" for some weeks before delivery has been exceptionally effective in minimizing labor pains, no doubt because it affords added nutrition to the overworked endocrines at this time.

**PROSTATE ENLARGEMENT:**

Two "Catalyn" and two vitamin E tablets per day, or three "Catalyn" tablets alone per day.

If the prostate condition does not show improvement in two weeks, supplement treatment with two vitamin F and one or two "V-P" Organic Mineral tablets per day for a couple of weeks.

**PURPURA HEMORRHAGICA (Scurvy):**

Four tablets daily of vitamin C. If the condition is critical or acute, one tablet every half hour for eight hours followed by four tablets per day.

**PYORRHEA:**

Three or four vitamin C tablets per day usually will cause a recalcification and consequent tightening of the teeth, which is perceptible within a week or ten days. Treatment should be continued until recalcificaiton is completed, which may require two or three months.

The vitamins will take care of the systemic situation, but naturally local conditions must be taken care of by the dentist according to the usual methods. There is usually infection to be treated and calculus to be removed.

VITAMIN NEWS

VITAMIN PRODUCTS CO. • MILWAUKEE, WISCONSIN

April 15, 1936 VOL. 4

## ALPHABETICAL TABLE OF RECOMMENDATIONS OF VARIOUS "V-P" CONCENTRATES USEFUL IN THE TREATMENT OF DISEASE – Continued

**RHEUMATIC PAINS: (Same schedule as for Neuritis)**

**RHINITIS:**

*Chronic:* Four "Catalyn" tablets together with four vitamin A tablets per day (one of each after each meal and before retiring) until the condition is controlled.

**RICKETS:**

One "Catalyn" tablet per day for children less than 7 years of age. Two "Catalyn" tablets per day for children 7 to 10 years of age. Three "Catalyn" tablets per day for children 10 years or over.

**SCURVY: (See Purpura Hemorrhagica and Pyorrhea.)**

**SINUS INFECTIONS:**

*Chronic:* Same schedule as for Rhinitis.

**STERILITY (Male or Female):**

Two "Catalyn" tablets and one "Cerol" capsule (or one vitamin E tablet) daily.

**THYROID DYSFUNCTION:**

Considered in the light of the theory which is becoming more and more accepted that the endocrines depend upon the vitamin intake for nutrition and that endocrines that are deprived of proper nutrition will act in one of two ways — they will either develop a compensatory enlargement, or their parenchymatous cells will die — it is not unreasonable to assume that the use of vitamins should theoretically be of importance in all endocrine disorders.

Iodine deficiency has been supposed to be the cause of most thyroid pathologies, but it is only a factor, and in the presence of the proper vitamin supply, much less iodine is normally necessary, whereas the absence of iodine aggravates the pathologies basically established by the vitamin shortage.

*Simple Goiter* (Non-functional Hypertrophy): One "Catalyn" tablet one-half hour before each meal if the patient is overweight; one tablet of "Catalyn" one-half hour after each meal if the patient is underweight. If the case is of long standing, there may be no effect, as the enlarged gland may have become infiltrated with connective tissue.

*Toxic Goiter:* Four "Catalyn" tablets per day for the first month, one after each meal and one at bedtime, reducing to three tablets per day thereafter. If the "Catalyn" is discontinued before three or four months treatment, you will notice that there is a tendency of the symptoms to return, so treatment should be considered over a period of four or five months at the least.

**TUBERCULOSIS:**

One "Catalyn" tablet and one vitamin C tablet after each meal and one each at bedtime. The value of "Catalyn" here is indirect, as a vitality and resistance builder.

There are two reactions to "Catalyn" in the average case of tuberculosis. One is that the usual susceptibility to colds is diminished, and the other is that the patient begins to show signs of gaining in weight.

For children, treatment should be started with one "Catalyn" tablet and one vitamin C tablet per day for the first week, and two each day thereafter should be given. Treatment may be increased to three tablets of each per day if satisfactory improvement is not evident at the end of two weeks.

**ULCERS:**

*Peptic (Gastric or Duodenal)*: Put the patient on a diet of nothing but orange juice and milk — a glass of each taken together as desired for a three day period — followed by an advised diet with four "Catalyn" tablets a day.

"Catalyn" alone for many ulcer patients may cause nausea unless the above procedure is followed. In fact, the nausea may be considered almost a diagnostic indication of peptic ulcers.

**VARICOSE VEINS:**

Two vitamin C tablets, two or three vitamin E tablets, and two "V-P" Organic Mineral tablets daily. Vitamin therapy in varicose veins usually is effective in controlling the tendency to inflammation, a tendency to scurvy being a common accompanying factor, which causes a breakdown of the endothelium, the primary factor in degeneration of the muscle fibers in the venous walls, which of course means permanent damage.

**LIST OF REACTIONS THAT MAY OCCUR WHEN VITAMIN CONCENTRATES ARE ADMINISTERED**

(1) Allergic Reactions:

Sometimes a rash is produced, similar to "strawberry rash" or the "bread rash" from whole wheat. Soon disappears on reduced dosage.

(2) Intestinal Reactions:

Patients who have an accumulation of stagnant material may experience rather severe gas pains within a few hours of their first dose of "Catalyn," immediately followed by an unusually malodorous evacuation.

(3) Stomach Reactions:

In presence of gastric ulcers, "Catalyn" may produce nausea. Three or four days on nothing but orange juice and milk — a glass of each taken together as desired — followed by an advised diet with four "Catalyn" tablets a day will usually control the ulcer situation. Guinea pigs soon develop ulcers in duodenum and stomach if deprived of vitamins B and C. (See *Vitamin News*, Vol. 2, No. 3.)

(4) Reactions from Old Chronic Infected Areas:

Bone ulcers, etc., immediately begin to exude pus — a positive indication of the institution of healing processes. Old infected areas that have apparently cleared up may be the source of neuralgic pains for some time after "Catalyn" is used, noted particularly in tooth abscesses. Never occurs where drainage exists.

(5) Reactions Due to Temporary Endocrine Unbalance:
Sometimes "Catalyn" seems to aggravate a functional disorder when its administration is commenced. This is because vitamins are the nutritional elements of the endocrine system (B and C, for instance, support the thyro-adrenal system), and cases are found where the activity of one endocrine organ is revived sooner than its balancing opponent; the one that has been underactive may be last to respond. The advised procedure here is to continue a small dosage of "Catalyn" until the normal balance is obtained.

(6) Reactions Due to Restoration of Normal Sensitiveness to Drugs:
"Catalyn" must not be given in large doses where digitalis has been or is being used in amounts of more than the normal dose. It immediately restores sensitiveness to this drug. "Catalyn" may also cause headaches in persons who habitually drink two or more cups of coffee at a meal, by restoring sensitiveness to caffeine. Sleeplessness can result from this as well.

**WHEN "V-P PHOSPHADE" IS ADMINISTERED:**
"V-P Phosphade," consisting of the acid class of food minerals (phosphoric acid and acid phosphates normally obtained by the enzymic reduction of the phytin components of cereals forming phosphoric acid and inosite as the first metabolic change in the body), can aggravate acidosis. Where this occurs, the dosage should be reduced to one-half teaspoonful per day (in water), and two tablets daily of the "V-P" Organic Minerals with two tablets of vitamin A added.

The use of "V-P Phosphade" is usually of vital importance (it is indicated in such serious conditions as arteriosclerosis, hypertension, and angina pectoris) so that where it is not well tolerated, the above schedule will be found helpful. The intolerance is a further consequence of other deficiencies and is not commonly noted except in the older and more evident cases of malnutrition.

**WHEN "V-P" ORGANIC MINERALS ARE ADMINISTERED:**
The Organic Mineral tablets, if taken by a normal adult in dosages of three or four tablets a day, can, in two weeks or so, result in such a sensitization of the nervous reflexes as to result in discomfort — better expressed in the vernacular as "heebie jeebies." Even one dose of one teaspoonful of the acid mineral — "V-P Phosphade" — will correct this situation. It is because of this action in restoring the normal reflexes, where they are weak, that the therapeutic merits of the Organic Minerals lie. We get too little of both the acid and basic minerals in our average diet.

# NOTES

# VITAMIN NEWS

VITAMIN PRODUCTS CO. • MILWAUKEE, WISCONSIN

January 15, 1936 VOL. 4

## VITAMINS

### A Review of Definitions and Principles

In any new science, a certain time must elapse before a sufficient background of facts can develop to permit a logical appraisal of the situation, which appraisal is indispensable before any basic principles can be laid down.

Premature conclusions are often incorrect. Persons of some scientific education in other fields have been prone to consider themselves competent to make arbitrary pronouncements that sound reasonable on their face, but which on consideration are found to be totally at variance with the facts.

Probably the most outstanding example of such witless comment is the statement that "any well balanced diet" will maintain health without the need of considering the vitamin intake.

The joker here is that what has always been considered a well balanced diet may be, and usually is, quite inadequate in view of our newer knowledge of nutrition; and the more we learn, the more inadequate it appears.

The new dictionaries are agreed on the following definition of a vitamin:

> "One of a class of substances of unknown composition, existing in minute quantity in natural foods and necessary to normal nutrition and growth, absence of which from the diet produces deficiency diseases, such as beriberi, scurvy and rachitis."

While considerable progress has been made on the investigation of the composition and chemical nature of the various vitamins, it is quite important that here, too, we avoid jumping at conclusions. Many of the past conclusions have proven faulty. The real test of a vitamin is its ability to cure deficiency diseases.

Two significant facts in particular are becoming apparent as follows:

1. Chemical purification of a vitamin principle may render it ineffective, known to be true of E[1], G[2] and B[3].
2. To produce the same vitamin effect in different species may require entirely different principles (chemically considered). (See appended reference[4] regarding this point in respect to vitamin D, and reference[5] in respect to vitamin C.)

It will be at once obvious that an assay of vitamins to be used for human therapy by means of animal test is of doubtful value until it is determined what relation there may exist between the effectiveness of the product under examination when used for the test animal and the human. Even assuming that this relation may be a constant coefficient (speaking now as regards Fact No. 22), the possibility remains that there may be associated or related principles in the animal economy differing from human metabolism that can alter the results in view of Fact No. 1. It is these considerations that have rendered it impossible for the clinician to depend upon unit content as determined by animal assay as an index of therapeutic merit.

With respect to vitamin A, the U.S.P. X. authorized its estimation in terms of carotene because of the naive theory that carotene was convertible at will into vitamin A in the human or animal organism. This was discontinued in the U.S.P. XI, a direct assay with test animals being required in which a comparison is made between the test sample and a standard reference cod liver oil. (No form of chemically pure vitamin A has as yet been made.) This also has been the approved method of making vitamin D assays according to both U.S.P. X and U.S.P. XI.

Such a test does just one thing. It standardizes the tested oil in terms of the reference oil with respect to its effect on the test animal. But suppose neither contained the principle that was necessary to perform as vitamin D in some species other than the rat, which was used as a test animal. They would be of no value in treating rickets in such an animal. As a matter of fact, the chicken must have a different substance to receive the vitamin D effect than is required in the rat[6] and we have precisely the situation described above. Highly concentrated forms of vitamin D (as determined by rat tests) have been found totally clueless (in fact, poisonous) to the chicken as a cure for rickets.

As to the applicability of the rat test to the human, we remain pretty much in the dark. There is evidence to show, however, that babies are more like the chicken in their reactions to the rat vitamin.

Primarily, a vitamin is a dietary essential that must be present to prevent some well defined deficiency disease or other. If various different species become afflicted with the same disease by reason of a deficiency of chemically different dietary principles that occur in such small amounts that it is difficult to find them, it becomes necessary, in speaking of a vitamin, to also specify the species for which it is effective.

Upon reflection, the reasonableness of these facts becomes more apparent. Each species has its own particular tissue chemistry — its own fatty acids, proteins and carbohydrates. The most suitable food for each species differs in the same manner — the cow can digest cellulose and form stearic acid; the pig can better handle cornstarch as carbohydrate, and forms from it mainly oleic acid. To assume that the same vitamin structures (molecularly speaking) serve all species in the same manner would, therefore, violate a primary principle of nutrition and metabolism.

Immunology has positively demonstrated the specific nature of the proteins of each species and has shown us how the chemical variation in blood proteins can be used to identify a blood stain as to its source, whether human or animal, and, if animal, what species. Many a murderer has been incarcerated, and, no doubt, some have suffered capital punishment on the acceptance of our courts of justice of such distinguishing tests. (I recall one case where the only evidence against a suspect was a tiny blood stain on a hunting knife, he claiming it to be rabbit blood. The laboratory technician found it to be human blood by immunological test, and after receiving a life sentence, the murderer confessed.)

It is such a reaction that causes a reversal of effect (antihormone reaction) when some hormone products are administered to a species other than the one that produced the hormone. Some time is required for the reaction to change from the positive to the negative, the hormone injections gradually losing their effect, finally having an opposite action.[7] Where the hormone administered is obtained from the same species as the animal to which it is administered, the normal effect continues undiminished when dosage is extended over a long period. (The hormone in question must be protein in nature to cause this immunological reaction.)

Because of this specific nature of hormones of each species, and because vitamins are to be considered the chemical precursors of the hormones, it is a reasonable conclusion to assume that there is a chemical difference in the vitamin principles that act most favorably as foods for the different species. The appended references show experimental evidence supporting this inference.

NOTE: More recent work has shown that vitamin G probably is specific in nature for the three species so far investigated – the rat, chick and human. (See references in the *Journal of Biological Chemistry*, 114:1, May 1936 by Lepkovsky and Jukes, pages 109-116; Jukes and Lepkovsky, pages 117-121.

## REFERENCES

[1] *Wheat Germ Oil*, page 10, The American Physician, Inc., New York (1935).

[2] *Biochemical Journal* (Discussion of complexity of vitamin B).

[3] Carter, Cyril W., *Biochemical Journal,* 25:933 (1934).

[4] Steenbock, Harry, *Journal of Biological Chemistry*, pp. 240-264, July, 1932.

[5] *Biochemical Journal*, 28:4, (1934).

[6] Bills, Charles E., *Physiological Reviews,* 15:1, 1-97 (See pages 45-46) Physiology of Sterols, Including Vitamin D.

> "In 1928, a solution of ergosterol, irradiated in this laboratory and standardized on rats, was administered to chickens by Dr. W. Carrick of Purdue University. Carrick found that as a preventive of rickets it compared very poorly with a rat-equivalent amount of cod liver oil (private communication). This led to a systematic investigation of the action of activated ergosterol in the chicken, the results of which were published in 1930. Under the conditions of their experiment, the vitamin D of cod liver oil appeared to be roughly 100 times as effective as that of irradiated ergosterol, the two preparations being standardized with rats. Works by various people amply confirmed the observation that the vitamin D of irradiated ergosterol is far less effective for the chicken than the rat-equivalent amount of vitamin D from cod liver oil. Or, to express it with equal accuracy, irradiated ergosterol is far more effective for the rat than the chicken-equivalent amount of cod liver oil.
>
> "From the investigation just mentioned and particularly from unpublished studies made in this laboratory, it appears that the observed differences between the two anti-rickets agents are not due to the presence or absence of vitamin A, nor to the nature of the oily vehicle. It is thus evident that the vitamin D of irradiated ergosterol is a different substance from that contained in cod liver oil."

Ibid (See pages 40-47).

> " ... It is noteworthy that, in spite of the almost immediate adoption of irradiated ergosterol as a therapeutic agent, nearly three years passed before evidence was obtained that a rat unit of this form of vitamin D exerts on the infant a quantitatively different effect than a rat unit of cod liver oil.

While this is not compliment to the preciseness of clinical medicine, it is doubtless explained in part by the fact that precise methods of standardization with rats were not in general use for either cod liver oil or activated ergosterol.

"Evidence that cod liver oil and irradiated ergosterol (Viosterol) in amounts equipotent for rats do not exert the same degree of antiricketic effect on children came largely from the studies of Hess, Lewis and Rivkin (1930) and Hess and Lewis (1932, 1933). These workers found that about 3 rat units of the ergosterol preparation were clinically equivalent to 1 rat unit of cod liver oil ...

"Bills suggested (1927) in the conclusion of a study on the synthesis of vitamin D by fish, that quite possibly vitamin D is not a single substance, but a mixture or series of substances as variable as the sterols with which it seems to be almost inseparably associated. It now appears, from the studies reviewed above, that the existence of at least three forms of vitamin D is established."

[7]Proceedings, Society of Experimental Biology and Medicine, 32:102 (1934) and Endocrinology, 20:311 (1935).

**Edited by Royal Lee**

VITAMIN NEWS

VITAMIN PRODUCTS CO. • MILWAUKEE, WISCONSIN

June 15, 1936 VOL. 4

# VITAMIN F

Vitamin F has been identified as linolenic and linoleic acid, or possibly the correct statement is to say that these fatty acids have been given the new name of vitamin F because of their newly discovered vitamin function.

Linoleic and linolenic acids are found in cereals, in especial abundance in flaxseed, but present in all to some extent. (Their abundance in flax is probably a matter of the high oil content of flax, the percentage in the oils of other cereals, rye and oats, probably being higher, but the cost of such oils is fifty to one hundred times that of flaxseed oil.) It has been shown that .001 milligram of linoleic acid produces definite improvement in deficient test animals, establishing the "vitamin" characteristics of minuteness of dosage.

In our first discussion of vitamin F (*Vitamin News*, Volume 3, No. 8, pages 57-58) we had not become aware of the fact that the investigators of the linolenic acid group were looking at another side of the same picture which we were describing in connection with our findings as to our "vitamin F." We were also under the same misapprehension as many others in assuming that linolenic acid was present in larger amounts in common foods (with apologies to those who believe that "any well balanced diet contains plenty of vitamins").

Matthews has called attention to the resemblance between the oxygen metabolism of linseed oil and protoplasm in the respect that some oxidative accelerator is required in each case, and Plimmer[1] pointed out the fact that the linolenic and linoleic acids present in linseed oil acted as the oxidative accelerator in the cereal oils.

Meyerhof[2] offers evidence to show that the linolenic acid group of fatty acids is the oxidative catalyst that brings about the oxygen transfers to the muscle cell. This, of course, supplies the theoretical hypothesis that explains the muscular atrophy and malfunction in Vitamin F deficiency, and also throws light on the findings of Zaicsek and Weiser of Budapest, who demonstrated that the feeding of rye to animals caused a muscular development in contrast to the fat accumulation produced by the feeding of wheat.

Our previous approach to the subject through the angle of calcium metabolism is, no doubt, merely another view of the same phenomenon, as oxygen metabolism and calcium metabolism have some important relation, since the control of oxygen metabolism by the thyroid is associated with a parallel control of calcium (when oxygen metabolism is enhanced by the administration of thyroxine, the serum calcium is also lowered) and the thyroid is now considered the physiological controller of tissue calcium content as well as the regulator of oxidation.

Of late, some other clinical uses for vitamin F besides its effect as a reducer of enlarged prostates have become outstanding. One is its action in correcting the common condition of "digestive distress" as characterized by hyperacidity, peptic ulcers, etc. Another is its action in relieving gall bladder trouble. Both of these conditions have been the great mysteries of pathology. It is probable that they both can be explained now on a common ground.

Sajous[3] indissolubly connected with oxygen metabolism the metabolic reactions of pepsin and trypsin. Trypsin excess in the bile has been, no doubt, correctly charged with initiating the gall bladder irritation of cholecystitis,[4] infection, no doubt, being a secondary consequence. So why not consider the same etiology for the irritation that sets the stage for peptic ulcer?

Here are the important facts. Pepsin and trypsin both are protein digesters, acting in series, pepsin in the stomach (in an acid media), trypsin in the small intestine where the reaction is alkaline (but it will act in either acid or alkaline surroundings), while pepsin will act only in the presence of acids. Now suppose there is a regurgitation of duodenal contents back into the stomach — a common occurrence. Irritation and a sensitiveness to the hydrochloric acid, which by reason of the irritation, may be overproduced, is the result. This acid now passes into the duodenum, able only to neutralize ordinary quantities, and more irritation results, to say nothing of the proteolytic effect of the excess trypsin on the mucosa.

The value of vitamin F in these cases is, no doubt, explainable by reason of its oxygenizing ability to combine the findings of Meyerhof and Sajous, by which less trypsin is required. To hypothecate, in the absence of enough vitamin F, an excessive amount of trypsin may be secreted (by reason of the well known compensative physiologic tendencies), and it may not only be responsible for local trouble in gall bladder, stomach and bowel, but may become a blood constituent in excess, with disastrous results. Why should not it start a proteolytic destruction of the vascular intima, and the typical case of arteriosclerosis develop? As corroborative evidence, we cite Joslin's statement that "The association of gall bladder disease and coronary sclerosis was striking" (among diabetics). He also states that "the amount and extent of coronary sclerosis in diabetic subjects examined postmortem is astonishingly great. Every one with a duration of diabetes of five years or more has shown some degree of coronary sclerosis."[5]

That is to be expected, according to our new hypothesis. Pancreatic overactivity is known to commonly accompany diabetes, the other pancreatic secretions being overproduced because of excessive sympathetic stimulus that should arouse the insulin-producing cells, too much trypsin thereby being secreted. The great incidence of gall bladder disease among diabetics is another significant point.

This may explain the success of our vitamin E tablet as a remedy for angina pectoris (usual dosage two or three vitamin E tablets a day with two or three "Catalyn" tablets). The vitamin E tablet contains considerable vitamin F as well as vitamin E, and the control of the hypertryptic condition may be the reason for its action. (A little "V-P Phosphade" and one vitamin D tablet daily often helps to hasten results.)

Further evidence of the correctness of this hypothesis is the fact that the vitamin F (linoleic acid) has been shown to have an anti-enzyme action against trypsin,[6] and linolenic acid has been shown to have an anti-peptic action (no doubt an exhibition of the same characteristic).[7] This will alter our theoretical assumption above, that in vitamin F deficiency more trypsin is secreted, but instead the normal quantity present becomes more active. Either way, however, we have a hypertryptic condition to cope with, and we have a new theory to explain some old and puzzling disorders, to say nothing of the results already definitely established in their treatment with vitamin F.

Keep in mind that vitamin F can bring about hypocalcemia if vitamin D and an ample supply of dietary calcium (raw milk) is not supplied, and that the use of the "V-P Phosphade" enables the patient to utilize his own pathological surplus of calcium carbonate.

Pacini[8] has given the following consequences of vitamin F deficiency as indicated by animal tests:

"1. A scaliness of the skin with a general affection of all the epidermal structures in which the hair becomes brittle and splits easily (fragilitans crinium), the finger nails ridge and split and may become eczematous (atrophia ungium) and the skin may become definitely dry with a tendency to exfoliate and later develop distinctly eczematous lesions.

"2. In the rat, a swelling of the extremities suggestive of angioneurotic edema occurs. In the dog, urticaria is the counterpart and in the human, giant hives.

"3. The hair fills with scurf and dandruff — a seborrheic dermatitis.

"4. The hair loosens and falls out readily — alopecia.

"5. Female animals show markedly impaired ovulation together with failures of reproduction and unusually long gestation periods.

"6. Males display disinclination to want to mate and eventually become completely sterile. Addition of vitamin F to the diet prevents or relieves this sterility.

"7. Animals eat the same amount of food, but drink twice the usual amount of water, suggesting involvement of the pituitary glands.

"8. Pronounced renal irritation as evidenced by the appearance of hematuria and albuminuria occurs.

"9. Growing animals fail to reach the full weight and remain stunted. Males reach about 70% and females about 80% of their adult weight."

## REFERENCES

[1] Plimmer, *Organic and Biochemistry*, page 163, Longmans Green & Co., 1933.

[2] Meyerhof, O., *Chemical Dynamics of Life Phenomena,* Lippincott, 1924.

[3] Sajous, *The Internal Secretions and the Principles of Medicine*, pages 852- 856, F. A. Davis, Co., Tenth Edition, 1922.

[4] Wakaman and Davison, *Enzymes*, page 71, Williams and Wilkins, 1926.

[5] Joslin, *Treatment of Diabetes Mellitus,* page 339, Lea & Febiger, 1935.

[6] Jobling, *Jol. Exp. Med.*, 19:239, 1914.

[7] Velluz, *Bull. Chim. Biol.*, 9:483, 1927.

[8] Pacini, *Brochure on Vitamin F.* Pharmaceutical Specialties Co., 1936.

# NOTES

VITAMIN NEWS

VITAMIN PRODUCTS CO. • MILWAUKEE, WISCONSIN

July 15, 1936 VOL. 4

# VITAMIN THERAPY IN DIABETES MELLITUS

The first account of the successful treatment of hyperglycemia with vitamin B concentrates was mentioned in these pages (Vol. 2, No. 5, page 29, paragraph 4). Vitamin B caused a slow but definite improvement in a majority of the cases treated. At that time, attention was called to the fact that diabetes with attendant hypertension also required vitamin C concentrate to get the best response according to clinical findings.

Diabetes with hypotension is a more evident case of vitamin B deficiency. Lack of B causes a characteristic loss of vascular tone due to the functional failure of the vascular innervation. In all probability the same functional failure of the pancreatic innervation can prevent the normal release of insulin after the ingestion of carbohydrates. In this case, the pancreas may be perfectly intact, as is known to be the case in many diabetics. The administration of vitamin B in such cases may result in immediate release of insulin (within 30 minutes according to the experience of a number of clinicians who have reported to us), and even symptoms of hypoglycemia — hyperinsulinism — may appear.

Hyperinsulinism after meals in otherwise healthy individuals is a not uncommon phenomenon. Strangely enough, the injection of insulin has proved a successful remedy in that it supplies insulin without arousing the pancreas, while if the pancreas is called on, it overdoes the job.

When vitamin B administration causes hyperinsulinism, it is probably a similar situation. Indeed, the failure of the nervous control would logically result in a loading up of the pancreas beyond the normal, and result in an abnormal amount being released on the repair of the nervous connection. Again, such loss of nervous control with no demand on the pancreas — or reduced demand — can logically result ultimately in pancreatic atrophy or degeneration. It is known that pancreatic alterations occur in avitaminosis B in test animals.[1]

The speed with which the administration of vitamin B in this type of case causes a resumption of insulin secretion has caused comment. It is no more speedy, however, than the cure of a paralyzed pigeon that has been prepared by withdrawal of vitamin B from its feed, when the vitamin concentrate is supplied. A bird that can neither stand nor fly is restored apparently to normal in a few minutes. The long continued partial avitaminosis to which human patients may be subjected, however, may not always respond as completely; the degenerations in such cases can be expected to be less easily restored. It is that fact that limits our success in both the nervous tissues as well as in the pancreas. Nothing but a clinical test on each patient will tell the story.

Diabetes accompanied with hypertension is a different matter. The hyperglycemia here may be due to the oversecretion of adrenin, which may also be causing the increased blood pressure. Adrenin has as one of its functions the release of glycogen from the liver. Too much adrenin may be due to avitaminosis C and B, as each of these vitamins is necessary to the proper function of the adrenals, especially the cortex, and in their absence a hypertrophy may result.[2] This hypertrophy often means a hypersecretion of the medulla with attendant hypertension — and diabetes if the pancreas is unable to take the extra load. The well-known effect of vitamins B and C (as

"Catalyn") to reduce hypertension in these cases depends on the effect on the adrenal gland. If the diabetic condition is due to adrenal stimulation, it also responds to this treatment.

The amount of adrenin that will cause hyperglycemia is less than that necessary to cause a rise in blood pressure.[3] Therefore, it is important to supply the vitamins B and C together in all cases, to see that vitamin C is tested in those cases where B alone fails to be of benefit. Under treatment with vitamin concentrates, the average diabetic patient improves so much in his general "sense of well being" that he is inclined to depart form his rigid diet, and that is the important thing to warn him against. A long continued schedule of increased vitamin and low carbohydrate intake is necessary for permanent benefit.

We must accept as a basic fact that most endocrine unbalance is a result of vitamin starvation. The outstanding feature of any chart of vitamin deficiency consequences is an appalling list of endocrine changes — atrophy or hypertrophy — parenchymatous death or "compensatory" enlargement.

Because the pancreas is often intact in severe diabetes, and because it has been found that the pituitary (both anterior and posterior) secretes hormones that cause hyperglycemia,[4] it has recently been suggested that pituitary disorder may be responsible for diabetes mellitus, and a control of the oversecretion of the diabetogenic hormones by means of X-ray treatments directed to the pituitary has been proposed, and some benefit reported in a few test cases.

But the production by the anterior pituitary of another pancreatropic hormone that stimulates the activity and growth of the Langerhansian Islets is known.[5] So, X-ray treatments are thereby ruled out. We know that avitaminosis B causes degeneration of the pituitary, and no doubt interferes with its normal hormone output, so the avitaminosis hypothesis of diabetes is further reinforced. The normal pituitary, no doubt, secretes a balanced output of glycemia regulators, with adrenin as a further factor. Such a set-up can reasonably be disturbed by vitamin deficiency in two ways:

1. Starvation of the endocrine involved.
2. Paralysis or reduced sensitivity of nervous controls.

An interesting news note recently stated that a South American honey bear in a zoo developed diabetes, requiring the administration of insulin. That means to us that the refined sweets that were fed the bear in place of its normal diet of honey merely did what could be expected. We know honey is one of the good sources of vitamin B. So is wheat — if we get it whole. But the use of vast amounts of refined carbohydrate separated from its normally accompanying vitamin that is necessary to insure it proper assimilation can only be expected to result in a rising curve of incidence of diabetes mellitus that exactly parallels the curve of rising volume of consumption of devitalized foods.

Diabetes mellitus is serious, not particularly because of the blood hyperglycemia, but because the lowered metabolism of glycogen brings about an automatic (defensive) reduction in the conversion of fat (normally stored in the liver) into glycogen, with a resultant damning up of fat in the blood and liver. It is this rise in blood fat that causes diabetic coma.

In diabetes mellitus we have this cycle of events:

1. Failure of the pancreas to supply insulin (for one reason or another).
2. Hyperglycemia and glycosuria.
3. An automatic reduction (defensive reaction to compensate for reduced glycogen metabolism) in

amount of reserve fat converted into glycogen.
4. Accumulation of fat in liver, as well as in tissues and in blood. (See *Vitamin News,* Dec. 15, 1935).
5. Diabetic coma because of high blood fat.

The susceptibility of the diabetic to infections and to gangrene can be combatted successfully with concentrates of vitamins C and D. In gangrene cases especially, the use of our vitamin C concentrate has produced spectacular results. The dosage should be one or two vitamin D tablets daily, with two to six vitamin C tablets.

## REFERENCES

[1] McCarrison, *Indian Journal of Medical Research*, 8:530-588, 1919.

[2] Sherman and Smith, *The Vitamins,* page 70. Second Edition, 1931.

[3] Houssay, B. A. and Di Benedetto, E., *Rev. Soc. Argent. De biol.*, 9:310, 1933.

The continuous injection of adrenaline into adrenalectomized dogs, in doses corresponding to the amount normally secreted or very slightly higher, simultaneously with injection of posterior pituitary extract, was followed by hyperglycemia ... It is deduced that the posterior pituitary hyperglycemia is due to a hemoral action of the liver requiring the secretion of adrenaline.

[4] Houssay, B. A. and di Benedetto, E., Ibid, 9:300, 1933.

Dogs anesthetized with chloralose received variable doses (1 to 2.5 and 5 to 10 mg. per kg.) of extract of standard powder of posterior pituitary gland. The injection was made intravenously, lasting 1 hour, 1 cc. of the solution being injected every minute. Blood sugar (Hagedorn and Jensen method) was determined up to 7 hours after the beginning of the experiment. An increase proportional to the dose injected was observed.

Lucke, *Arch. F. exper. Path. U Pharmakol.*, 170:166, 1933. (abstracted in Phys. Abata., 19:56)

A hormone produced in the anterior pituitary is specifically concerned with carbohydrate metabolism, acts as an antagonist to insulin, and is therefore so designated.

[5] Anselmino, K. J., Herold, J. and Hoffman, F., *Klin. Wschnschr.*, 12:1435-1436, 1933.

The authors interpret their findings as evidence that the anterior lobe extract has increased the functional activity of the insular tissue.

The authors conclude that the anterior pituitary factor acts by way of the pancreas where it caused an increase in insulin output.

Geiger, E., *Arch. F. exper. Path. U Pharmakol.*, 172:295, 1933.

The autonomic innervation of the pancreatic islets has been demonstrated and the vagus shown to carry fibers that cause insulin discharge.

Houssay, B. A., Biasatti, A. and Rietti, C. T., *Rev. Soc. Argent. de biol.*, 9:489, 1933.

**Edited by Royal Lee**

VITAMIN NEWS

VITAMIN PRODUCTS CO. • MILWAUKEE, WISCONSIN

August 15, 1936 VOL. 4

## VITAMINS, ENDOCRINOLOGY AND OLD AGE

We get old not because of the effects of time alone, but because our endocrine system is arranged to operate a given period of time and "runs down" like an eight-day clock. That is illustrated by the fact that a pigeon dies of senile degeneration in 10 years, while a parrot, physically similar and supplied with the same food, normally reaches five or more times that age.

We are compelled to conclude that the life period is determined by the vagaries of evolution, being a hereditary characteristic that is beyond ordinary influences. We know that certain occupations shorten the life period, and others are conducive to longevity. Life insurance statistics show that deep-sea fishermen live the longest, watch-makers ranking next. About the only thing in common between these two fields of activity is that in each the worker has little occupational cause for worry. It offers supporting evidence to the old axiom that "worry kills more people than work."

The physician, according to the statistics, has a relatively low position in the longevity scale. By reason of his ability to prolong the lives of others, we should expect a different rating. Personally, I am of the opinion that the reason the phsyician is short-lived is because he, being familiar with the use of drugs and other means of stimulating the hormone output of his endocrine apparatus in an emergency, prematurely consumes his vital reserves. Ultimately, no doubt, the time will arrive when there will be a general knowledge of vitamin therapy, so that the course will be followed of replenishing the nutrition of the endocrines in emergencies instead of prodding them into reluctant activity with stimulants.

It is also highly probable that with our rapidly expanding knowledge of endocrinology, we shall soon be able to replace with some success the vital hormones that now become deficient, and maintain functions that cease otherwise, thereby permitting the gradual development of the characteristics of old age. Vitamin therapy is limited to preventing the premature senility that is a result of endocrine starvation, but it cannot prolong life beyond the normal physiological limits. Even intelligent vitamin therapy, however, can quite possibly increase the average life span 20 per cent or more.

Endocrine recession begins at the age of 25 to 30. This is demonstrated by the fact that a prize fighter is at his physical peak within these time limits. The physical changes for about 20 years are usually quite insignificant, however. But this may be because we do not look deep enough. There is a gradual increase in calcium content of the connective tissue, the increase in blood vessel walls, according to Hesse (1929), being as follows:

2 years — .16 per cent,
34 years — .38 per cent,
56 years — 1.97 per cent.

It is a peculiar fact that as age advances, the arteries become less elastic, and the veins more so.[1] This nullifies the normal function of arteriole "stop cock" control of blood to the capillary beds of the muscular and other tissues that brings in immediate reserves of nutrition in emergencies, at the call of the nervous controls.

Hugo Schulz[2] in 1902 called attention to the fact that the elasticity of connective and elastic tissues was proportional to the silicic acid content, and that the silicic acid content was greatest in the young subject, and gradually dropped as age advanced, following an opposite course to the calcium content.

Other investigations have shown that treating excised animal tissue with soluble silicates measurably increases the elastic response (reduces the "hysteresis" loss).[3]

Also, success is reported in treating arteriosclerosis with internal dosage of sodium silicate,[4-a] and in treating skin diseases of senility[4-b], again silicic acid content of tissue fluids has been found to prevent excessive alkalinity (a condition necessary to cancer development).[4-c]

No doubt some as yet unsuspected hormone, or group of hormones, controls the silica metabolism just as the metabolism of calcium is regulated. It would be reasonable to suspect thyroid, and the anterior pituitary hormones, particularly the growth principle, as we shall see later.

## REFERENCES

[1] Clark, Janet, Elasticity of Veins, *American Journal of Physiology*, 105:426, 1934.

[2] Schulz, Hugo, Further Communications on Silicic Acid, Much. *Med. Wochenschr.*, 49:440-444, 1902; Schulz, Hugo, Silicic Acid in Animal and Human Organs, *Pflugers Archives*, 84:67-100, 1901.

[3] Kochmann, M. and Maier, L., *Biochme. Zeitschr.*, 223:243-248, 1930.

> "Elasticity — measured in terms of changes in tension and relaxation and tested in similar pieces of skin from white mice — is increased by the presence of silicic acid ...
>
> "Similar sized pieces of skin from white mice, immersed for various periods in silicic acid, show a greater elasticity than skin preparations from control animals.
>
> "In both cases, the momentary shift in elasticity and the elastic after-effects are smaller; momentary elasticity is shorter and elastic after-effect shortening is greater."

[4-a] Guede, Therapeutic Value of Silicate of Sodium: Its Anti-sclerotic Action, *J. Med. Paris*, 54:151, February 15, 1934.

> "Scleroses of certain areas, especially arterial sclerosis, and above all, those of the coronary arteries, with one of the clinical manifestations — angina pectoris, are very responsive to silicious therapy. There seems to be a selective action ... which the facts show sufficiently

clearly. Arterial hypertension, fortunately, is improved ... Experimental data led to trying silicious therapy in certain asthma cases, in tubercular diabetes (a case of Kuhn showed disappearance of its acidosis), and in pregnancy (to aid in the development of the fetus). In conclusion, all conditions calling for an active re-mineralization (fractures, bone affections) generally show the necessity of silicious therapy.

"Results are very encouraging; in atheroma, in the beginning, functional troubles are ameliorated; vertigos, the "algias," and circulatory, cephalic and precordial conditions disappear, while simultaneously a return of vitality is felt. There is a greater elasticity of the arteries and especially diureses in amelioration of the circulatory conditions. Functional disorders are improved in arterial hypertension. Marked sedative effects are demonstrated in angina crises. The effect in reducing arterial tension, although recorded by numerous authorities, is not as definite as the action in improving the subjective symptoms. But what is the purpose of systematically lowering a high arterial tension? Except for certain cases, it seems a truly defensive action, an adaptation to a state for which its rise is no longer responsible. It must be tried, all the more to reduce it, without disturbing the equilibrium between cardiac forces and peripheral resistance. In short, the aim here is to lower and still to maintain it at the useful minimum, which is often below normal.

"Conclusion: Experimentally silica was found to possess indisputable anti-atheroma properties. Its metabolism undergoes profound modifications in old age and in the course of certain diseases. The facts warrant its use therapeutically without fear of harm, and it ameliorates many afflictions very interestingly. It may be given a trial, too, in a certain number of ailments whose etiologies are still obscure, or whose treatment by other means is difficult."

[4-b] Luithlen, F., *Wien. Med. Woch.*, 1923. Kuhn, A., *Munch. Med. Woch.*, 1921.

[4-c] Murata, M., Matsumoto, T., Variations in Hydrogen Ion Concentration in Organs under Sodium Silicate Administration, *Tr. Soc. Path. Jap.*, 23:266, 1933.

# NOTES

VITAMIN NEWS

VITAMIN PRODUCTS CO. • MILWAUKEE, WISCONSIN

September 15, 1936 VOL. 4

## VITAMINS, ENDOCRINOLOGY AND OLD AGE — Continued

The degenerations and changes of advancing years should be classified, if possible, into primary and secondary phenomena. They are probably all secondary to endocrine changes. The endocrine changes are in all probability (in the light of our present incomplete conceptions) mainly secondary to changes in the gonads and pituitary.

> We know that wrinkles, obesity, edema and a grossness of the features follow thyroid hypoactivity.[5]
>
> Pancreatic changes and an oversecretion of trypsin bring about (among innumerable other things) cirrhosis of the liver, vascular damage (visible as facial telangiectases), hemorrhoids, and we suspect, arteriosclerosis.[6]
>
> Gray hair, baldness and obesity result mainly from a defection of pituitary hormones.
>
> Various symptoms of nerve degeneration and atrophy occur (so that some medical writers have considered nerve degeneration the basic cause of senility).

It is probable that each endocrine has its antagonist, or rather its synergist, that must be present to maintain a balance. The thyroid is a calcium eliminator, but without the thymus and parathyroid, too much thyroid will result in serious trouble, for there will be no calcium assimilation.

In senility, all the endocrines regress and the ideal case is the one that meanwhile maintains a physiologic balance. To know how to prevent the regression will require further investigations along lines that are being intensely studied today as to the various hormonic relations of gonad and pituitary. For instance, it was recently shown that the growth hormone of the anterior pituitary prevented the normal senile tissue degeneration in rats.[7]

To attempt the use of gland extracts to ward off senility is not as simple as the explanation. Dr. Lorand in his once-popular book — *Old Age Deferred* — extolled thyroid as a preserver of youth. But any physician knows the unsatisfactory, to say the least, consequences of ill-advised thyroid medication. It is apparent that the thyroid in most cases had "compensatively" regressed. If it had not reduced its activity, it would have caused toxic effects, which are often observed along with the above signs of hypothyroidea. (Without the synergists of the thyroid, it is possible to have simultaneous symptoms of both hypo- and hyperthyroidea. These synergists include pituitary, parathyroid, thymus, gonad, spleen and liver (bile acids), at least. Probably they include all calcium metabolizers, and all protein metabolizers.) Evidently, an endocrine balance has been lost in these cases. It is obvious that some synergists of the thyroid are lacking.

To run down these synergists will not answer the question, as it would, in all probability, be a chase of the will-o-the-wisp that would take us to each of the endocrines in turn.

Pituitary hormones are known to maintain the activity and integrity of thyroid, parathyroid, suprarenals, gonads, pancreas, etc., for instance. It is probable that the pituitary controls the endocrines in a double manner, through the nervous system as described by Sajous — the normal and facile method — but elaborates specific hormones, that stimulate the development of the parenchyma of each endocrine as well to insure the presence of the hormone to be released by nerve impulses. In our Vitamin News issue of July 1936, we showed that insulin-secreting cells owed their regenerating properties to a hormonic stimulus from the posterior pituitary, and also that sympathetic nerve fibers are present to enable the pituitary — the "test organ" of Sajous — to originate a nerve impulse to the Islets of Langerhans when the insulin content of the blood drops below normal. Sajous established the presence of continuous nerve fibers from the pituitary to the adrenals. Also, we have the pituitary adrenotropic hormone and its nervous control. The same situation is known to be true of parathyroid and thyroid. Sajous, from his anatomic and physiologic studies, doubted the existence of pituitary hormones because of the obvious fact that the pituitary is a part of the brain mechanism, and histologically composed mainly of nerve cells. He was, no doubt, correct in assuming that the major and basic function of the pituitary is to act as a nervous control of the other endocrines, but it also has an "executive department" which has a function of sending "endocrinotropic" principles through the blood stream to the various endocrines to see that a stock of the necessary hormones are being made and are ready for telegraphic orders. We attempted to show in the July 1936 *Vitamin News* that diabetes mellitus could occur both from a breakdown of the telegraph (vitamin B deficiency) as well as from other causes and that the pituitary supplied both a stimulating and an inhibitory hormone to the pancreas, one of which caused regeneration; the other an atrophy of the Islets.

The need of both a stimulating and an inhibiting factor is apparent when we accept the theory of separate nervous control and hormone maintenance of supply apparatus. A sensitive governing device must have just as efficient a braking means as power-applying means, if designed for the control of a mechanism that is self maintaining — a mechanism that once started may not stop when the initiating influence ceases to act.

To summarize, then, we may say that, in the light of present knowledge, senile degenerations occur because of endocrine failure (physiological regression). This loss of function can be, and usually is, hastened considerably by reason of vitamin deficiency and the key or master endocrine is the pituitary, because it issues hormones that regulate the growth and activity of the other endocrines, lacking which stimulus endocrine activity ceases. And it is probably true that the particular pituitary hormone that specifically prevents tissue degeneration is the growth hormone, possibly acting through the media of its effect upon the thyroid or gonads.

The importance of growth principle is evident when we realize that senility is a condition where destructive influences are uncombated by vigorous cell proliferation. Brailsford-Robertson in 1923[8] pointed out that any culture of cell life, whether protozan or metazoan, was characterized by two facts:

1. A substance accumulates in the nutritive media that progressively reduces cell proliferation.

2. Replacement of the old nutritive media with fresh brings about a renewed cycle of mitotic activity.

He has in detail described to us the mechanism that causes senescence — whether protozan or metazoan — the accumulation in the cell nucleus of the "autocatalyst." Endocrinology offers the promise of showing us the mechanism that opposes the effects of the accumulation of the "autocatalyst" — in all probability through the medium of a hormone that will ultimately be commercially available.

## REFERENCES

[5] French, *Differential Diagnosis,* Fifth Edition, Wm. Wood and Co., page 499, 1936.

[6] Ibid, page 46; page 65; Sajous, *The Internal Secretions and the Principles of Medicine*, Tenth Edition, page 43, 1923.

[7] Evans, H.M. *Journal of the American Medical Association*, 104;1232, 1935.

"... The study of Lee and Schaffer showed that treated animals do not possess the characteristic age changes that normal rats exhibit (decreases in the proportion of water, nitrogen, fat-free dry tissue and ash, and increases in the percentage of fat), but retained with considerable exactitude their initial composition in certain chemical constituents. This propulsion of growth in the rat's adult life is therefore associated with the retention of certain juvenile chemical characteristics in the tissue produced, and the question naturally arises as to whether the 'youthfulness' of this tissue indicates 'youthfulness' of the animal with regard to expectance of a correspondingly longer life span ... "

Abstracted in *Endocrinology*, 19:618, 1935.

[8] Brailsford-Robertson, *The Chemical Basis of Growth and Senescence*, Lippincott, 1923.

**Edited by Royal Lee**

# NOTES

# VITAMIN NEWS

VITAMIN PRODUCTS CO. • MILWAUKEE, WISCONSIN

October 15, 1936 VOL. 4

## A REVIEW OF ESSENTIAL FACTS IN CALCIUM METABOLISM

We have previously pointed out in these pages the fact that in all probability, every vitamin had an influence on the metabolism of calcium.

To recapitulate, vitamin A deficiency is known to cause a precipitation of calcium as kidney stones, indicating that it is instrumental in maintaining calcium in solution or in organic combination[1].

Vitamin B deficiency is known to cause pathology only when accompanied by a calcium deficiency[2]. The cramps and convulsions of beriberi are, no doubt, a result of the lowered blood calcium. Howe, in his studies on dental caries in 1921, found that vitamin B deficiency caused atrophy of the parathyroids. A high-protein diet can bring on convulsions if the vitamin B intake is low,[3] an indication that the presence of vitamin B is necessary to the maintenance of the normal blood calcium level. The vitamin B requirement is also known to be higher when the thyroid is overactive,[4] in the absence which thyrotoxic symptoms appear sooner (Note that the thyroid is the physiologic calcium eliminator).[5]

Vitamin C deficiency is characteristically known to result in a decalcification of bone, loosened teeth being a primary indication of scurvy.[6]

Vitamin D, of course, is known by all to result in a lowered affinity of blood serum for calcium with attendant reduced assimilation.

Vitamin E is the only vitamin that has not been shown to have a direct connection with calcium metabolism up to the present time.

Vitamin F can be considered an important factor in calcium assimilation because it reduces blood calcium by increasing its diffusion into the tissues, and cooperates with vitamin D by unloading the blood of its calcium load, probably mainly into muscle cells which are probably the greatest consumers of this element in the adult body (In the immature economy, vitamin C is important in its effect of facilitating the deposition of blood calcium in bone). Vitamin F may also be important in aiding the formation of bone, for it definitely hastens the formation of the hypertrophic processes in arthritis, if given alone, while vitamin C has the opposite effect. It quickly reduces excess blood calcium and is an antidote for hypervitaminosis D, as in sunstroke.

Vitamin G is another factor in maintaining the solubility of calcium for in its absence, vitamin D has little or no effect. In hypovitaminosis G in test animals, cataracts of they eyes quickly form from precipitated calcium. An important clinical use of vitamin G is in the treatment of arthritis, its merit here, no doubt, being its cooperative effect with vitamin D, and the use of massive doses of vitamin D, being, in our opinion, necessary only because of the lack of knowledge that the synergist vitamin G is deficient.

One important fact to be kept in mind is that the blood calcium may be high and still the patient may be deficient in that element. The tissues may be starved even though the transportation system be loaded excessively if those vitamins be lacking that are necessary to cause the diffusion through the vascular walls. A not infrequent cause of kidney disease in children is the hypercalcemia due to overdosage of vitamin D preparations, and the resultant albuminuria can only be successfully controlled with a regular dosage of vitamin A. We have a number of such case histories in our files. In one, a boy of nine who had been heavily dosed with vitamin D concentrate all winter, developed a nephritis in the spring, and was diagnosed as hypervitaminosis D by the attending physician. The parents were warned to keep the youngster out of the sun, which advice was disregarded, and a few hours on the beach in bathing suit proved fatal through an attack of acute nephritis with toxicosis from sunburn. (See Reference [7] for further details on toxicity of vitamin D.)

The toxicity of vitamin D is a result of the high level of blood calcium, and in pregnancy and lactation when the calcium requirement is greater, a correspondingly larger dosage of vitamin D can be tolerated.[8] The greatly increased requirement of all the vitamins in pregnancy and lactation is, no doubt, due mainly to the enhanced calcium metabolism. As we have often emphasized, one of the most spectacular results of vitamin administration is the treatment of the ills of pregnancy.

Authorities agree that we are all in danger of receiving too little calcium in our food. Milk is often pointed out as a carrier of calcium that can compensate for its absence in other foods, such as bread. The pasteurization of milk, however reduces its assimilable calcium to the point that it fails to contain enough for the growing child.[9]

Add to this a vitamin deficiency that reduces the efficiency of assimilation and we have ample reason for the evidences of calcium starvation to be seen on every hand, beginning with maldevelopment of the bones and teeth in the infant, low resistance and susceptibility to dental caries, colds, children's diseases, etc. in the child ending with a million consequences of these continuing factors, endocrine imbalance, etc. in the adult.

Northen has demonstrated that this calcium deficiency even extends to the soil on which vegetable crops are grown.[10] He even claims that insect parasites refuse to touch plants (tomato and cucumber) that are grown on soil containing all necessary mineral elements — even though intertwined with vines fed from deficient soil that were alive with bugs, showing that this matter of "resistance" includes insect as well as bacterial parasites. This recalls the comment made to me in all seriousness by a veterinarian that he noticed that fleas would often leave a dog that was receiving his vitamins (as "Catalyn").

## REFERENCES

[1] Osborne and Mendel, *J.A.M.A.*, lxix, 32, (1917); Also McCarrison, *Brit. Med. J.*, 717 (1927); and Fujimaki, *Japan Med. World*, vi, 29 (1926) through Chemical Abstracts, xxiv, 5802.

Bergulund, Medes, Huber, Longcope, and Richards, pages 147-149, *The Kidney in Health and Disease* (1935).

"One of the most important and striking recent advances in the pathology of nutrition is the demonstration of urolithiasis through vitamin A deficiency. Osborne and Mendel discovered urinary or renal calculi in about ten per cent of their rats on diets deficient in vitamin A, while no calculi were found in the controls on normal diet. This result has been abundantly confirmed by Fujimaki and McCarrison, especially in rats on diets deficient in other factors in addition to vitamin A. In some cases, the vesical calculi (visible by the roentgen-rays) disappeared when the animals were placed on normal diet. Similar results were obtained by Van Leersum, Perlman and Weber and Tyson and Smith, working on vitamin A-free diets.

"The work of Van Leersum is of especial interest and importance, because he could find no cystitis, but traced the pathogenesis of the calculi to the kidney. In 88 per cent of his test animals, sections showed numerous small calcareo-fatty granular concretions or casts in the renal tubules and ducts. (These somewhat resemble the above-mentioned changes resulting from fat deficiency.) He concluded that degeneration of the renal epithelium caused the calcareous deposits, and that these were carried to the bladder, where they grew to form the larger concretions. Recently, Tyson and Smith have likewise noted that renal calculi frequently appear in rats on low vitamin A diets. When obstruction to urinary outflow is present, pyonephrosis develops. They conclude that there is no metaplasia of the renal pelvic epithelium without infection, which is present from the beginning in all cases. Furthermore, this abnormal epithelium, with acute or chronic renal infection, may persist following an apparent cure by the addition of vitamin A (in cod liver oil) to the diet."

[2] Tohoku, *Jol. Exper. Med.*, 184, January, 1935.

[3] Mathews, *Physiological Chemistry*, 4th Edition, page 855, William Wood and Co., 1923.

[4] Cowgill and Palmeieri, *American Journal of Physiology*, page 146, July 1933.

[5] Eggs, F., *Deutsche Ztschr. F. Chir.*, 242:321, 1934; Chem. Abstracts, 29:2585.

[6] Szent - Gyorgy (quoted from *Modern Living,* page 236, November, 1934) states:

"Under normal conditions, you see, there is very little scurvy among human beings. But I began to change my mind when it was shown that the absence of vitamin C produced the destruction of teeth before the symptoms of scurvy set in."

[7] Harris, *British Medical Journal*, 2:367-73, August 26, 1933.

[8] Kozelka, Hart and Bohstedt, *Jol. Biol. Chem.*, 61:225 (1924).

[9] Daniels and Stearns, *Jol. Biol. Chem.*, 61:225 (1924).
Sherman and Smith, *The Vitamins,* Second Edition, page 152 (1931).

[10] Beach, Rex, Modern Miracle Men, *Cosmopolitan,* page 60-61, 175-178, June 1936.

VITAMIN NEWS

VITAMIN PRODUCTS CO. • MILWAUKEE, WISCONSIN

November 15, 1936 VOL. 4

## A REVIEW OF ESSENTIAL FACTS IN CALCIUM METABOLISM (Continued)

We begin to see why wheat deserves its place as the "king of cereals" among those used as human food. It refuses to grow on soil that is deficient in calcium and phosphorus, whereas rye, for example, will grow on the most impoverished land and will contain far less of the essential minerals. Unless we make use of the wheat in its entirety as food, we lose this great benefit, of course. The reason that the minerals and vitamins are in the outer layer of the wheat berry is because they are water-soluble, and as the kernel ripened, by the evaporation of sap, these elements were of necessity left in that location. That explains the location of the germ, or embryo, in the outer layer as well.

The blood serum contains calcium ions, phosphate ions and potassium ions in a delicate physiological balance, maintained by hormonic influences, if not by both vitamin and hormonic influences together. The outstanding influence is the effect of the parathyroid, which is nearly parallel in effect to vitamin D (it being proven that the vitamin D can be substituted successfully for the hormone in maintaining serum calcium).[11]

It is probable that a physiological saturation of both serum calcium and phosphate ions exist, and any increase of either must result in excretion of the other (or its deposition in the bone reserves).[12] This explains the value of phosphate in the treatment of rickets; it promotes deposition of calcium in the bone, and explains the finding that most rickets is rather due to phosphate shortage than a low calcium intake. In fact, the probability is that if a proper balance of mineral salts is present in the food intake, a low mineral diet only causes a delayed growth[13].

Muscular cramps, convulsions (tetany) are a consequence of an excessively lowered calcium-phosphate balance, and are aggravated by alkalosis.[14] The administration of acids or phosphate (as "V-P Phosphade") permits the mobilization of calcium necessary to relief.

The balance existing between the calcium and potassium ions is in all probability important in the maintenance of a balance between the sympathetic and parasympathetic nervous systems, potassium promoting activity or sensitiveness of the latter, calcium the former.[15]

Potassium is utilized in the body mainly in organic combination as contrasted with sodium which is usually in the inorganic form. Excessive intake of sodium chloride causes elimination of calcium and potassium, the more important minerals from a cell activity standpoint.[16] Sodium chloride seems to have the function of maintaining the osmotic balances, and the level is controlled mainly by the cortical hormone of the adrenals, a shortage of this hormone resulting in a concentration of the blood to a point of extreme viscosity (Addison's Disease), relieved either by the administration of sodium chloride or the cortical hormone.

Potassium found in organic (protein) combination in raw green leaf vegetables, is rendered inorganic by cooking, (as is the calcium of raw milk), and is available in concentrated form as "V-P" Organic Mineral tablets.

This matter of maintaining the proper balance between the sympathetic and parasympathetic systems is of major importance, for it has been shown that they oppose one another in the control of many functions (just as two reins are necessary to keep a horse in the middle of the road), and an interference with the operation of either by reason of a deficiency of calcium on one hand and organic potassium on the other can bring about such conditions as, for example, gastric ulcers (because of either low calcium or low organic potassium intake, the former rendering the sympathetics more sensitive and the latter the parasympathetics less sensitive), for which the cutting of the left branch of the vagus has been found a surgical remedy.[17]

Both vitamin F and the "V-P" Organic Mineral tablets have been independently used successfully for the relief of this type of gastrointestinal trouble. The vitamin F is, no doubt, of benefit because it increases the calcium diffusion to the nerve cell, thereby reducing the sympathetic hyperactivity, and the "V-P" Mineral revives the parasympathetic function. The benefits here, as usual, preceded the explanation.

The known benefits of vitamins C and F in angina pectoris can be explained on similar grounds in view of the recent findings that most cases of that malady are really cases of esophagus cramp,[18] probably due to calcium deficiency in hypersensitizing the vagus.

The surgical remedy in this disease is the removal of the thyroid, here explainable on the ground that thyroid is a powerful calcium eliminator, and its influence is bad where the intake is already deficient.

## REFERENCES

[11] Kozelka, Hart and Bohstedt, Growth, Reproduction and Lactation in Absence of Parathyroid Gland, *J. Biol. Chem.*, 100:715-729, May 1933.

[12] Peters and Van Slyke, *Quantitative Clinical Chemistry*, Volume 1, Interpretations, page 812, Williams and Wilkins Co., Baltimore, 1935.

"If it is assumed that bone is in chemical contact with serum and tissue fluids, not only the formation of bone, but its very existence would be impossible if these fluids were not saturated with the salts of which bone is composed, because a solid remains undissolved in the presence of a liquid in which it is soluble only when the latter has become saturated with the solid. Although it will become evident in the subsequent discussion that all the known facts at present can not be brought into agreement with such a theory, the general conception that serum and other fluids which contain calcium and phosphorus are normally in a state of effective or biological saturation with $Ca_3(PO_4)_2$, affords the best explanation of the reactions of these ions."

[13] Toepfer and Sherman, The Effect of Liberal Intakes of Calcium or Calcium and Phosphorus on Growth and Body Calcium, *Jol. Biol. Chem.*, 115, 3:685, October, 1936).

[14] Peters and Van Slyke, *Quantitative Clinical Chemistry*, Volume 1, Interpretations, page 828, Williams and Wilkins Co., Baltimore, 1935.

[15] Cantarow, *Calcium Metabolism and Calcium Therapy*, Second Edition, page 78, Lea and Febiger, 1933.

"... It appears probable that calcium ions are concerned with sympathetic activity and potassium ions with parasympathetic activity ... "

[16] Mathews, *Principles of Biochemistry*, page 323, Williams and Wilkins Co., 1936.

"... And in general, protoplasm of all cells of the body contain more potassium than sodium ... "

"From this, we may conclude that potassium is generally in union with the organic substances, the proteins and phospholipides, etc., while sodium is usually in inorganic union ... "

[17] Cushing, H., *Pituitary Body, Hypothalmus and Parasympathetic Nervous System*, page 211-212, Charles C. Thomas, Baltimore, 1932.

"... On these general principles is based the surgical division of the left branch of the vagus as it passes to the stomach wall — a procedure advocated for ulcer patients showing high preoperative free acidity with hypermotility, and routinely practiced by some surgeons both in this country and abroad with results said to be, at least temporarily, excellent."

Klein, E., Left Vagus Section and Partial Gastrectomy for Duodenal Ulcer with Hyperacidity, *Ann. Surg.*, xc, 65-68, 1929.

[18] Jackson and Jackson, *J. Lab. and Clin. Med.*, September, 1936.

Abstracted in *News Week,* page 23, September 5, 1936.

"Air — trapped in esophagus or stomach by acute spasmodic, incoordinate contractions of these organs — may become highly compressed. Then it exerts distending forces responsible for the ailment's characteristic pain.

..............................................................

"At the esophageal orifice of the stomach, the irritating currents (electrical) caused dog hearts to beat with a wild, uncontrolled rhythm. 'Stimulation within ... the esophagus at most points above the level of the opening of the heart (produced) vigorous muscular movements in some areas of the chest, or in the forelimbs, neck, abdomen, or other parts of the body.'"

**Edited by Royal Lee**

# NOTES

VITAMIN NEWS

VITAMIN PRODUCTS CO. • MILWAUKEE, WISCONSIN

December 15, 1936 VOL. 4

# INSTRUMENTAL EVIDENCES OF RESULTS WITH VITAMIN THERAPY

The object of this publication has been to arouse the interest of the physician in the use of vitamin concentrates for therapeutic purposes and to offer, where possible, sound theoretical reasons for the results obtainable from such use.

The medical profession has been historically apathetic to new departures in treatment, no doubt, because of the host of "false alarms" that are constantly springing up under high commercial pressure, and which have developed the doctor's sales resistance to the highest degree.

Nevertheless, most physicians strive to follow the policy of not being "the last to drop the old, nor the first to adopt the new." It requires much accumulated experience to establish the merits of new methods and materials, as far as procedure in the treatment of disease is concerned.

Today, there is much activity in the field of the development of instrumental means for determining the clinical need of and response to vitamin treatment. One of the devices useful for this purpose is the new electric sphygmograph*. This machine will visually and unmistakably demonstrate the marked improvement that follows the administration of any remedy that improves the heart action or affects the blood pressure.

The effect of vitamin concentrates in normalizing the heart action and blood pressure is evident from a study of the two sets of sphygmograms illustrated on the next page.

One effect of the deficiency of vitamin B alone is a vascular dilation that slows the heart. But, indirectly, vitamin B deficiency, coupled with vitamin A and vitamin C deficiency, may be a factor (along with iodine deficiency) in causing hyperthyroidea with its accompanying racing heart. Therefore, we usually find in the heart patient a composite picture of these factors, which obviously means not only a greater load (by reason of vascular atony), but more speed as well, because of the thyroid involvement, so we put a strain on the heart comparable to the effect on an automobile engine when we open the throttle wide on a hill so steep as to prevent acceleration of speed. That is why we see such spectacular improvement when we supply vitamin concentrates to the heart patient. We reduce the load (contract to normal the dilated vessels), and slow the speed (by normalizing the thyroid).

From our limited experience with the use of this new instrument, we believe it to be possible to demonstrate some improvement in almost any kind of a heart case with vitamin concentrates. Naturally, anyone familiar with what autopsies show in heart patients knows that there are plenty of incurable forms of degeneration. But why penalize the remaining functional tissue by not giving vitamins?

We attribute the change in the first case to a functional improvement in the nervous control of the heart action mainly by reason of the vitamin B content. (Tests have shown that this is the only single concentrate to cause a marked improvement in 15 to 30 minutes.) This parallels animal tests, where a paralytic avitaminotic pigeon is restored in 20 minutes by an injection of vitamin B.

It will be noted that there was no increase in the pulse rate, but a more steady and regular action. Were this a case of uncomplicated vitamin B deficiency, the initial pulse rate would be below normal, and would be brought up to normal by vitamin B administration. But a clear case of single vitamin deficiency is seldom seen. The rapid improvement shown by the administration of vitamin B, however, is indicative that the result obtained is through the medium of bettering the nervous functions, which is the specific action of the vitamin B.

In the second case, sphygmograms taken at intervals have shown a progressive improvement in the case of the 74-year-old patient. (Our available space permits only the two to be shown.)

These are typical cases; it is not necessary to select special patients to show the favorable results of vitamin treatment. On the other hand, it is the great exception to find a heart case that does not show very definite changes for the better.

It is not our intention to convey the idea that vitamin concentrates are a substitute for other therapeutic measures which the physician has found useful, but the use of such concentrates is a supplementary treatment that will correct a causative factor that has heretofore been unsuspected.

*Made by Cameron Heartometer Co., 666 West Division St., Chicago, Illinois, U.S.A.

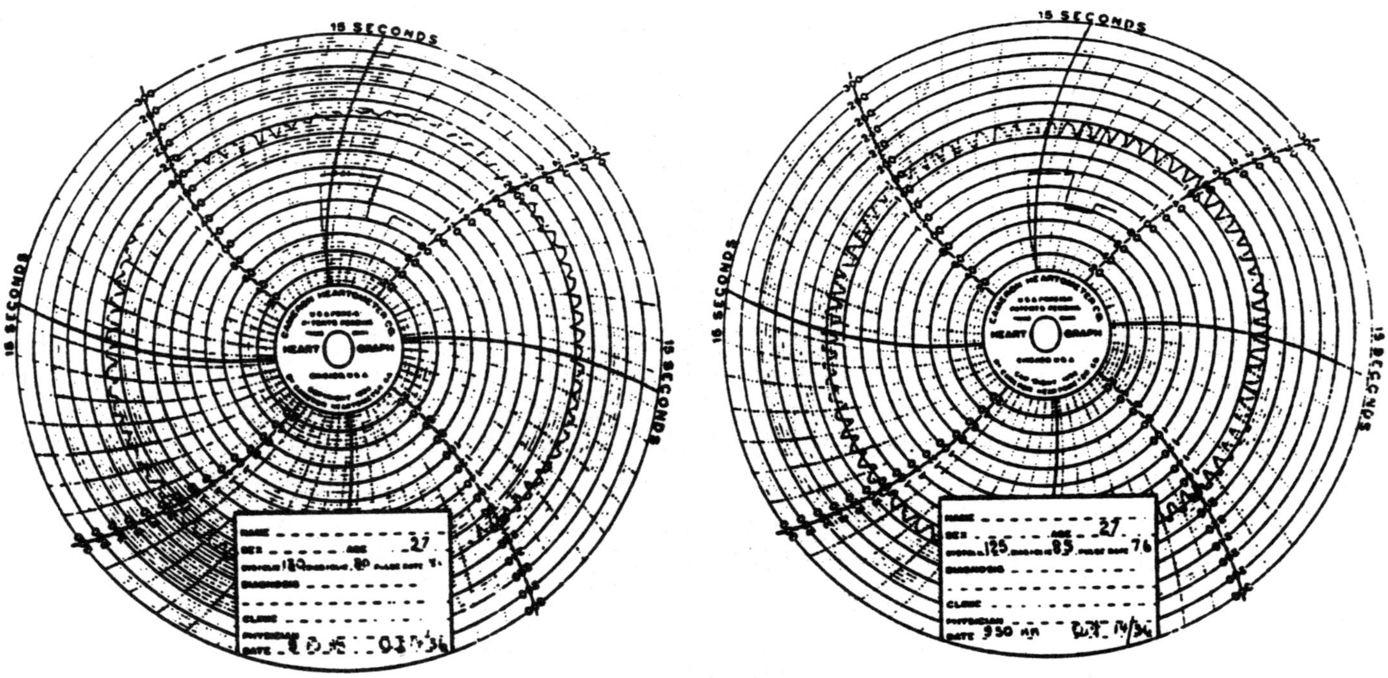


Case 1. The improvement in regularity and power of pulse after the administration of two vitamin B tablets. Sphygmograms taken ten minutes apart, vitamin B tablets given at time of the first test.

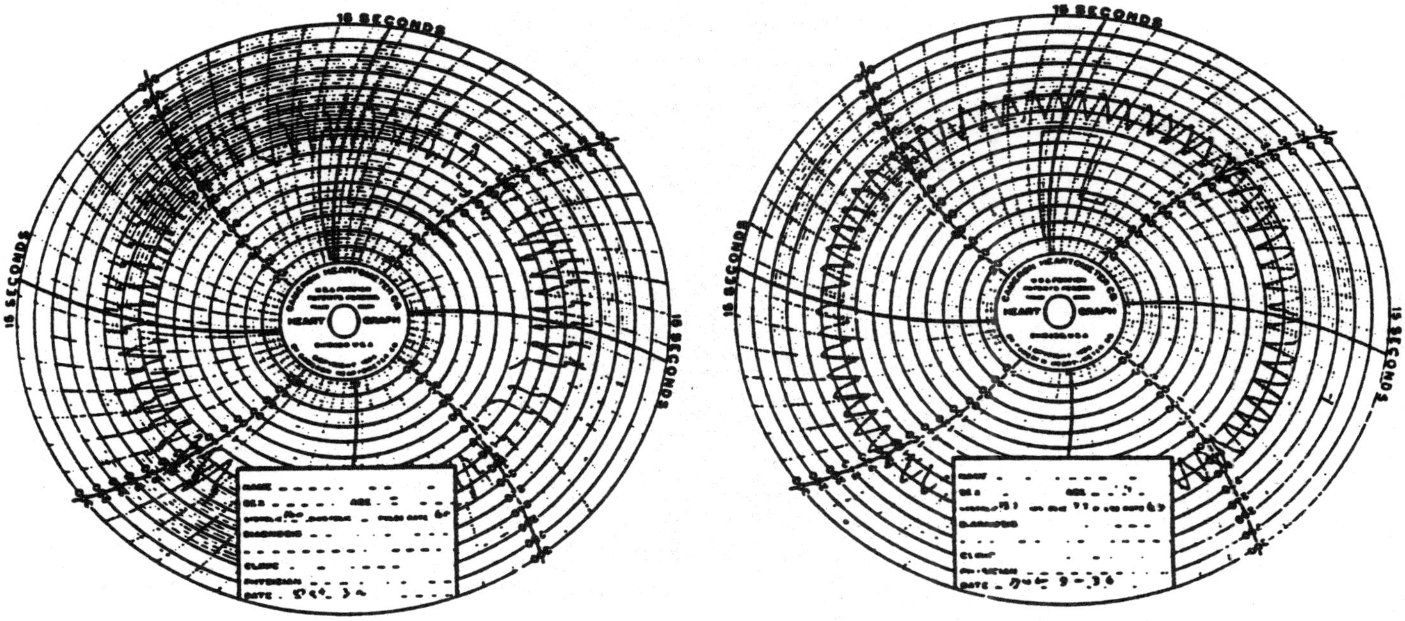

Case 2. Improvement in what is apparently an arteriosclerotic patient (age 74). Tests made 37 days apart. "Catalyn" administered meanwhile, four tablets daily. First sphygmogram shows the extremely low elasticity of vessels as indicated by sudden rise and fall of pressure.

**Edited by Royal Lee**

# NOTES

# VITAMIN NEWS

VITAMIN PRODUCTS CO. • MILWAUKEE, WISCONSIN

January 15, 1937 VOL. 5


## "V-P" ORGANIC MINERAL TABLETS

"V-P" Organic Mineral tablets supply the basic alkali minerals (mainly organic potassium) as distinguised from the acid mineral phosphorus. The phosphoric radical is supplied normally in the diet by the compound phytin in bran. This is broken down in the blood stream or in digestion by an enzyme into inosite and phosphoric acid. This phosphoric acid is at once neutralized by combination with alkalies, and is responsible for the normal elimination of calcium carbonate from the tissues that tends otherwise to collect and cause various symptoms of disease. Our "V-P Phosphade"** is an efficient supplementary source of the phosphoric radical.

The alkali minerals — sodium, potassium, magnesium and calcium — also if deficient, cause many of the symptoms of vitamin deficiency. This is because, in general, the function of vitamins is to promote mineral metabolism. A deficiency of necessary minerals may result in the same evidence of mineral starvation as is found in certain forms of vitamin deficiency.

"V-P" Organic Mineral tablets should be used to supplement "Catalyn"* wherever there is a delay in obtaining expected results. One tablet a day is sufficient, with a somewhat reduced dosage of "Catalyn."

A specific action of "V-P" Mineral tablets is to improve the function of the parasympathetic nervous system. The bowel elimination may be improved through this effect in that the reflex reaction to colonic pressure may be greatly enhanced, and it appears that we have here a very effective remedy for "lazy colon." In fact, an overdosage of these tablets can bring about a temporary condition of oversensitiveness of the entire parasympathetic system. A few doses of "V-P Phosphade" have been of immediate effect in correcting this oversensitiveness.

Potassium is known to be necessary to the maintenance of function of the parasympathetic nervous system, and calcium to be necessary to function of the sympathetics.[1]

Potassium must be in organic combination to be useful in the body.[2]

The sympathetic and parasympathetic systems oppose one another and maintain a functional balance in human physiology.[3]

Overactivity of the vagus (a parasympathetic) nerve can be a factor in the causation of gastric ulcer with hyperacidity.[4]

Vitamin F and "V-P" Organic Mineral tablets act to mobilize both calcium and potassium in the tissue fluids and restore a normal balance of power between the sympathetics and parasympathetics. This probably explains the benefit of this treatment for both gastrointestinal disorders that lead to ulcers, and the obvious benefits in most angina pectoris cases, for the latter has been identified as a condition of irritability of areas supplied by the vagus, and quite recently, substantial evidence has been offered to show that the pain attacks in angina pectoris are really cramps of the esophagus.

For either of these conditions, one Organic Mineral Tablet and one vitamin F tablet is recommended with the noon and evening meal (two of each per day) (preferably with two "Catalyn" tablets daily).

Since a lowered calcium supply to the nerve cell (as is a consequence of vitamin D and F deficiency) causes a hypersenstiveness of the motor nerves, and a reduced organic potassium supply paralyzes the parasympathetic nerves, it is clear how the normal balance between the opposing effect of these systems is overthrown in the same direction by a reduced supply of either organic potassium, or vitamin F.

"V-P" Organic Minerals are a concentrate of the organic mineral compounds in green leaf vegetable juice. The concentration is made without heat, and by the removal of undesirable materials, the possible dosage is increased to a point where definite and immediate results are obtainable. To take enough watercress, spinach or alfalfa tea to get the same amount of mineral salts may result in toxic effects from other compounds present that could more than offset the benefits from the minerals.

## ANALYSIS of "V-P" ORGANIC MINERAL TABLETS

| | | | |
|---|---|---|---|
| Aluminum (as $Al_2O_3$) | 0.36 | Iodide (as I) | none |
| Iron (as $Fe_2O_3$) | trace | Sulfate (as $SO_3$) | 3.52 |
| Manganese (as $Mn_3O_4$) | 2.91 | Silicate (as $SiO_2$) | 0.05 |
| Calcium (as CaO) | 4.76 | Phosphate (as $P_2O_5$) | 0.71 |
| Magnesium (as MgO) | 1.61 | Nitrogen (as N) | 4.50 |
| Potassium (as $K_2O$) | 8.86 | Sugars (as glucose) | none |
| Chloride (as Cl) | 0.33 | Water | 7.60 |
| Bromide (as Br) | none | Unidentified Organic Matter | 60.78 |

[1] Cantarow, Abraham, *Calcium Metabolism and Calcium Therapy,* Second Edition, page 78, Lea & Febiger, 1933.

[2] Mathews, Albert P., *Principles of Biochemistry,* page 323, Williams and Wilkins Co., 1936.

[3] Cantarow, Abraham, *Calcium Metabolism and Calcium Therapy*, Second Edition, page 78, Lea & Febiger, 1933.

[4] Cushing, Harvey, *Pituitary Body, Hypothalmus and Parasympathetic Nervous System*, page 211-212, Charles C. Thomas, Baltimore, 1932.

[5] Klein, E., Left Vagus Section and Partial Gastrectomy for Duodenal Ulcer with Hyperacidity, *Ann. Surg.*, xc, 65-68, 1929.

* "Catalyn" tablets are a combination of concentrates of all the vitamins, intended to supply a "balanced ration" of vitamins for therapeutic purposes as well as for use to supplement the diet.

** "V-P Phosphade"—A phosphoric acid and alkali phosphate combination for correcting the phosphate deficiency resulting from too little of the cereal roughage in the diet.

VITAMIN NEWS

VITAMIN PRODUCTS CO. • MILWAUKEE, WISCONSIN

February 15, 1937 VOL. 5

## VITAMINS AND DENTISTRY

(Continued from Page 17)

As references of interest to the dentist in affording a more up-to-date picture of the relationships of vitamins A, B, C and D to dental disease we offer the following extracts from

[1] *Vitamins: A Survey of Present Knowledge* (British Medical Research Council), 1932.

[2] *The Vitamins and Their Clinical Application*, Stepp, Kuhnaus and Schroeder, Germany, 1936.

[1] Pages 90-91:

"VITAMIN D IN RELATION TO THE TEETH. The investigations carried out by M. Mellanby (1918-30) have included animal experiments and clinical investigations on man. The former have demonstrated the importance of specific dietetic factors in controlling the development of the teeth, and in determining their reactions to harmful stimuli ...

> "Young puppies fed on diets deficient in vitamin D exhibit obvious defects in the development of their teeth and jaws, the most important of which are the following:
>
> 1. Delay in the eruption of the permanent teeth, affecting particularly those teeth which normally erupt at a late period.
> 2. Thickening of the jaw bones and irregularity in the arrangement of the teeth, most noticeable in the lower incisors.
> 3. Irregularly formed and poorly calcified enamel, the surface of which is pitted and grooved and frequently pigmented.
> 4. Defective development and irregular calcification of the dentine, which can be satisfactorily studied only by microscopic examination of ground sections of the teeth.
> 5. Abnormal development of the calcified tissues at the gingival margin and hence irregularity of the periodontal membrane.

Page 93:

"EFFECT OF THE MINERAL SUPPLY ON THE STRUCTURE OF THE TEETH. The absolute or relative amounts of calcium and phosphorus in an experimental diet were found to influence the degree and character of the calcification of the teeth. When there was little or no vitamin D in the diet, extra supplies of calcium in the form of carbonate resulted in a slight but distinct improvement in the structure of the teeth. The effect of adding phosphates under these conditions was variable, but the beneficial effect sometimes observed was only slight. The addition of calcium salts, the carbonate, phosphate, or hydrogen phosphate, to diets containing butter resulted usually in great improvement in the calcification of the teeth. When liberal quantities of vitamin D were given, the addition of calcium salts to a diet otherwise containing very little of this element sometimes resulted in the production of an increased amount of dentine, though the structure was always perfect or nearly perfect even when the diet contained only small amounts of calcium. In the presence of sufficient quantities of vitamin D, the ratio of calcium to phosphorus could also be varied within considerable limits without producing any effect on the development of the teeth. It therefore appears safe to conclude that an adequate supply of vitamin D is of greater importance in determining the perfect development of the teeth than an abundant or carefully balanced supply of calcium and phosphorus (M. Mellanby, 1923, 1299)."

Pages 100-102:

"PERIODONTAL DISEASE. Dogs, especially pet dogs, are, like man, very susceptible to periodontal disease. These animals were therefore chosen by M. Mellanby for an extensive study of the etiology of this disease of the tissues surrounding the teeth. It was found that dogs could be kept under laboratory conditions for periods up to 8 years and so long as the diet was complete from birth onwards, they remained free from periodontal disease. If, however, the diet was deficient in vitamins A and D and rich in cereals, especially during the period of growth in the early months of life, this disease ultimately developed. These dietetic defects acted in two ways, by allowing the abnormal development of periodontal tissues, and by allowing these abnormally formed tissues to change their anatomical relations to the teeth and become subject to invasion by micro-organisms.

"VITAMINS A AND D IN RELATION TO THE STRUCTURE OF PERIODONTAL TISSUES. Experiments on puppies brought up on diets rich and poor respectively in both vitamins A and D, or deficient in either vitamin A or D only, showed that vitamin A primarily controls the normal development of the soft periodontal tissues, including the sub-gingival epithelium and the underlying connective tissues, while, as might be expected, vitamin D is largely responsible for the normal calcification of the alveolar bone and the other hard tissues.

"Thus, if the diet is deficient in both fat-soluble vitamins A and D, as for instance when olive oil replaces cod-liver oil, the following abnormalities develop:

1. Thickening of the gingival region.
2. Imperfect development of the alveolar bone, particularly of the alveolar crest, and of the laminae durae, with the inclusion of osteoid tissue and poorly calcified bone.
3. Imperfection of the epithelial attachment to the hypoplastic enamel.
4. Poor calcification of the laminae durae.
5. Hypertrophy of the sub-gingival epithelium with the development of finger-like processes.
6. Abnormal arrangement of the connective tissue of the corium, with connective tissue reaction and cell infiltration.
7. Irregular thickness of the periodontal membrane.

"Irregular alignment of some of the teeth and tilting of the teeth in relation to the jaw are also sometimes found when the diets are deficient in vitamins A and D.

"VITAMINS A AND D IN RELATION TO PERIODONTAL DISEASE. The term 'periodontal disease,' which is susceptible of various meanings, is here used in its widest sense, that is to say, to denote any morbid condition affecting the tissues surrounding the teeth, ranging from simple gingivitis to 'pyorrhoea alveolaris' with extensive absorption of bone.

"McCollum, Simmonds, Kinney and Grieves (1922) found that they term 'attaching-tissue' lesions after death in some rats fed on experimental diets, especially when these were low in calcium, phosphorus and fat-soluble vitamins.

"In M. Mellanby's experiments (1930) the majority of the dogs used were about 2 months old when the experiments were begun, and in some cases were born in the laboratory from mothers whose diets were controlled throughout pregnancy and lactation. In a few experiments in which curative, rather than prophylactic measures, were tested, the animals were several years old when brought to the laboratory suffering from periodontal disease.

"The periodontal tissue of dogs kept in kennels in a laboratory and fed from the time of weaning for 8 years on a diet containing, among other ingredients, white bread and a liberal supply of vitamins A and D are rendered very resistant to periodontal disease. On the other hand, the periodontal tissues of animals kept under similar conditions of diet and environment, but receiving comparatively little vitamins A and D for the first 6½ years, are very susceptible to the disease.

"These experiments stress the fundamental importance of including vitamins A and D in the diet during the early developmental period of the periodontal tissues are to resist disease. A large supply of these vitamins given later, even from the fifth month onwards, does not entirely compensate for a deficiency during the early period of life, although vitamin A given in large doses may then prevent the spread of the pathological condition. Conversely, the addition of a liberal supply of vitamins A and D to a diet composed largely of white bread, for nearly a year after weaning (i.e. for the full developmental period), renders the periodontal tissues resistant to disease in later life, even when the diet of the adult animal is deficient in these vitamins for long periods.

"It will be noted that hyperplasia of the squamos epithelium adjoining the teeth produced by vitamin A deficiency in the developing period of growth is a special instance of the general effect of this deficiency. The susceptibility to bacterial infection of this hyperplastic epithelium of the gums or gingival margin is a condition which would also be expected from other known instances, in which infective foci and epithelial overgrowth are commonly associated with a deficient intake of this vitamin. Just as the administration of vitamin A in such conditions tends to correct the pathological changes of the epithelium and to heal the septic foci, so also in pyorrhea alveolaris in dogs massive vitamin A therapy seems to increase the resistance of the gum tissues to microorganisms to the extent that the exudate of pus is greatly diminished and may even be suppressed.

"VITAMIN C AND DENTAL TISSUES. One of the earliest investigations on the influence of the diet on the teeth was that of Zilva and Wells (1919), who fed guinea-pigs on a scorbutic diet of oats, bran, and autoclaved milk. Ground and decalcified sections of the teeth showed defects in the pulp, odontoblasts and dentine. In the pulp, various degrees of degeneration of a type designated as 'fibroid' were found, and in the dentine an irregular 'osteoid' condition. Changes in the teeth were observed even in the mildest degree of scurvy, but never when a sufficiency of vitamin C was added to the basal diet.

"Howe (1919, 1921, 1923) has also carried out much experimental work on guinea-pigs and monkeys, primarily, however, with a view to establishing the relation of diet, and in particular of vitamin C to caries. He concludes that a deficiency of this vitamin leads to decalcification of the teeth. Toverud (1923, 1926) made a histological and chemical examination of some of the teeth of Howe's guinea-pigs and found the defects described by Zilva and Wells, Robb and collaborators (1921) found similar changes in the teeth of guinea-pigs on a scorbutic diet.

"Extensive investigations by Hojer (1924, 1926, Hojer and Westin 1925) and others have also emphasized the importance of vitamin C in determining the structure of the teeth in guinea-pigs. They summarize the defects that follow vitamin C deficiency as follows:

1. The gradual change and disappearance of the odontoblastic layer.
2. The amorphous calcification of the 'predentine' and the absence of canals in this layer.
3. The previously calcified dentine becomes porous.
4. The dilatation of the vessels in the pulp.
5. The production of nerve lesions and oedema of the pulp tissues.

"As a result of these investigations, a method was devised for the estimation of the antiscorbutic value of foods."

[2] Page 44:

" ... In rats, dental caries is produced by withdrawal of vitamin $B_1$. Food rich in vitamin $B_1$ prevents acid reaction upon enamel. Upon regeneration of bone and formation of callus, vitamin $B_1$ has favorable effect, the nature of which is still unknown. An essential anti-infectious activity is not possessed by vitamin $B_1$ ... "

Sajous has stated that vitamin C deficiency results in a loss of bactericidal power of the mouth fluids, as vitamin B and vitamin C are cooperative in most of their functions, a deficiency of either causing an aggravation of symptoms due to a deficiency of the other. We can, thereby, see why orange juice is only partly effective in the control of caries. The deficiencies of vitamin C and vitamin A seem to be the basic factors in setting the stage for pyorrhea, deficiency of vitamin A causing a degeneration and overgrowth of periodontal epithelial structures, while vitamin C deficiency is responsible for capillary fragility and consequent tendency to hemorrhage, to say nothing of the decalcification of supporting bone resulting from the same cause. Loose teeth can usually be restored to usefulness by administration of vitamin C concentrate alone.

VITAMIN NEWS

VITAMIN PRODUCTS CO. • MILWAUKEE, WISCONSIN

March 15, 1937 VOL. 5

# A REVIEW OF OUR PAST COMMENTS IN THE LIGHT OF LATER FINDINGS

It has been the purpose of *Vitamin News* to bring to the attention of the physician the therapeutic merits of vitamin products, particularly those supplied under the "V-P" trademark. Many statements have been made which at the time were not supportable by any recognized scientific research, but which were based only on results obtained that had been reported to the writer.

The readers of *Vitamin News* are entitled to know how many of these scientifically unsubstantiated statements suggesting therapeutic uses of vitamin concentrates have later, by more detailed research, been found correct, and a partial account is offered below.

Any credit due your humble servant for first recognizing an explanation for many of these facts can be considerably discounted in view of the newness of vitamin science in general, in which any practical minded person with some knowledge of biochemistry could not fail to see the obvious.

It should be emphasized that the statements made here were inspired by the results of clinical therapeutic experiences in connection with the use of "V-P" single vitamin concentrates and "Catalyn," representing the vitamins in their natural associated "complexes," while scientific proof had to wait for the preparation of the chemically pure vitamins with which tests were made, in most cases on test animals. It is obvious that scientific work must be chemically purified and identifiable in order to be able to positively attribute the effects in question to a specific influence.

Also, an opinion that may be the result of a very highly developed ability of judgement is only a guess from a scientific viewpoint until the properly controlled tests are made, which may be years subsequent to the expression of opinion, even though such opinions may be verified in a more practical, if less scientific way by clinical tests.

And the scientific test, in positively establishing the relation between cause and effect, is only a small step forward. To go the whole way we have a long road to follow yet, to know from a biochemical viewpoint all that takes place. As yet, this represents an almost entirely closed book.

As a short cut, to enable present-day sufferers to receive the relief that may be available by use of vitamin concentrates, we have followed the course of publishing clinical findings that were consistently reproducible, for in many cases no relief was possible otherwise, according to the best medical authorities.

The fact that many of the important attributes of vitamins herein described were first noted to exist by clinical users of "V-P" products long before any mention was made of the effect in the scientific literature should be convincing evidence to the physician of the superiority of the "natural complex" concentrate over the chemically-purified and animal-tested product..

Animal tests, we have repeatedly stated (*Vitamin News*, pages 45, 52 and 75) should be used only to suggest deficiency syndromes, not to make standardization tests, because of the fact that many of the purified vitamins are specific for species.

We have always found our vitamin C concentrate more outstanding in performance than the findings of clinical investigations of ascorbic acid warranted. So has Szent-Gyorgi, the original discoverer of ascorbic acid. In his clinical tests, he found that some other factor was responsible for the prevention of vascular fragility.

> *Los Angeles Times*, New Lemon Vitamin Cure for Bleeding, Sunday, March 14, 1937, Editorial Section, Part II, page 1 and page 3.
>
> " ... In repeated tests, he (Szent-Gyorgi) found that his Citrin or vitamin P from lemons or red pepper in fourteen days would clear up a hemorrhagic condition when pure vitamin C from some other source was useless.
>
> "As he describes it: 'The extracts were fractionated. The active substance (vitamin P) was found in the end in a fraction consisting of practically pure flavon or flavonal glycoside. Forty milligrams of this fraction given daily intravenously to man, restored in a fortnight, regularly, the normal capillary resistance. Spontaneous bleeding ceased, the capillary walls lost their fragility towards pressure differences and no more plasma protein left the vascular system on increased venous pressure.'"

Does the "V-P" Vitamin C concentrate control vascular fragility? The following case is authentic:

> Diagnosis – Purpura Hemorrhagica with Blood Findings Similar to Secondary Anemia.
>
> Patient – Female, age 55.
>
> Case of 15 years standing, of gradually increasing intensity to cause complete physical breakdown. Usual routine followed; taken to hospital where 5 blood transfusions were given. Patient did not respond.
>
> Treatment: "V-P Catalyn" and "V-P" Vitamin C Complex given at the rate of one tablet of each per hour. After the third day, patient showed signs of returning vitality. Fourth day dosage reduced to four tablets of "Catalyn" and four tablets of Vitamin C complex per day. Eighth day, patient was able to sit up in bed. Same dosage continued. Twelfth day, patient up in convalescent's chair. Dosage continued at four "Catalyn" and four Vitamin C complex tablets per day. At the end of third week, patient resumed light household duties. Dosage continued at four "Catalyn" and four Vitamin C complex tablets per day.
>
> Treatment was begun eighteen months ago.
> Patient now is active and in very good health.

Why this difference? Our vitamin C concentrate was developed by testing vitamin C extracts made by various methods for treating pyorrhea and scurvy as exhibited by mouth lesions; the one found most effective was the one commercialized. Its chemical nature and complexity are matters that can be fussed over by future investigations. It is effective and commercially available and *has been* for five years. The human race devoured foods for how many thousands of years before any of us became endowed with sufficient curiosity to start a chemical investigation of them — not but what such efforts are laudable and valuable, but, why starve to death waiting for complete knowledge? We haven't yet even mastered the chemistry of plain sugar metabolism. It was as late as 1920 that the molecular construction of our commonest carbohydrate, cane sugar, was first mapped (Irvine and Steele, *J. Chem. Soc.*, 117:1474. 1920). And synthesis of it was not accomplished until 1928 (Pictet and Vogel, *Comp. Rend.*, 186:727, 1928). We still are in the dark as to how it is assimilated. If we have had to wait for a knowledge of sugar chemistry that long, is it reasonable to expect a complete knowledge of vitamin chemistry before making use of them therapeutically?

It is the physician's duty to *test* products offered and to watch critically for results — either good or bad. Failure to watch for untoward results after accepting a manufacturer's word has resulted in much harm in the case of vitamin D of synthetic origin. The irradiated vitamin D first made was not vitamin D at all, but mainly toxisterol* ("Vigantol" in Germany and a proprietary vitamin D, which is a household word in this country, promoted by one of our leading pharmaceutical firms). It invariably caused renal damage if continued for any length of time. We have seen many cases of hematuria and albuminuria in children where overdosage with this so-called vitamin D was responsible. The remedy? Plenty of vitamin A (preferably "V-P" Vitamin A complex). Some cases has so little renal parenchyma left that only continuous dosage with vitamin A maintained a normal function.

These toxic effects have even been attributed to vitamin D itself:

> Eddy, W. H., and Dalldorf, Gilbert, *The Avitaminoses: The Chemical, Clinical and Pathological Aspects of The Vitamin Deficiency Diseases*, page 228, Williams and Wilkins Company, 1937.
>
> "By further adjustments of the dose of vitamin D, Collazo and Kohler were able to produce nephrosclerosis which progressed to kidney insufficiency and death. Albuminuria and tubular casts were present in the urine. The larger arteries were sclerotic. Other manifestations of vitamin D intoxication of this degree are metastatic calcification, phosphaturia and polyuria as well as hypercalcemia and phosphatemia. According to Collzo and Kohler, these effects may be produced at will in various species and in man."

* The belief has grown in recent years that ... and that some of the earliest instances of toxicity were due to toxic products (toxisterol) developed by too prolonged irradiation of ergosterol." — Eddy and Dalldorf, *The Avitaminoses,* page 229, 1937.

**Edited by Royal Lee**

# NOTES

VITAMIN NEWS

VITAMIN PRODUCTS CO. • MILWAUKEE, WISCONSIN

April 15, 1937 VOL. 5

# A REVIEW OF OUR PAST COMMENTS IN THE LIGHT OF LATER FINDINGS (Continued)

1. VITAMINS AND HYPERTHYROIDISM. One of the first syndromes in which the multiple vitamin product ("Catalyn") was found of great value was in the condition of hyperactivity of the thyroid. If the disease had progressed to the state of thyroid enlargement, it was usually even possible not only to correct the toxicosis, tachycardia, and the general symptomatic situation, but also to reduce the glandular enlargement.

It is now five years since we announced the value of vitamin concentrates in the treatment of hyperthyroidea.

It is thirteen years since we called attention to the obvious fact that the health of the endocrines depended primarily upon vitamin nutrition. (See Lee, R., *The Systemic Causes of Dental Caries*, page 2, 1923.)

In *Vitamin News* of November 13, 1933, we made the following seemingly bold statement:

> "'Catalyn' is the first specific remedy that can be depended upon to produce immediate results in all uncomplicated cases of toxic goiter. It is effective purely because it contains all the vitamins in such proportions as to as nearly as possible correct the deficiencies resulting from our present-day methods of food preparation.
>
> "The iodine deficiency that so far has received the entire blame for goiter conditions is only a contributory factor. It becomes important only when a vitamin deficiency is present. Iodine alone will not cure goiter, but the vitamin treatment does."

These statements, based only on consistent clinical results, are now supported by the following references, which show that vitamins A, B, C, D and E are all concerned in the maintenance of a normal thyroid function.

> Stepp, W., Kuhnau, J. and Schroeder, H., *Die Vitamine (The Vitamins and Their Clinical Application)*, Ferdinand Enke, Stuttgart, Germany, 1936.
>
> "The law that all vitamins form a functional unit, none of them unfolding its physiological effect independent of the others, is especially apparent in the close correlations existing between vitamin $B_1$ and the rest of the vitamins. The relation of vitamin A to vitamin $B_1$ is antagonistic insofar as by generous vitamin A supply, the symptoms of lack of vitamin $B_1$ are increased and inversely an A hypervitaminosis is favorably influenced by vitamin B feeding (Yonechy, Chevallier). On the other

hand, vitamin A as well as vitamin $B_1$ oppose thyroxin and vitamin D (Jusatz)... "

" ... The exact determination of the daily vitamin $B_1$ requirement in man is difficult since it is largely dependent upon the intensity of the metabolic processes (Cowgill) (Palmierie). If the general metabolism is increased by the administration of thyroid or thyroxine, the vitamin $B_1$ requirement rises. It is true, therefore, that symptoms of a vitamin $B_1$ deficiency develop with thyroid administration along with an ordinarily sufficient vitamin $B_1$ supply, and conversely the clinical syndromes of hyperthyroidism may be favorably influenced by an abundant vitamin $B_1$ administration (Himwich, Goldfarb, Cowgill) (Sure and Smith).

"The administration of extracts of yeast affect symptoms of Basedow favorably (Abelin). Conversely, with lack of vitamin $B_1$ the production of thyroxin is restricted. Usually with vitamin $B_1$ avitaminosis atrophy of the thyroid is found and likewise clinically symptoms of hypothyroidism (Verzar, Pighini, Kihn). Because of this fact, a chronic vitamin $B_1$ hypovitaminosis has been made responsible for endemic goiter besides the iodine deficiency. It has been shown in regions in Switzerland where goiter is rampant, that the nutrition of the people is markedly deficient in vitamin $B_1$. In cows kept in barns during the winter and given vitamin-poor feed, colloid goiters appeared, which were reduced as well with feed rich in vitamin $B_1$ as with iodine (Fischer). In view of the close relationship between fat metabolism, iodine and thyroid (Chidester) the restorative action of vitamin $B_1$ is possibly due to the fact that vitamin $B_1$ may normalize the fat absorption and the lipoid economy."

Sure and Smith, Hyperthyroidism and Nutrition: Vitamin B and Thyroxin, *J. Nutrition,* 7:548, 1934. (Abstract)

"It has been found that the albino rat can tolerate large doses of thyroxine for relatively long periods of time when adminstered orally to the full-grown animal on diets abundant in vitamin B. Collapse, however, takes place readily when the ration is deficient in this dietary essential. Subcutaneous injection of thyroxin is decidedly more toxic than oral administration. It has been found that a highly concentrated Vitamin B extract from rice polishings exerts a remarkable influence in experimentally produced hyperthyroidism in the rat, and it is suggested to the clinician that oral or preferably parenteral administration of potent standardized vitamin B concentrate may be indicated in toxic goiter, particularly in non-operative cases."

Svirbely, Joseph L., The Effect of Desiccated Thyroid, a — Dinitrophenol and Cortical Hormone Extract on the Vitamin C Content of Some Organs of the Guinea Pig Fed Graded Doses of Ascorbic Acid, *Journal of Biological Chemistry*, 111, 1:147-154, September 1935.

"Large amounts of ascorbic acid promote the general vitality and appearance of guinea pigs on a thyroid diet. The vitamin C content of organs depends on the amount of ascorbic acid fed and decreases as the metabolic rate of the tissues is increased."

This finding that dinitrophenol destroys the tissue content of vitamin C fits in very well with the discovery made by users of "Catalyn" that cataracts caused by dinitrophenol can be eliminated by the administration of that product, no doubt, mainly because of its content of vitamin C complex.

Deutsch, H., Reed, C. I., and Struck, H. C., The Role of the Thyroid in the Calorigenic Action of Vitamin D, *American Journal of Physiology*, 117:1, 1936. (Abstracted in *Endocrinology,* page 307, March 1937.)

"Experiments carried out on two dogs show that after complete thyroparathyroidectomy, large doses of vitamin D produce no significant increase in the metabolic rate. Previous work has shown that the calorigenic action of Vitamin D on normal animals is not due to action on the parathyroids. The authors therefore conclude that the thyroid plays an important part in this reaction. Variation in metabolic rate roughly paralleled changes in body weight."

Singer, Eleanore, Effects of Vitamin E Deficiency on the Thyroid Gland of the Rat, *Journal of Physiology,* 87:287, 1936. (Abstracted in *Endocrinology,* pages 311-312, March 1937.)

"Absence of vitamin E from the diet changes the normal active rat thyroid to one with much colloid and low cuboidal cells. The normal appearance was restored by E extracts or wheat germ oil, and partially by alkaline anterior pituitary extracts. Iodine administration for four to ten days did not affect the histological appearance, nor did seven days of pregnancy. The table lists eleven types of experiments on fifty-seven rats and there are two plates with photographs of the thyroid sections."

2. DIABETES MELLITUS. The value of "Catalyn" and vitamin B concentrate in improving the condition of the diabetic, with usually a definite reduction in the hyperglycemia, was soon noted when these products were first made available to the physician. The probability of an etiologic relationship between vitamin B deficiency and diabetes was suggested in the 1923 article — "The Systemic Causes of Dental Caries," before mentioned. The present opinion is best stated in the words of Stepp et al.

" ... The close relationship of the vitamin $B_1$ to carbohydrate metabolism has stimulated the use of it in the therapy of diabetes mellitus. The hyperglycemia and glycosuria-reducing effect peroral yeast administration have been known for a long time and in animal experimentation, at least, assured beyond objection (Beckel et al). Twenty years ago, v. Euler and Svanberg established the antidiabetic effect of yeast extracts, and that has also been observed in man. It has been submitted that daily doses of dry yeast (10 to 30 gm.) in cases of diabetes of medium grade may entirely or partially replace Insulin (Vogt, Hoepfner-Klotz, Melcer, Mansberg, Winter-Smith). V. Driglaski alone failed with yeast with his diabetics. The reason may be found in the length of time he used the yeast (eleven days), while Melcer, Gringoire et al insist on giving it for six to eight weeks before success may be expected. The effect lasts much longer than that of Insulin. One might explain that with the necessity of refilling the depleted vitamin depots. Further investigation is necessary. Whether the Insulin-like substance of the yeast (v. Euler) is identical with vitamin $B_1$ has not been determined so far with certainty. In pigeon beriberi, almost constantly a rise of blood sugar and blood lactic acid is found, which is removed by $B_1$ (and allegedly by insulin. On the other hand, as has been (continued) ...

# VITAMIN NEWS

VITAMIN PRODUCTS CO. • MILWAUKEE, WISCONSIN

May 15, 1937 VOL. 5

## A REVIEW OF OUR PAST COMMENTS IN THE LIGHT OF LATER FINDINGS (Continued)

mentioned, the point of attack of vitamin $B_1$ in the sugar economy is entirely different from that of Insulin. That does not speak against the possibility of an Insulin-like effect of vitamin $B_1$ since we know that the radiation products of ergosterin (vitamin D and A. D. 10) may entirely replace the parathyroid hormone, however different their working mechanism may be. Clinical trials with crystallized vitamin $B_1$ have not shown any positive results so far. Purified vitamin $B_1$ preparations in the hands of Sainton, Mills, and Labbe have proven to be strongly effective in diabetes. While Stepp failed to influence the blood sugar in health and diabetes, Williams and coworkers have reported frank successes with large doses of pure vitamin $B_1$ in diabetes. It is evident that dosage plays a considerable role. Further investigations in this direction are urgently desired, because of the possibility that we may possess in vitamin $B_1$ for the first time a true and physiologically vital peroral anti-diabeticum in an isolated and chemically homogenous form. Since thyroxin increases the need of vitamin $B_1$, as mentioned, the danger of symptoms arising from vitamin $B_1$ deficiency in hyperthyroidism is real. Care is, therefore, necessary in morb. Basedow to procure an adequate supply of vitamin $B_1$ (besides vitamin A)."

3. VITAMINS AND THE HEART. Since loss of muscular vigor is a characteristic of both beriberi and scurvy, to say nothing of the paralysis resultant from vitamin E or vitamin F deficiency, and the specific damage to heart function due to the effects of vitamin B deficiency on the nervous system, it is now clear why "Catalyn" was found to be so beneficial in many forms of heart disease, whether organic or functional.

Since our recommendations in "Catalyn" literature five years ago regarding the value of the produce for cardiac disease, the following references have become available.

*Cleveland Plain Dealer*, "Reveal New Forms of Heart Disease," April 20, 1937.

"St. Louis, April 19. A hitherto unrecognized form of heart disease in the United States caused by malnutrition and a specific treatment for it were described today before the annual meeting of the American College of Physicians.

"Dr. Soma Weiss and Dr. Robert W. Wilkins of Boston reported that in 120 of their patients, enough to make it 'relatively common,' the specific form of heart disease was found and traced readily to nutritional deficiency.

> "A 'rapid and often spectacular cure' resulted from the simple administration of vitamin B.
>
> "In the northeastern part of the nation at least 'the disease occurs principally among alcoholics, diabetics, food cranks and pregnant women,' the Boston physician declared.
>
> "'In its pure form it develops in persons without organic heart disease,' but when the two occur together, 'failure of the heart is often precipitated or aggravated' leading to disintegration of the circulation and death if not treated."

In the December 15, 1936 issue of *Vitamin News,* we offered as evidence of the effectiveness of our vitamin B concentrate a sphygmogram of a patient before and after taking two tablets, a very definite improvement in regularity being shown within ten minutes.

Herewith, we show a still more striking improvement occurring in 15 minutes in a patient where the nervous system balance was still more out of control. The third chart (after six days treatment) indicates approximately a normal nervous function.

None of our other concentrates alone has the slightest action in 15 minutes, according to sphygmograph tests. They do contribute, however, very much over a period of time to the resumption of normal physiological balances where the heart abnormality has been adding to the difficulty of other organs in accomplishing their functions. A reduced blood supply obviously aggravates a low nutritional supply, whether it be vitamins or other food elements required by each organ. In this manner a multiple vitamin deficiency may develop in the patient with cardiac disease. That is the probable explanation for the remarkable tonic action of "Catalyn" in these cases. Vitamin B deficiency is a key factor here, too, in that one of the first signs of its lack is a reduction of assimilative efficiency through the debilitation of the alimentary mucosa, to say nothing of the frequent loss of appetite also due to this cause. Now follow this with a breakdown of the nervous structures that control the heart and you will realize what an important "staff of life" vitamin B is — and it normally would occur in ample quantities in our bread if we used only that made from unbleached flour, or better, that made from fresh whole wheat.

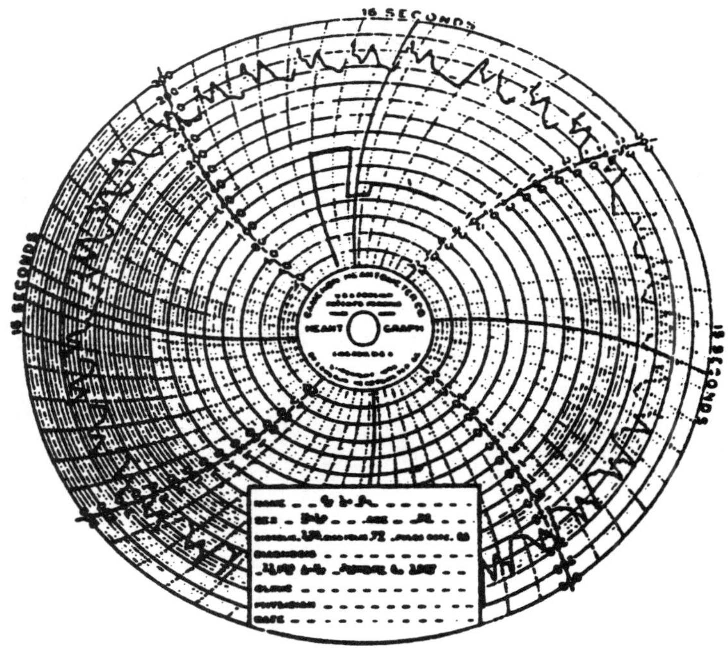

Before Treatment

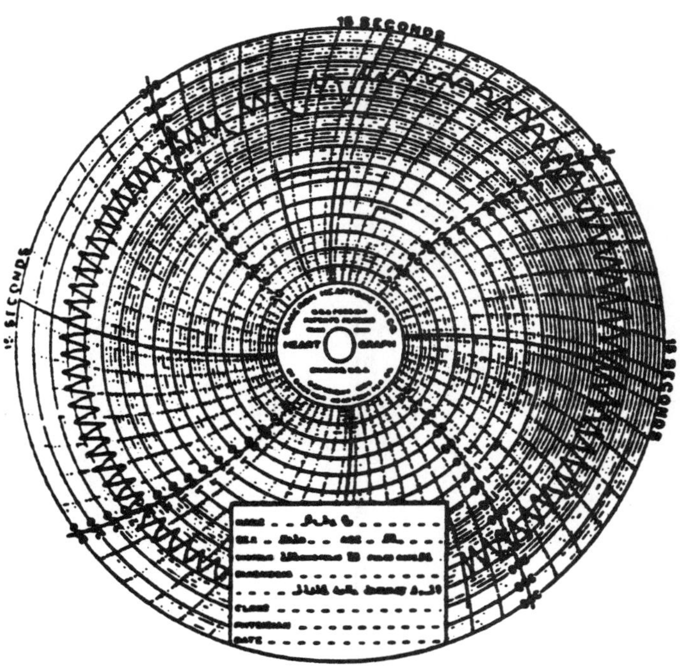

Fifteen minutes after taking two tablets of "V-P" Vitamin B complex.

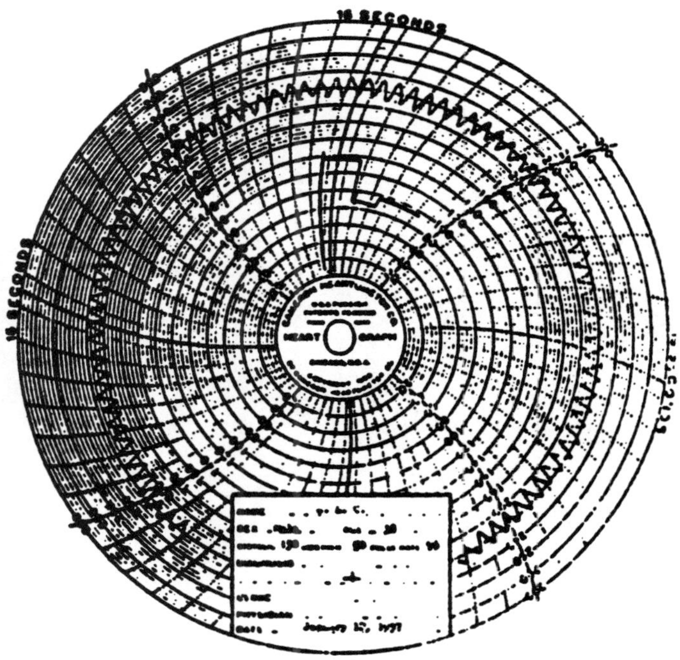

Six days later, four tablets of "V-P" Vitamin B complex per day being taken meanwhile.

Edited by Royal Lee

# NOTES

VITAMIN NEWS
VITAMIN PRODUCTS CO. • MILWAUKEE, WISCONSIN

June 15, 1937 VOL. 5

# VITAMIN CHART

## VITAMIN A COMPLEX

**Apparent Function:**

1. Necessary to normal function and integrity of:
   - Tissues of epiblastic origin;
   - Epithelial tissues (wound-healing hastened, resistance to infections raised);
   - Nervous system.
2. Necessary to maintenance of normal cell metabolism, such as:
   - Cell respiration;
   - Blood cell generation (platelets).
3. Necessary to formation and integrity of periodontal tissue.
4. Promotes growth, feeling of well-being and longevity.
5. Essential to successful reproduction.
6. Prevents keratinization of tissues.

**Possible Results of Deficiency:**

7. Retarded appetite, growth and development (due to interference with assimmilation).
8. Disturbed dental and bone development (atrophy).
9. Susceptibility to infections as well as slow healing of the following:
   - Reticulo-endothelium;
   - Epithelium, due to degenerative change in structures of skin and mucosa.
10. Presence (due to lowered resistance) of:
    - Infections of eye (corneal ulcers) and degeneration of eyes (xerophthalmia, keratomalacia, night blindness, total blindness);
    - Infections of ear (otitis media);
    - Infections of genitourinary tract;
    - Infections of mucous tract (tonsilitis);
    - Infections of respiratory tract (penumonia, tuberculosis);
    - Infections of gastrointestinal tract (diarrhea);
    - Infections of sinuses.
11. Presence of keratinizations and metaplasia of:
    - Epithelium;
    - Genitourinary tract (making for difficult delivery of young);
    - Mucous tract;
    - Respiratory tract;
    - Glands.
12. Interference with successful reproduction and lactation (loss of sex impulse):
    - Sterility in the female by failure of ovulation or resorption of fetus;

– Sterility in the male by temporary injury to seminiferous epithelium;
– Prolonged gestation, retained and diseased placenta, difficult delivery.

13. Development of:
   – Pernicious anemia;
   – Secondary anemia;
   – Rickets (in conjunction with vitamin D deficiency);
   – Gastritis;
   – Bronchitis.
14. Development of kidney and bladder disorders (metaphasias) and renal dysfunction:
   – Formation of stones (calculi);
   – Nephritis;
   – Cystitis.
15. Excessive growth of lymphoid tissue.
16. Degeneration of the nervous system — dulling or perversion of special senses.

**Results of Absence:**

17. Atrophy of organs and glands (testes, liver, spleen, thyroid, pituitary and salivary).
18. Degenerative skeletal muscle lesions develop.
19. Ophthalmia, xerophthalmia, keratomalacia, conjunctivitis or keratoconjunctivitis.
20. Death.

---

## VITAMIN B COMPLEX

**Apparent Function:**

1. Stimulates and promotes appetite and normal digestion.
3. Promotes optimal growth (increases height and vigor).
3. Necessary to maintenance of normal metabolic processes such as:
   – Carbohydrate metabolism (lactic acid excesses);
   – Cell respiration.
4. Necessary to normal pregnancy and lactation.
5. Maintains nervous function.
6. Stimulates digestive secretions, including insulin.
7. Necessary to maintenance of muscle tonus.
8. Prevents toxicosis from protein components in high meat diets.

**Possible Results of Deficiency:**

9. Susceptibility to infections due to lowered resistance.
10. Disturbed carbohydrate metabolism (diabetes mellitus) (lactic acid excesses, slow or labored respiration).
11. Functional disorders, atrophy or pathological enlargement of adrenals, brain, gonads, heart (heart block and bradycardia), kidneys liver, ovaries, pancreas, pituitary gland, spleen, testes, thymus and thyroid glands — goiter.
12. Tendency to functional gastrointestinal disorders (Intestinal immobility, loss of tonus, constipation, lack of gastric secretions, ulcers, impaired appetite [anorexia] and digestion).
13. Tendency to muscle paralysis (loss of tone).
14. Loss of weight and vigor, stunted growth and emaciation.

15. Tendency to edematous conditions.
16. Fall in body temperature.
17. Degeneration of central nervous system (impaired nerve function, convulsions, tetany).
18. Anemia.
19. Disturbances of reproductive cycle (sterility — atrophy of seminiferous tubules, loss of libido, anestrus — hemorrhage at partus and abortions).
20. Dental caries.
21. Predisposes to allergic conditions.

**Results of Absence:**

22. Beriberi.
23. Peripheral and other forms of neuritis (polyneuritis).
24. Death.

---

## VITAMIN C COMPLEX

**Apparent Function:**

1. Essential to health and integrity of endothelial tissues (raises resistance to infections).
2. Essential to proper development of teeth.
3. Essential to oxygen metabolism.
4. Regeneration of blood cells.
5. Maintains proper blood-clotting time.

**Possible Results of Deficiency:**

6. Tendency to structural tissue changes:
   - (a) Diseases of blood vessels and capillaries (fragility, hemorrhages, tendency to bruise easily, "black and blue spots," purpura hemorrhagica), (varicosities).
   - (b) Diseases of gums (hemorrhage, sore gums), (pyorrhea).
   - (c) Tooth degeneration (necrosis, caries).
   - (d) Joint and bone changes (decalcification, friability).
   - (e) Mucous membrane hemorrhages.
   - (f) Destruction of bone marrow.
7. Tendency to epithelial lesions (ulcerations of mouth, intestines, etc.).
8. Increased susceptibility or reduced resistance to infections.
9. Retarded growth and loss of weight.
10. Physical weakness, depression and irritability.
11. Rapid respiration and heart action.
12. Blood degeneration (Tendency to certain types of anemia, reduced hemoglobin, destruction of bone marrow).
13. Development of heart weakness.
14. Increased weight and enlargement of spleen, liver, stomach, intestines and kidneys.
15. Atrophy or hypertrophy of glands:
   - (a) Reduced secretion of adrenals;
   - (b) Morbid secretion of thyroid (toxic goiter).
16. Development of arthritis (rheumatic tendency).

17. Development of edematous conditions.
18. Complications of pregnancy and lactation as well as ill effects to new born (abortions).
19. Tendency to raised temperature.
20. Possible sterility.
21. Lowered glucose tolerance.
22. Cataract.
23. Predisposes to allergic conditions.

**Results of Absence:**

24. Scurvy.
25. Sprue.
26. Death.

---

## VITAMIN D COMPLEX

**Apparent Function:**

1. Essential to proper mineral metabolism; absorption from alimentary tract, utilization (health and calcification of bone and teeth) (antirachitic action) and excretion of calcium and phosphorus.
2. Necessary to successful pregnancy and lactation.
3. Necessary for normalizing and reducing time of labor.
4. Necessary to maintain blood platelets at normal level.
5. Maintains normal coagulation time of blood.
6. Maintains growth (longitudinal bone growth).
7. Aids in maintaining muscle tone.
8. Increases strength of capillaries.
9. Related to hormonal function.
10. Increases resistance to infections (especially against tuberculosis).
11. Necessary to normal respiratory function.

**Possible Results of Deficiency:**

12. Rickets and osteomalacia (improper calcification of bone).
13. Growth retarded.
14. Enlargement of liver, kidney and spleen.
15. Instability and irritability of nervous system and tissues.
16. Decreases resistance to infections.
17. Muscular weakness, constipation and reduced mobility of gastrointestinal tract.
18. Increased tendency to dental caries and defective teeth (improper calcification) (pyorrhea).
19. Parathyroid dysfunction (enlargement).
20. Menstrual disorders, cessation of ovulation, uterine atrophy, difficult childbirth due to deformities in pelvic development.

**Results of Absence:**

21. Osteoporosis.
22. Rickets.

## VITAMIN E

**Apparent Function:**

1. Necessary to reproduction in both male and female (necessary to prevent irreparable sterility in male).
2. Necessary to maintenance of mental altertness.
3. Necessary to growth and vigor.
4. Possibly to prevent carcinoma.
5. Necessary to resistance to infections.
6. Possibly to prevent paralysis of young (from E-deficient mothers).
7. Vermifuge (possibly due to associated priniciples).
8. Some influence on the endocrines (pituitary, anterior pituitary).

**Possible Results of Deficiency:**

9. Loss of weight, retarded growth, weakness.
10. Wasting of muscles, paralysis.
11. Lowered resistance in infections (particularly to infantile paralysis).
12. Sterility (Temporary in female — interference placental function). (Permanent in male — irreparable semin iferous epithelial injury).

**Results of Absence:**

13. Severe paralysis.
14. Disturbances of latter stages of pregnancy, producing sterility (fetal resorption and habitual abortion).
15. Roughness, falling out (alopecia) and altering of the texture of the hair.
16. Possible tendency to malignancies.

---

## VITAMIN F

**Apparent Functions:**

1. Necessary to healthy epidermis (protection against infection).
2. Maintains normal growth and reproduction.
3. May be necessary to maintain normal blood sugar (possibly related to insulin secretion).
4. Necessary to cell respiration.
5. Necessary to hair health.
6. Necessary to brain function and probably to function of other nerve tissue.

**Possible Results of Deficiency:**

7. Epidermal manifestations (ridged and split fingernails, eczematous conditions, dermatitis — infantile and allergic, scurf, dandruff and hemorrhagic spots on the skin).
8. Brittleness and falling out of hair (alopecia).
9. Involvement of endocrine glands (pituitary in particular).
10. Involvement of visceral organs (particularly kidneys).
11. Lowers resistance to allergies.
12. Susceptibility to vitamin D poisoning.

13. Loss of sex instinct.
14. Lowered resistance to infections (tuberculosis, in particular).

**Results of Absence:**

15. Cessation of growth and subsequent death.
16. Severe renal manifestations (hematuria, albuminaria, and severe nephritis).
17. Sterility (Impaired and irregular ovulation with interference with mechanism of labor in the female), loss of sex potentia with eventual sterility in the male).

---

## VITAMIN G COMPLEX

**Apparent Function:**

1. Necessary to growth and development.
2. Necessary to cell respiration.
3. As growth stimulus, promotes normal repair processes and thereby delays senility.
4. Necessary to blood regeneration.

**Possible Results of Deficiency:**

5. Underdevelopment and retarded growth from malnutrition.
6. Eye disorders (conjunctivitis).
7. Incipient pellagra.
8. Abnormally slow regeneration of erythrocytes (secondary anemia).
9. Cutaneous changes (pellagric symptoms, mild dermatitis).
10. Nerve lesions and irritability (Neuritis).
11. Loss of hair (alopecia).
12. Sprue
13. Interferes with normal skin respiration.
14. Alimentary tract disorders (Gastroenteritis, stomatitis, digestive disturbances).
15. Fatty infiltration and degeneration of the liver.
16. Renal manifestations (cystitis, Hemorrhagic conditions of the urine, stones — renal calculi).

**Results of Absence:**

17. Gastrointestinal disturbances (gastroenteritis, stomatitis, ulcerative colitis, diarrhea, nausea, vomiting, achlorhydria).
18. Cessation of growth.
19. Eye disorders (keratinization, severe conjunctivitis, ophthalmia, cataracts).
20. Severe pellagra.
21. Severe nerve and spinal degeneration. (Mental disorders, hyperirritability).
22. Death.

---

NOTE: This chart is based on a bibliography of over three hundred references.
VITAMIN PRODUCTS COMPANY MILWAUKEE, WISCONSIN.

**Edited by Royal Lee**

# VITAMIN NEWS

VITAMIN PRODUCTS CO. • MILWAUKEE, WISCONSIN

July 15, 1937 VOL. 5

## BIBLIOGRAPHY FOR VITAMIN CHART

### (VITAMIN A)

1. Gardner, E. and Gardner, F., *American Journal of Diseases of Children*, 47:1261, 1934.
— Harris, L. J., *Vitamins in Theory and Practice*, page 158, Cambridge University Press, 1935.
— *Journal of the American Medical Association*, Editorial, 97:783, 1931.
— Mathews, Albert P., *Principles of Biochemistry*, page 411, William Wood & Co., Baltimore, 1936.
— Medical Research Council, *Vitamins; A Survey of Present Knowledge,* page 90, London, 1932.
— Mellanby, E. and Green, H. H., *British Medical Journal*, 1929.
— Quigley, Daniel, Thomas, *Notes on Vitamins and Diets*, pages 16-17, 43, Consolidated Book Publishers, Inc., Chicago, 1933.
— Sherman, H. C., and Smith, S. L., *The Vitamins*, Second Edition, Monograph Series, No. 6, pages 280, 282, The Chemical Catalogue Co., Inc., New York, 1931.
— Shibata, M., *Jap. Journal of Experimental Medicine*, 9:21, 1931.
— Stepp, W., Kuhnau, J. and Schroeder, H., *The Vitamins and Their Clinical Application*, Ferdinand Enke, Stuttgart, Germany, 1936.
— United States Department of Agriculture, *Circular No. 84*.
— *Washington, (D.C.) Star,* Vitamin A Lack Held Stone Cause, January 11, 1935.

2. Mathews, Albert P., *Principles of Biochemistry*, page 411, William Wood & Co., Baltimore, 1936.
— McCollum, E. V., and Simmonds, N., *The Newer Knowledge of Nutriton*, Fourth Edition, pages 495-496, The MacMillan Co., New York, 1929.
— Stepp, W., Kuhanu, J. and Schroeder, H., *The Vitamins and Their Clinical Applications*, Ferdinand Enke, Stuttgart, Germany, 1936.

3. Macleod, J. J. R., *Physiology in Modern Medicine*, Seventh Edition, page 752, C. V. Mosby Co., St. Louis, 1935.
— Medical Research Council, *Vitamins: A Survey of Present Knowledge*, page 90, London, 1932.
— Shibata, M., *Jap. Journal of Experimental Medicine*, 9:21, 1931.

4. Eddy, W. H. and Dalldorf, G., *The Avitaminoses*, pages 31, 64, The Williams and Wilkins Co., Baltimore, 1937.
— Howell, William H., *A Textbook of Physiology*, Twelfth Edition, Revised, pages 967, 968-969, W. B. Saunders Co., Philadelphia, 1933.
— Mathews, Albert P., *Principles of Biochemistry*, page 411, William Wood & Co., Baltimore, 1936.
— McClendon, J. F., *A Manual of Biochemistry*, page 3, John Wiley & Sons, Inc., New York, 1934.
— Sherman, H. C., and Smith, S. L., *The Vitamins*, Second Edition, Monograph Series, No. 6, pages 287, 292, The Chemical Catalogue Co., Inc., New York, 1931.

— Sure, Barnett, *The Vitamins in Health and Disease*, page 23, The Williams and Wilkins Co., Baltimore, 1933.

5. Eddy, W. H., and Dalldorf, G., *The Avitaminoses*, page 64, The Williams and Wilkins Co., Baltimore, 1937.
— Mathews, Albert P., *Principles of Biochemistry*, page 411, William Wood & Co., Baltimore, 1936.
— McClendon, J. F., *A Manual of Biochemistry*, page 3, John Wiley & Sons, Inc., New York, 1934.
— Sherman, H. C., and Smith, S. L., *The Vitamins*, Second Edition, Monograph Series, No. 6, page 291, The Chemical Catalogue Co., Inc., New York, 1931.
— United States Department of Agriculture, *Circular No. 84*.

6. McClendon, J. F., *A Manual of Biochemistry*, page 3, John Wiley & Sons, Inc., New York, 1934.
— Stepp, W., Kuhnau, J. and Schroeder, H., *The Vitamins and Their Clinical Application*.

7. Barborka, Clifford J., Diet and Preventive Dentistry, *Journal of the American Dental Association,* 23, 6:977-985, June, 1936.
— Eddy, W. H., and Dalldorf, G., *The Avitaminoses*, page 54, The Williams and Wilkins Co., Baltimore, 1937.
— Howell, William H., *A Textbook of Physiology*, Twelfth Edition, Revised, page 968, W. B. Saunders Co., Philadelphia, 1933.
— Macleod, J. J. R., *Physiology in Modern Medicine*, Seventh Edition, pages 730-731, C. V. Mosby Co., St. Louis, 1935.
— Mathews, Albert P., *Principles of Biochemistry*, pages 416-417, William Wood & Co., Baltimore, 1936.
— Medical Research Council, *Vitamins: A Survey of Present Knowledge*, page 25, London, 1932.
— Sherman, H. C., and Smith, S. L., *The Vitamins*, Second Edition, Monograph Series, No. 6, pages 273-274, 278, The Chemical Catalogue Co., Inc., New York, 1931.
— United States Department of Agriculture, *Circular No. 84*.

8. Eddy, W. H., and Dalldorf, G., *The Avitaminoses*, page 52, The Williams and Wilkins Co., Baltimore, 1937.
— Medical Research Council, *Vitamins: A Survey of Present Knowledge*, page 192, London, 1932.
— Smith, M. C., and Lantz, E. M., *Journal of Home Economics*, 25:411, 1935.
— Stepp, W., Kuhnau, J., and Schroeder, H., *The Vitamins and Their Clinical Application*, Ferdinand Enke, Stuttgart, Germany, 1936.

9. Barborka, Clifford J., *Diet and Preventive Dentistry, Journal of the American Dental Association,* 23, 6:977-985, June, 1936.
— Eddy, W. H., and Dalldorf, G., *The Avitaminoses*, pages 59-60, The Williams and Wilkins Co., Baltimore, 1937.
— Green and Mellanby, *British Medical Journal*, ii, 691, 1928.
— Howell, William H., *A Textbook of Physiology*, Twelfth Edition, Revised, page 968, Saunders Co., Philadelphia, 1933.
— Medical Research Council, *Vitamins: A Survey of Present Knowledge*, page 33, London, 1932.
— Sherman, H. C., and Smith, S. L., *The Vitamins*, Second Edition, Monograph Series, No. 6, pages 274, 280, 281, 287, The Chemical Catalog Co., Inc., New York, 1931.
— Stepp, W., Kuhnau, J. and Schroeder, H., *The Vitamins and Their Clinical Application*, Ferdinand Enke, Stuttgart, Germany, 1936.

10. Eddy, W. H. and Dalldorf G., *The Avitaminoses*, pages 33, 34, 38-39, 40, 57, 258, The Williams and Wilkins Co., Baltimore, 1937.
— Macleod, J. J. R., *Physiology in Modern Science*, Seventh Edition, pages 731, 732, C. V. Mosby Co., St. Louis,

1935.
— Mathews, Albert P., *Principles of Biochemistry*, pages 415-416, William Wood & Co., Baltimore, 1936.
— Quigley, Daniel Thomas, *Notes on Vitamins and Diets*, pages 16, 98, Consolidated Book Publishers, Inc., Chicago, 1933.
— Rosslene, A. H., *Journal of Nutrition*, 8:75, 1934.
— Sherman, H. C., and Smith, S. L., *The Vitamins*, Second Edition, Monograph Series, No. 6, pages 274, 278, 286-287, The Chemical Catalog Co., Inc., New York, 1931.
— Sure, Barnett, *The Vitamins in Health and Disease*, page 23, The Williams and Wilkins Co., Baltimore, 1933.

11. Eddy, W. H. and Dalldorf, G., *The Avitaminoses*, pages 47, 51, 258, The Williams and Wilkins Co., Baltimore, 1937.
— Harris, L. J., *Vitamins in Theory and Practice*, page 158, Cambridge University Press, 1935.
— Howell, William H., *A Textbook of Physiology*, Twelfth Edition, Revised, page 968, W. B. Saunders Co., Philadelphia, 1933.
— Macleod, J. J. R., *Physiology in Modern Medicine*, Seventh Edition, page 732, C. V. Mosby Co., St. Louis, 1935.
— Mathews, Albert P., *Principles of Biochemistry*, page 411, William Wood & Co., Baltimore, 1936.
— McClendon, J. F., *A Manual of Biochemistry*, page 3, John Wiley & Sons, Inc., New York, 1934.
— Medical Research Council, *Vitamins: A Survey of Present Knowledge*, pages 29, 33, London, 1932.
— Sherman, H. C., and Smith, S. L., *The Vitamins*, Second Edition, Monograph Series, No. 6, pages 280, 289, The Chemical Catalog Co., Inc., New York, 1931.
— Stepp, W., Kuhnau, J., and Schroeder, H., *The Vitamins and Their Clinical Application*, Ferdinand Enke, Stuttgart, Germany, 1936.

12. Eddy, W. H. and Dalldorf, G., *The Avitaminoses*, pages 49, 50, 51, 64-65, The Williams and Wilkins Co., Baltimore, 1937.
— Howell, William H., *A Textbook of Physiology*, Twelfth Edition, Revised, pages 968, 974, W. B. Saunders Co., Philadelphia, 1933.
— Mason, K. E., Differences in Testis Injury and Repair After Vitamin A Deficiency, Vitamin E Deficiency, and Inanition, *American Journal of Anatomy,* 52:153-240, 1933.
— Mason, K. E., *Reproductive Function in Female Rats on Low Levels of Vitamin A, Anatomical Record,* 58, 4, Suppl. 80, 1934.
— McClendon, J. F., *A Manual of Biochemistry*, page 3, John Wiley & Sons, Inc., New York, 1934.
— Medical Research Council, *Vitamins: A Survey of Present Knowledge*, pages 33-34, 112, London, 1932.
— Sherman, H. C. and Smith, S. L., *The Vitamins*, Second Edition, Monograph Series, No. 6, pages 289, 336, The Chemical Catalog Co., Inc., New York, 1931.
— Stepp, W., Kuhnau, J. and Schroeder, H., *The Vitamins and Their Clinical Application*, Ferdinand Enke, Stuttgart, Germany, 1936.
— Sure, Barnett, *The Vitamins in Health and Disease*, page 23, The Williams and Wilkins Co., Baltimore, 1933.
— United States Department of Agriculture, *Circular No. 84*.

13, DeSanctis, Adolph and Craig, John D., A Five-Year Clinical Study of the Prophylactic Value of Antirachitic Agents, *New York State Journal of Medicine,* 34, 16:712-714, 1934.
— Eddy, W. H. and Dalldorf, G., *The Avitaminoses*, page 34, The Williams and Wilkins Co., Baltimore, 1937.
— Mathews, Albert P., *Principles of Biochemistry*, pages 415-416, William Wood & Co., Baltimore, 1936.
— McCollum, E. V., and Simmonds, N, *The Newer Knowledge of Nutrition*, Fourth Edition, page 495, The MacMillan Co., New York, 1929.
— Stepp, W., Kuhnau, J. and Schroeder, H., *The Vitamins and Their Clinical Application*, Ferdinand Enke, Stuttgart,

Germany, 1936.

14. Berglund, Medes, Huber, Longcope and Richards, *The Kidney in Health and Disease*, pages 147-149, 253-255, Lea & Febiger Co., Philadelphia, 1935.
— Eddy, W. H. and Dalldorf, G., *The Avitaminoses*, pages 34, 49, 56, 64, 258, The Williams and Wilkins Co., Baltimore, 1937.
— Fujimaki, *Jap. Med. World*, vi, 29, 1926.
— Mathews, Albert P., *Principles of Biochemistry*, page 417, William Wood & Company, Baltimore, 1936.
— McCarrison, R., *British Medical Journal*, 1:717, 1927.
— McCarrions, R., *Ibid*, 2:159-160, 1927-1928.
— Medical Research Council, *Vitamins: A Survey of Present Knowledge*, page 237, London, 1932.
— Sherman, H. C. and Smith, S. L., *The Vitamins*, Second Edition, Monograph Series, No. 6, pages 278, 292, The Chemical Catalog Co., Inc., New York, 1931.
— Washington (D. C.) Star, *Vitamin A Lack Held Stone Cause*, January 11, 1935.

15. Eddy, W. H., and Dalldorf, G., *The Avitaminoses*, page 54, The Williams & Wilkins Co., Baltimore, 1937.
— McCollum, E. V., and Simmonds, N., *The Newer Knowledge of Nutrition*, Fourth Edition, page 495, The MacMillan Co., New York, 1929.

16. Eddy, W. H. and Dalldorf, G., *The Avitaminoses*, pages 41-42, 52-53, The Williams and Wilkins Co., Baltimore, 1937.
— Harris, L. J., *Vitamins in Theory and Practice*, pages 166-167, Cambridge University Press, 1935.
— Macleod, J. J. R., *Physiology in Modern Medicine*, Seventh Edition, page 732, C. V. Mosby Co., St. Louis, 1935.
— Mathews, Albert P., *Principles of Biochemistry*, pages 415-416, William Wood and Company, Baltimore, 1936.
— Stepp, W., Kuhnau, J. and Schroeder, H., *The Vitamins and Their Clinical Application*, Ferdinand Enke, Stuttgart, Germany, 1936.

17. Eddy, W. H. and Dalldorf, G., *The Avitaminoses*, page 51, The Williams and Wilkins Co., Baltimore, 1937.

18. Eddy, W. H. and Dalldorf, G., *The Avitaminoses*, page 54, The Williams and Wilkins Co., Baltimore, 1937.

19. Eddy, W. H. and Dalldorf, G., *The Avitaminoses*, pages 34, 40, The Williams and Wilkins Co., Baltimore, 1937.
— Howell, William H., *A Textbook of Physiology*, Twelfth Edition, Revised, page 968, W. B. Saunders Co., Philadelphia, 1933.
— Jeghers, H., Night Blindness Due to Vitamin A Deficiency: A Consideration of Its Importance in Traffic *Problems, New England Journal of Medicine,* 216:51-56, January 14, 1937.
— Mathews, Albert P., *Principles of Biochemistry*, page 411, William Wood & Co., Baltimore, 1936.
— McClendon, J. F., *A Manual of Biochemistry*, page 3, John Wiley & Sons, Inc., New York, 1934.
— Sherman, H. C. and Smith, S. L., *The Vitamins*, page 274, Second Edition, Monograph Series, No. 6, The Chemical Catalog Co., Inc., New York, 1931.
— Stepp, W., Kuhnau, J. and Schroeder, H., *The Vitamins and Their Clinical Application*, Ferdinand Enke, Stuttgart, Germany, 1936.

20. Macleod, J. J. R., *Physiology in Modern Medicine*, Seventh Edition, page 731, C. V. Mosby Co., St. Louis, 1935.
— Mathews, Albert P., *Principles of Biochemistry*, pages 416-417, William Wood & Co., Baltimore, 1936.
— Medical Research Council, *Vitamins: A Survey of Present Knowledge*, pages 25, 29, London, 1932.

— Sherman, H. C. and Smith, S. L., *The Vitamins*, Second Edition, Monograph Series, No. 6, pages 273-274. The Chemical Catalog Co., Inc., New York, 1931.

Eddy and Dalldorf, *The Avitaminoses*, pages 52-53, Williams and Wilkins Co., 1937.

> "Degenerative changes in the nervous system also occur in vitamin A deficiency. Mellanby has observed such lesions in the dog, rabbit, rat and birds.
>
> "The lesions in the cord are disseminated, chiefly of the ascending fibers and, therefore, more extensive in the upper levels of the cord. The dorsal spino-cerebellar tracts are affected even at low levels. The nerve cells, chiefly those of the posterior root ganglia, Clarke's column and dentate nucleus, also show degenerative changes, and sometimes disappear. In the peripheral nerves, the afferent fibers are frequently degenerated. Such lesions are found in the optic, trigeminal, and sciatic nerves. Mellanby reports a dog on a deficient diet for seven years which was completely blind, due to optic nerve degeneration.
>
> "Zimmerman has studied the nervous lesions in A deficiency with similar results except for the changes in the optic nerve. The distribution of the lesions was similar to that described by Mellanby. Zimmerman observed the persistence of nerve lesions after recovery. The lesions manifest themselves first by a clumsy in-coordination, and finally, spasticity. Mellanby related the eye lesions to the degeneration of the trigeminal nerve, considering the former due to the degeneration. This is an interesting theory, which is, as yet, unsupported by similar pathologic processes familiar to us, or by other observations of the lesions in vitamin A deficiency."

*Dental Survey*, 10, 12:62, December, 1937.

> "Principal findings of their (De Sanctis and Craig) evaluation of antirachitic agents were: that rickets are due to a deficiency of vitamin A as well as of vitamin D; ... "

Mathews, *Principles of Biochemistry*, page 411, William Wood and Co., 1936.

> "FUNCTIONS OF VITAMIN A IN THE BODY. Vitamin A is necessary for proper growth of young mammals and other animals; and it is necessary probably for the continued health of all tissues of epiblastic origins. Thus it is needed by the brain and central nervous system, the retina of the eye, the skin and all skin glands such as the tear, sweat, sebaceous, salivary and other skin glands; for the mucous membranes of the mouth and vagina, both of these being of epiblastic origin. Its presence in the liver indicates that it fulfills some function in that organ. There is some evidence that it is needed for the health of the mucous membrane of the intestine. It seems to play also some part in fertility and the processes of reproduction. Whether it is necessary for the blood-forming or hematopoietic system is doubtful, but some observations indicate that it is.

"The absence of the vitamin in the diet causes certain definite and specific diseases and predisposes to general infections."

Booth and Hansen, *Present Day Status of Vitamins*, Journal Lancet, 57, 12:532-533, December, 1937.

"Chief Symptoms of Avitaminosis A

A. In Man.

1. Night blindness (nyctolopia or hemeralopia), and xerophthalmia (keratomalacia) eventually leading to partial or complete blindness. Bitot's spots, opaque whitish deposits in the scleral conjunctive, are the most characteristic signs.
2. Keratinization of epithelial cells in various parts of the body frequently associated with respiratory, gastrointestinal and genitourinary disturbances.
3. Cornification and eruption of the skin with papular and pustular lesions.
4. Retarded growth, weakness and loss of weight.
5. Increased susceptibility to infections of mucous membranes (claimed by some, denied by others). Only true where supply of vitamin A has been inadequate or its storage in the body depleted."

Macleod, *Physiology in Modern Medicine*, page 732, C. V. Mosby Co., 1935.

"A definite structural change occurs in the epithelial surfaces when the diet is deficient in vitamin A. This consists in substitution of stratified keratinizing epithelium for the normal epithelium in the respiratory, digestive, and genitourinary tracts, and it is possible that it is on this account that these become more susceptible to infections. In any case, such changes in the alimentary canal must interfere with food absorption and, as we have seen, it is on this account and not because of any specific growth-promoting properties that the body weight falls in absence of this vitamin."

# VITAMIN NEWS

**VITAMIN PRODUCTS CO. • MILWAUKEE, WISCONSIN**

**August 15, 1937** **VOL. 5**


## BIBLIOGRAPHY FOR VITAMIN CHART

### (VITAMIN B)


1. Eddy, W. H. and Dalldorf, G., *The Avitaminoses*, pages 79, 115, The Williams and Wilkins Co., Baltimore, 1937.
— McClendon, J. F., *A Manual of Biochemistry*, page 4, John Wiley & Sons, Inc., New York, 1934.
— Sherman, H. C. and Smith, S. L., *The Vitamins*, Second Edition, Monograph Series, No. 6, pages 72, 73, The Chemical Catalog Co., New York, 1931.
— Sure, Barnett, *Vitamins in Health and Disease*, pages 39, 41, The Williams and Wilkins Co., Baltimore, 1933.

2. Eddy, W. H. and Dalldorf, G., *The Avitaminoses*, page 79, The Williams and Wilkins Co., Baltimore, 1937.
— Howell, William H., *Textbook of Physiology*, Twelfth Edition, Revised, page 969, W. B. Saunders Co., Philadelphia, 1933.
— Medical Research Council, *Vitamins: A Survey of Present Knowledge*, pages 128-129, London, 1932.
— Morgan, A. F. and Barry, M. M., *American Journal of Diseases of Children*, 39:933, 1930.
— Quigley, D. T., *Notes on Vitamins and Diets*, page 41, Consolidated Book Publishers, Inc., Chicago, 1933.
— Ross, J. R. and Summerfeldt, P., *American Journal of Diseases of Children,* 49:1185, 1935.
— Summerfeldt, P., *American Journal of Diseases of Children*, 45:284, 1932.
— Sure, Barnett, *Vitamins in Health and Disease*, page 39, The Williams and Wilkins Co., Baltimore, 1933.

3. Eddy, W. H. and Dalldorf, G., *The Avitaminoses*, pages 81-82, The Williams and Wilkins Co., Baltimore, 1937.
— Howell, Wm. H., *Textbook of Physiology*, Twelfth Edition, Revised, page 101, W.B. Saunders Co., Philadelphia, 1933.
— Macleod, J. J. R., *Physiology in Modern Medicine*, Seventh Edition, page 744, C. V. Mosby Company, St. Louis, 1935.
— Mathews, Albert P., *Principles of Biochemistry*, pages 56, 58, 429, William Wood and Co., Baltimore, 1936.
— Medical Research Council, *Vitamins: A Survey of Present Knowledge*, page 133, London, 1932.
— Quigley, D. T., *Notes on Vitamins and Diets*, page 54, Consolidated Book Publishers Co., Inc., Chicago, 1933.
— Stepp, W., Kuhnau, J. and Schroeder, H., *The Vitamins and Their Clinical Application*, Ferdinand Enke, Stuttgart, Germany, 1936.
— Wiggers, Carl J., *Physiology in Health and Disease*, page 961, Lea and Febiger Co., Philadelphia, 1934.

4. Eddy, W. H. and Dalldorf, G., *The Avitaminoses*, pages 111, 112, 117, 119, The Williams and Wilkins Co., Baltimore, 1937.
— Mathews, Albert P., *Principles of Biochemistry*, page 420, William Wood & Co., Baltimore, 1936.
— Medical Research Council, *Vitamins: A Survey of Present Knowledge*, pages 132-133, 139, London, 1932.
— Quigley, D. T., *Notes on Vitamins and Diets*, pages 36-39, The Consolidated Book Publishers Co., Inc., Chicago, 1933.
— Sherman, H. C. and Smith, S. L., *The Vitamins*, Second Edition, Monograph Series, No. 6, The Chemical Catalog

Co., New York, 1931.
— Stepp, W., Kuhnau, J. and Schroeder, H., *The Vitamins and Their Clinical Application*, Ferdinand Enke, Stuttgart, Germany, 1936.

5. *Chicago Tribune*, Find Way to Synthesize Second Vitamin: Aid to Insanity, January 28, 1935.
— Eddy, W. H. and Dalldorf, G., *The Avitaminoses*, page 105, The Williams and Wilkins Co., Baltimore, 1937.
— Gildea, M. C. L., Castle, W. B., Gildea, E. F., and Cobbs, S., Neuropathology of Experimental Vitamin Deficiency, *American Journal of Pathology,* 11, 65:669, July, 1935.
— Quigley, Daniel Thomas, *Notes on Vitamins and Diets*, page 43, Consolidated Book Publishers Co., Inc., Chicago, 1933.
— Schuler, R., Chemistry and Physiology of Vitamin B,. *Drug & Cosmetic Industry*, 39, 2:180, August, 1936.

6. Mathews, Albert P., *Principles of Biochemistry*, page 59, William Wood & Co., Baltimore, 1936.
— Webster and Armour, *Proceedings of Society for Experimental Biology and Medicine*, January, 1934.

7. Stepp, W., Kuhnau, J. and Schroeder, H., *The Vitamins and Their Clinical Application*, Ferdinand Enke, Stuttgart, Germany, 1936.

8. Mathews, Albert P., *Physiological Chemistry*, Fourth Edition, page 855, William Wood & Co., Baltimore, 1925.

9. Eddy, W. H. and Dalldorf, G., *The Avitaminoses*, page 264, The Williams and Wilkins Co., Baltimore, 1937.
— Mathews, Albert P., *Principles of Biochemistry*, page 421, William Wood Co., Baltimore, 1936.
— McCollum, E. V. and Simmons, Nina, *The Newer Knowledge of Nutrition*, Fourth Edition, page 499, Macmillan Co., New York, 1929.
— Medical Research Council, *Vitamins: A Survey of Present Knowledge*, page 137, London, 1932.

10. Eddy, W. H. and Dalldorf, G., *The Avitaminoses*, pages 81, 116, 117, The Williams and Wilkins Co., Baltimore, 1937.
— Harris, L. J., *Vitamins in Theory and Practice*, pages 64-67, Cambridge University Press, London, 1935.
— Howell, William H., *A Textbook of Physiology*, Twelfth Edition, Revised, page 930, W. B. Saunders Co., Philadelphia, 1933.
— Labbe, Nepreux and Gringoire, *Bull. Acad. De Med.*, Paris, 109:689-702, 1933.
— MacLeod, J. J. R., *Physiology in Modern Medicine*, Seventh Edition, page 744, C. V. Mosby Co., St. Louis, 1935.
— Mathews, Albert P., *Principles of Biochemistry*, page 57, Williams Wood & Co., Baltimore, 1936.
— McCollum, E. V. and Simmons, Nina, *The Newer Knowledge of Nutrition*, Fourth Edition, page 223, Macmillan Co., 1929.
— Medical Research Council, *Vitamins: A Survey of Present Knowledge*, pages 133-134, 1932.
— Schrader, G. A., *Alabama Agricultural Experimental Station*, Forty-second Annual Report, page 35, 1931.
— Sherman, H. C. and Smith, S. L., *The Vitamins*, Second Edition, Monograph Series, No. 6, pages 70, 81, The Chemical Catalog Co., Inc., New York, 1931.
— Stepp, W., Kuhnau, J. and Schroeder, H., *The Vitamins and Their Clinical Application*, Ferdinand Enke, Stuttgart, Germany, 1936.
— Sure, B., *Vitamins in Health and Disease*, page 41, The Williams and Wilkins Co., Baltimore, 1933.
— Vorhaus, M. G., Williams, R. R. and Waterman, R. E., Studies and Crystalline Vitamin $B_1$: Observations in Diabetes, *American Journal Of Digestive Diseases and Nutrition*, 2, (:541-557, November, 1935.
— Wiggers, Carl J., *Physiology in Health and Disease*, page 961, Lea and Febiger, Philadelphia, 1934.

11. Barborka, C. J., Diet and Preventive Dentistry, *Journal of the American Dental Association*, 23, 8:977-985, June, 1936.
— Eddy, W. H. and Dalldorf, G., *The Avitaminoses*, pages 84, 106-107, The Williams and Wilkins Co., Baltimore, 1937.
— Harris, L. J., *Vitamins in Theory and Practice*, pages 65-67, Cambridge University Press, London, 1935.
— Howell, W. H. A., *Textbook of Physiology*, Twelfth Edition, Revised, page 970, W. B. Saunders Co., Philadelphia, 1933.
— Macleod, J. J. R., *Physiology in Modern Medicine*, Seventh Edition, pages 744-745, C. V. Mosby Co., St. Louis, 1935.
— Mathews, Albert P., *Principles of Biochemistry*, pages 58, 59, 421, William Wood & Co., Baltimore, 1936.
— McCollum, E. V. and Simmons, Nina, *The Newer Knowledge of Nutrition*, Fourth Edition, pages 231-232, Macmillan Co., 1929.
— Medical Research Council, *Vitamins: A Survey of Present Knowledge*, pages 134-137, London, 1932.
— Sherman, H. C. and Smith, S. L., *The Vitamins*, Second Edition, Monograph Series, No. 6, pages 70, 81, 82, The Chemical Catalog Co., Inc., New York, 1931.
— Stepp, W., Kuhnau, J. and Schroeder, H., *The Vitamins and Their Clinical Application*, Ferdinand Enke, Stuttgart, Germany, 1936.
— Sure, Barnett, *Vitamins in Health and Disease*, page 41, The Williams and Wilkins Co., Baltimore, 1933.
— Tahoka Journal of Experimental Medicine, page 184, 1935.
— Vorhaus, M. G., Williams, R. R. and Waterman, R. E., Studies on Crystalline Vitamin $B_1$: Observations in Diabetes, *American Journal of Digestive Diseases and Nutrition*, 2, 9:541-557, November, 1935.
— Wiggers, C. J., *Physiology in Health and Disease*, page 960, Lea & Febiger Co., Philadelphia, 1934.
— Barborka, C. J., Diet and Preventive Dentistry, *Journal of the American Dental Association,* 23, 6:977-985, June, 1936.
— Eddy, W. H. and Dalldorf, G., *The Avitaminoses*, pages 79-80, 94, 105-106, 112-114, 116, The Williams and Wilkins Co., Baltimore, 1937.
— Fitts, J. B., Motor and Secretory Dysfunction of the Gastro-intestinal Tract and the Vitamin B Factor: A Clinical Study, *Southern Medical Journal,* 28:920-923, October, 1935.
— Howell, W. H., *Textbook of Physiology*, Twelfth Edition, Revised, page 970, W. B. Saunders Co., Philadelphia, 1933.
— Marks, H. E., *Medical Journal and Record*, March 2, 1932.
— Mathews, Albert P., *Principles of Biochemistry*, page 423, William Wood & Co., Baltimore, 1936.
— McCollum, E. V. and Simmons, Nina, *The Newer Knowledge of Nutrition*, Fourth Edition, pages 227, 231-232, Macmillan Company, 1929.
— Medical Research Council, *Vitamins: A Survey of Present Knowledge*, pages 131, 134-135, 137, London, 1932.
— Rowlands, M. J. and Browning, E., *Lancet*, 1:180, 1928.
— Sherman, H. C. and Smith, S. L., *The Vitamins*, Second Edition, Monograph Series, No. 6, pages 70-71, 74-75, The Chemical Catalog Co., Inc., New York, 1931.
— Sparks, M. I. and Collins, E. N., The Role of Vitamin $B_1$ in Tonus of the Large Intestine, *American Journal of Digestive Diseases and Nutrition,* 2, 10:618-620, December, 1935.
— Stepp, W., Kuhnau, J. and Schroeder, H., *The Vitamins and Their Clinical Application*, Ferdinand Enke, Stuttgart, Germany, 1936.
— Sure, B., *Vitamins in Health and Disease*, page 40, The Williams and Wilkins Co., Baltimore, 1933.
— Wiggers, Carl J., *Physiology in Health and Disease*, pages 961-962, Lea & Febiger Co., Philadelphia, 1934.

13. Calais, J. A., *Became. Ztschr.*, 134:194-214, 1922.
— Drummond, J. C. and Marrian, G. F., The Physiological Role of Vitamin $B_1$, the Relationship of Vitamin B to

Tissue Oxidation, *Biochemical Journal,* 20:1229-1255, 1926.
— Eggleton, R. and Gross, L., A Note on the Blood Sugar Levels of Rats Fed With Complete Diets and Diets Deficient in Vitamin B., *Biochemical Journal*, 19:633-637, 1925.
— McCollum, E. V., and Simmons, Nina, *The Newer Knowledge of Nutrition*, Fourth Edition, page 493, Macmillan Co., 1929.
— Sherman, H. C. and Smith, S. L., *The Vitamins*, Second Edition, Monograph Series, No. 6, page 83, The Chemical Catalog Co., Inc., New York, 1931.
— Stepp, W., Kuhnau, J. and Schroeder, H., *The Vitamins and Their Clinical Application*, Ferdinand Enke, Stuttgart, Germany, 1936.
— Sure, B., *Vitamins in Health and Disease*, page 40, The Williams and Wilkins Co., Baltimore, 1933.

14. Barborka, C. J., Diet and Preventive Dentistry, *Journal of the American Dental Association,* 23, 6:977-985, June, 1936.
— Eddy, W. H. and Dalldorf, G., *The Avitaminoses*, page 80, The Williams and Wilkins Co., Baltimore, 1937.
— Howell, William H., *Textbook of Physiology*, Twelfth Edition, Revised, page 970, W. B. Saunders Co., Philadelphia, 1933.
— Marks, H. E., *Medical Journal and Record*, March 2, 1932.
— Mathews, Albert, P., *Principles of Biochemistry*, page 421, William Wood & Co., Baltimore, 1936.
— Medical Research Council, *Vitamins: A Survey of Present Knowledge*, page 129, London, 1932.
— Sherman, H. C. and Smith, S. L., *The Vitamins*, Second Edition, Monograph Series, No. 6, pages 70, 72, 83, The Chemical Catalog Co., Inc., New York, 1931.
— Shipley, P. G., McCollum, E. V. and Simmons, N., Studies in Experimental Rickets, IX, Lesions in the Bones of Rats Suffering from Uncomplicated Beriberi, *Journal of Biological Chemistry,* 49:399-410, 1921.
— Stepp, W., Kuhnau, J. and Schroeder, H., *The Vitamins and Their Clinical Application*, Ferdinand Enke, Stuttgart, Germany, 1936.
— Sure, B., *Vitamins in Health and Disease*, pages 53-54, The Williams and Wilkins Co., Baltimore, 1933.
— Wiggers, Carl J., *Physiology in Health and Disease*, pages 961-962, Lea & Febiger Co., Philadelphia, 1934.

15. Delafield, F. and Prudden, T. M., *Textbook of Pathology*, Fifteenth Edition, page 496, William Wood & Co., New York, 1931.
— Mathews, Albert P., *Principles of Biochemistry*, page 423, William Wood & Co., Baltimore, 1936.
— Stepp, W., Kuhnau, J. and Schroeder, H., *The Vitamins and Their Clinical Application*, Ferdinand Enke, Stuttgart, Germany, 1936.

16. Howell, William H., *Textbook of Physiology*, Twelfth Edition, Revised, page 970, W. B. Saunders Co., Philadelphia, 1933.
— Macleod, J. J. R., *Physiology in Modern Medicine*, Seventh Edition, page 744, C. V. Mosby Co., St. Louis, 1935.
— Medical Research Council, *Vitamins: A Survey of Present Knowledge*, page 131, London, 1932.
— Sherman, H. C. and Smith, S. L., *The Vitamins*, Second Edition, Monograph Series, No. 6, page 70, The Chemical Catalog Co., Inc., New York, 1931.
— Stepp, W., Kuhnau, J. and Schroeder, H., *The Vitamins and Their Clinical Application*, Ferdinand Enke, Stuttgart, Germany, 1936.

17. Delafield, F. and Prudden, T. M., *Textbook of Pathology*, page 496, Fifteenth Edition, William Wood & Co., Baltimore, 1931.
— Eddy, W. H. and Dalldorf, G., *The Avitaminoses*, pages 103-105, The Williams and Wilkins Co., Baltimore, 1937.

— Gildea, M. C. L., Castle, W. B., Gilbea, E. F. and Cobb, S., Neuropathology of Experimental Vitamin Deficiency, *American Journal of Pathology,* 11, 65:669, July, 1935.
— Harris, L. J., *Vitamins in Theory and Practice*, page 67, Cambridge University Press, London, 1935.
— Howell, William H., *Textbook of Physiology*, Twelfth Edition, Revised, page 970, W. B. Saunders Co., Philadelphia, 1933.
— Mathews, Albert P., *Principles of Biochemistry*, pages 59, 419-420, William Wood and Co., Baltimore, 1936.
— Sherman, H. C. and Smith, S. L., *The Vitamins*, Second Edition, Monograph Series, No. 6, page 70, The Chemical Catalog Co., Inc., New York, 1931.
— Stepp, W., Kuhnau, J. and Schroeder, H., *The Vitamins and Their Clinical Application*, Ferdinand Enke, Stuttgart, Germany, 1936.
— Wiggers, C. J., *Physiology in Health and Disease*, pages 960-962, Lea & Febiger Co., Philadelphia, 1934.

18. Haden, R., *American Journal of Digestive Diseases and Nutrition*, 1:628, 1934.
— Hutter, A. M., Middleton, Wm. S. and Steenbock, H., *Journal of the American Association*, 101:1305, 1925.
— Macleod, J. J. R., *Physiology in Modern Medicine*, Seventh Edition, pages 744-745, C. V. Mosby Co., St. Louis, 1935.
— McCollum, E. V. and Simmons, Nina, *The Newer Knowledge of Nutrition*, Fourth Edition, page 223, MacMillan Co., 1929
— Medical Research Council, *Vitamins: A Survey of Present Knowledge,* page 137, London, 1932.

19. Eddy, W. H. and Dalldorf, G., *The Avitaminoses*, page 107, The Williams and Wilkins Co., Baltimore, 1937.
— Frank, R. T., *The Female Sex Hormone*, page 123, Charles C. Thomas, Baltimore, 1929.
— Hitsuko, Chin., *Journal Chosen Medical Association*, 23:968.
— Mathews, Albert P., *Principles of Biochemistry*, page 423, William Wood & Co., Baltimore, 1936.
— MacLeod, J. J. R., *Physiology in Modern Medicine*, Seventh Edition, page 745, C. V. Mosby Co., St. Louis, 1935.
— Medical Research Council, *Vitamins: A Survey of Present Knowledge*, page 136, London, 1932.
— Moore, Carl R. and Samuels, L. J., *American Journal of Physiology*, 96:278, 1931.
— Carl R. and Samuels, L. J., *American Journal of Physiology*, 96:278, 1931.
— Medical Research Council, *Vitamins: A Survey of Present Knowledge*, page 127, London, 1932.
— Stepp, W., Kuhnau, J. and Schroeder, H., *The Vitamins and Their Clinical Application*, Ferdinand Enke, Stuttgart, Germany, 1936.

20. Stepp, W., Kuhnau, J. and Schroeder, H., *The Vitamins and Their Clinical Application*, Ferdinand Enke, Stuttgart, Germany, 1936.

21. Mathews, Albert P., *Principles of Biochemistry*, pages 918-919, William Wood and Co., Baltimore, 1925.

22. Barborka, Clifford J., Diet and Preventive Dentistry, *Journal of the American Dental Association*, 23, 6:977, June 1936.
— Cutter, Irving S., How to Keep Well: Scurvy and the Onset of Arthritis, *Chicago Daily Tribune,* January 21, 1936.
— Eddy, W. H. and Dalldorf, G., *The Avitaminoses*, pages 79, 90, 97, The Williams and Wilkins Co., Baltimore, 1937.
— Mathews, Albert P., *Principles of Biochemistry*, page 419, William Wood and Co., Baltimore, 1936.
— Medical Research Council, *Vitamins: A Survey of Present Knowledge*, page 127, London, 1932.

23. Delafield, F. and Prudden, T. M., *Textbook of Pathology*, page 496, Fifteenth Edition, William Wood & Co.,

Baltimore, 1931.
— Eddy, W. H. and Dalldorf, G., *The Avitaminoses*, pages 89, 103-105, The Williams and Wilkins Co., Baltimore, 1937.
— Mathews, Albert P., *Principles of Biochemistry*, pages 419-420, William Wood and Co., Baltimore, 1937.

24. Gildea, M. C. L., Castle, W. B., Gilbea, E. F. and Cobb, S., Neuropathology of Experimental Vitamin Deficiency, *American Journal of Pathology*, 11, 65:669, July, 1935.
— Mathews, Albert P., *Principles of Biochemistry*, pages 419-420, William Wood and Co., Baltimore, 1936.
— Medical Research Council, *Vitamins: A Survey of Present Knowledge*, page 129, London, 1932.
— Sherman, H. C. and Smith, S. L., *The Vitamins*, Second Edition, Monograph Series, No. 6, page 83, The Chemical Catalog Co., Inc., New York, 1931.

Medical Research Council, *Vitamins: A Survey of Present Knowledge*, page 122, London, 1932.

> "There is now a general consensus of opinion that beriberi is a disease of dietetic origin...
>
> "Beriberi may appear in two well-marked forms. In one ('dry' type) there is great muscular wasting, anesthesia of the skin, and finally paralysis of the legs, and in some cases of the arms, diaphragm and intercostal muscles. There is an associated degeneration of the peripheral nerves involving both motor and sensory fibres..."

Peters, Biochemical Lesion in Vitamin $B_1$ Deficiency, *Lancet*, 1:1161, May 23, 1936.

> "Upon this absence of an important factor ($B_1$) in the development of energy from carbohydrates would be sufficient to stop normal functioning of some groups of nerve cells. Those which normally had the most work to do might be expected to run out of their supply of the catalyst vitamin $B_1$ sooner than others. In other words, interrupt the normal metabolism of glucose at any stage, and brain cells do not function properly..."

Booth and Hansen, The Present Day Status of the Vitamins, *Journal Lancet,* 57, 12:534, December, 1937.

> "Chief Symptoms of Avitaminosis $B_1$.
>
> A. In Man.
>
> 1. Beriberi
>    (a) Peripheral neuritis with paralysis of extremities and muscular atrophy or edema.
>    (b) Vasomotor symptoms: heart palpitations, dyspnea, enlargement of right side of heart.
> 2. Retarded growth and development.
> 3. Polyneuritis, especially of alcoholic origin; also in pregnancy, in diabetes, and in malnutrition in children, and in the malnutrition associated with chronic diseases or some primary alimentary disease.
> 4. Gastrointestinal disturbances: atrophy of lingual papillae, achlorhydria, intestinal hypotonicity.
> 5. Ocular disorders: retinal hemorrhages, optic neuritis.
> 6. Anorexia.
> 7. Impaired carbohydrate metabolism.
> 8. Failure of lactation."

Ibid, page 535.

"Clinical Applications of Vitamin $B_1$.

1. Prevention and cure of beriberi.
2. Promotion of normal growth in children.
3. Anorexia due to avitaminosis B.
4. In chronic alcoholism with Vitamin B-deficiency polyneuritis.
5. In pernicious vomiting and polyneuritis of pregnancy.
6. For nutrition in lactating women.
7. Valuable in concentrated form in conditions where ordinary foods are poorly utilized.
8. In diabetic neuritis.
9. In cardiovascular disease (Weiss and Wilkins — 1936. Sure and Jones — 1937)."

Sure, *Vitamins in Health and Disease*, page 41, Williams and Wilkins Co., 1933.

# NOTES

// VITAMIN NEWS

VITAMIN PRODUCTS CO. • MILWAUKEE, WISCONSIN

September 15, 1937 VOL. 5

## BIBLIOGRAPHY FOR VITAMIN CHART

### (VITAMIN C)

1. Eddy, W. H., and Dalldorf, G., *The Avitaminoses*, page 169, The Williams and Wilkins Co., Baltimore, 1937.
— Findlay, G. M., The Relation of Vitamin C to Bacterial Infection, *Journal of Pathology and Bacteriology,* 26:1-18, 1923.
— Hess, A. F., *American Journal of Diseases of Children*, November, 1927.
— *Medicine*, 13:205, 1934.
— *Proceedings of Society of Experimental Biology and Medicine*, page 1157, April, 1935.
— Quigley, Daniel Thomas, *Notes on Vitamins and Diets*, page 126, Consolidated Book Publisihers Inc., Chicago, 1933.
— Wiggers, C. J., *Physiology in Health and Disease*, page 987, Lea & Febiger, Philadelphia, 1934.

2. Eddy, W. H. and Dalldorf, G., *The Avitaminoses*, page 169, The Williams and Wilkins Co., Baltimore, 1937.
— Medical Research Council, *Vitamins: A Survey of Present Knowledge*, page 102, London, 1932.
— *Vitamin D Milk,* 2, 1:2, January, 1935.

3. Eddy, W. H. and Dalldorf, G., *The Avitaminoses*, pages 168-169, 185, The Williams and Wilkins Co., Baltimore, 1937.
— Harris, L. J., *Vitamins in Theory and Practice*, page 106, Cambridge University Press, 1935.
— Wiggers, C. J., *Physiology in Health and Disease*, pages 967-968, Lea & Febiger, Philadelphia, 1934.

4. Stepp, W., Kuhnau, J. and Schroeder, *The Vitamins and Their Clinical Application,* Ferdinand Enke, Stuttgart, Germanay, 1936.

5. Stepp, W., Kuhnau, J. and Schroeder, *The Vitamins and Their Clinical Application*, Ferdinand Enke, Stuttgart, Germany, 1936.

6. Barborka, C. J., Diet and Preventive Dentistry, *Journal of the American Dental Association,* 23, 6:977-985, June, 1936.
— Delafield, F. and Prudden, T. M., *A Textbook of Pathology*, Fifteenth Edition, pages 495-496, William Wood & Co., New York, 1931.
— Drummond, J. C. and Marrian, G. F., The Physiological Role of Vitamin B., I. The Relation of Vitamin B to Tissue Oxidation, *Biochemical Journal,* 20:1229-1255, 1926.
— Eddy, W. H. and Dalldorf, G., *The Avitaminoses*, pages 169, 175, 178, 185, The Williams and Wilkins Co., Baltimore, 1937.
— Findlay, G. M., The Blood and Blood Vessels in Guinea Pig Scurvy, *Journal of Pathology and Bacteriology,* 24:446-454, 1921.

— Hanke, M. T., *Journal of Nutrition*, 3, 4:448, January, 1931.
— Harris, L. J., *Vitamins in Theory and Practice*, pages 106, 212, 213, Cambridge University Press, 1935.
— *Journal of the American Medical Association*, 103, 13:1022, September 29, 1934.
— Macleod, J. J. R., *Physiology in Modern Medicine*, Seventh Edition, pages 747, 749, C. V. Mosby, St. Louis, 1935.
— McClendon, J. F., *A Manual of Biochemistry*, pages 4, 87, John Wiley & Sons, Inc., New York, 1934.
— Medical Research Council, *Vitamins: A Survey of Present Knowledge*, pages 90, 102, 192-193, London, 1932.
— Plimmer, R. H. B. and Plimmer, V. G., *Foods, Health, Vitamins,* Third Edition, page 18, Longmans Green & Co., New York, 1928.
— Quigley, Daniel Thomas, *Notes on Vitamins and Diets*, pages 120, 126-127, Consolidated Book Publishers, Inc., Chicago, 1933.
— Quigley, D. T., *Vitamin Chart*, Consolidated Book Publishers, Inc., Chicago, 1933.
— Sherman, H. C., *Chemistry of Food & Nutrition*, Fifth Edition, page 441, The Macmillan Co., New York, 1937.
— Sherman, H. C. and Smith, S. L., *The Vitamins*, Second Edition, Monograph Series, No. 6, pages 162-163, 164, 166, 172, The Chemical Catalog Co., Inc., New York, 1931.
— Stepp, W., Kuhnau, J. and Schroeder, H., *The Vitamins and Their Clinical Application*, Ferdinand Enke, Stuttgart, Germany, 1936.
— Sure, B., *Vitamins in Health and Disease*, page 79, The Williams and Wilkins Co., Baltimore, 1933.
— Wiggers, C. J., *Physiology in Health and Disease*, pages 967-968, Lea & Febiger, Philadelphia, 1934.

7. *Archives of Internal Medicine*, 51:426.
— Quigley, D. T., *Notes on Vitamins and Diets*, page 43, Consolidated Book Publishers, Inc., Chicago, 1933.

8. *Drug Trade News, 10, 9:35, April, 1935.*
— Eddy, W. H. and Dalldorf, G., *The Avitaminoses*, page 177, The Williams and Wilkins Co., Baltimore, 1937.
— *Proceedings of Society of Experimental Biology and Medicine*, page 1089, April, 1935.
— Sherman, H. C. and Smith, S. L., *The Vitamins*, Second Edition, Monograph Series, No. 6, pages 163-164, The Chemical Catalog Co., Inc., New York, 1931.
— Stepp, W., Kuhnau, J. and Schroeder, H., *The Vitamins and Their Clinical Application*, Ferdinand Enke, Stuttgart, Germany, 1936.
— Wiggers, C. J., *Physiology in Health and Disease*, page 969, Lea & Febiger, Philadelphia, 1934.

9. Eddy, W. H. and Dalldorf, G, *The Avitaminoses*, page 177, The Williams and Wilkins Co., Baltimore, 1937.
— Sherman, H. C. and Smith, S. L., *The Vitamins*, Second Edition, Monograph Series, No. 6, pages 171-172, The Chemical Catalog Co., Inc., New York, 1931.
— Stepp, W., Kuhnau, J. and Schroeder, H., *The Vitamins and Their Clinical Application*, Ferdinand Enke, Stuttgart, Germany, 1936.
— Wiggers, C. J., *Physiology in Health and Disease*, page 967, Lea & Febiger, Philadelphia, 1934.

10. Eddy, W. H. and Dalldorf, *The Avitaminoses*, page 175, The Williams and Wilkins Co., Baltimore, 1937.
— Quigley, D. T., *Vitamin Chart*, Consolidated Book Publishers, Inc., Chicago, 1933.

11. Eddy, W. H. and Dalldorf, G., *The Avitaminoses*, page 175, The Williams and Wilkins Co., Baltimore, 1937.
— Quigley, D. T., *Vitamin Chart*, Consolidated Book Publishers, Inc., Chicago, 1933.
— Wiggers, C. J., *Physiology in Health and Disease*, page 968, Lea & Febiger, Philadelphia, 1934.

12. Archives of *Diseases of Childhood*, 8:117-144, 1933.
— Delafield, F. and Prudden, T. M., *A Textbook of Pathology*, Fifteenth Edition, pages 495-496, William Wood & Co., New York, 1931.
— Eddy, W. H. and Dalldorf, G., *The Avitaminoses*, page 179, The Williams and Wilkins Co., Baltimore, 1937.

13. Quigley, D. T., *Notes on Vitamins and Diets*, page 126, Consolidated Book Publishers, Inc., Chicago, 1933.
— Stepp, W., Kuhnau, J. and Schroeder, H., *The Vitamins and Their Clinical Application*, Ferdinand Enke, Stuttgart, Germany, 1936.

14. Berglund, Medes, Huber, Longcope and Richards, *The Kidney in Health and Diseases*, pages 150-151, Lea and Febiger Co., Philadelphia, 1935.
— Eddy, W. H. and Dalldorf, G., *The Avitaminoses*, page 179, The Williams and Wilkins Co., Baltimore, 1937.
— Medical Research Council, *Vitamins: A Survey of Present Knowledge*, pages 192-193, London, 1932.
— Sherman, H. C. and Smith, S. L., *The Vitamins*, Second Edition, Monograph Series, No. 6, page 166, The Chemical Catalog Co., Inc., New York, 1931.

15. Eddy, W. H. and Dalldorf, G., *The Avitaminoses*, pages 190, 202, The Williams and Wilkins Co., Baltimore, 1937.
— Medical Research Council, *Vitamins: A Survey of Present Knowledge*, pages 192-193, London, 1932.
— Sherman, H. C. and Smith, S. L., *The Vitamins*, Second Edition, Monograph Series, No. 6, page 166, The Chemical Catalog Co., Inc., New York, 1931.

16. Cutter, Irving S., How to Keep Well, *Chicago Daily Tribune,* Chicago, January 21, 1936.
— Eddy, W. H. and Dalldorf, G., *The Avitaminoses*, page 176-178, 274-275, The Williams and Wilkins Co., Baltimore, 1937.
— Rinehart, James F., *Annals of Internal Medicine*, December, 1935.

17. Eddy, W. H. and Dalldorf, G., *The Avitaminoses*, page 177, The Williams and Wilkins Co., Baltimore, 1937.

18. Eddy, W. H. and Dalldorf, G., *The Avitaminoses*, pages 203-204, The Williams and Wilkins Co., Baltimore, 1937.
— *Journal of the American Medical Association*, 103:78, 1934.
— Medical Research Council, *Vitamins: A Survey of Present Knowledge*, page 194, London, 1932.
— Sherman, H. C. and Smith, S. L., *The Vitamins*, Second Edition, Monograph Series, No. 6, The Chemical Catalog Co., Inc., New York, 1931.
— Stepp, W., Kuhnau, J. and Schroeder, H., *The Vitamins and Their Clinical Application*, Ferdinand Enke, Stuttgart, Germany, 1936.

19. Eddy, W. H. and Dalldorf, G., *The Avitaminoses*, pages 175, 177-178, The Williams and Wilkins Co., Baltimore, 1937.

20. Eddy, W. H. and Dalldorf, G., *The Avitaminoses*, page 190, The Williams and Wilkins Co., Baltimore, 1937.

21. Sigal, A. and King, C. G., The Relationship of Vitamin C to Glucose Tolerance in the Guinea Pig, *Journal of Biological Chemistry,* 116, 2:489-492, December, 1936.

22. Josephson, E., *Ascorbic Acid in Cataract*, Science, 82:222-223, September 6, 1935.

23. Mathews, Albert P., *Physiological Chemistry*, pages 918-919, William Wood & Co., Baltimore, 1925.

24. Barborka, C. J., Diet and Preventive Dentistry, *Journal of the American Dental Association*, 23, 6:977-985, June, 1936.
— Eddy, W. H. and Dalldorf, G., *The Avitaminoses*, pages 174-184, The Williams and Wilkins Co., Baltimore, 1937.
— Stepp, W., Kuhnau, J. and Schroeder, H., *The Vitamins and Their Clinical Application*, Ferdinand Enke, Stuttgart, Germany, 1936.

25. Stepp, W., Kuhnau, J. and Schroeder, H., *The Vitamins and Their Clinical Application*, Ferdinand Enke, Stuttgart, Germany, 1936.

26. Eddy, W. H. and Dalldorf, G., *The Avitaminoses*, page 185, The Williams and Wilkins Co., Baltimore, 1937.
— Macleod, J. J. R., *Physiology in Modern Medicine*, Seventh Edition, page 747, C. V. Mosby Co., St. Louis, 1935.
— Quigley, D. T., *Notes on Vitamins and Diets*, page 126, Consolidated Book Publishers, Inc., Chicago, 1933.

Medical Research Council, *Vitamins: A Survey of Present Knowledge*, page 102, London, 1932.

> "Extensive investigations of Hojer and others have also emphasized the importance of vitamin C in determining the structure of the teeth in guinea pigs. They summarize the defects that follow vitamin C deficiency as follows:
>
> 1. The gradual change and disappearance of the odontoblastic layer.
> 2. The amorphous calcification of the 'predentine' and the absence of canals in this layer.
> 3. The previously calcified dentine becomes porous.
> 4. The dilatation of the vessels in the pulp.
> 5. The production of nerve lesions and edema of the pulp tissues."

Eddy and Dalldorf, *The Avitaminoses*, page 169, 1937.

> " ... In the absence of vitamin C, certain cells are no longer able to perform their function properly, and this is why in scurvy the blood vessels become too weak and bleeding results, and why the teeth also, for example, lose their normal structure and become diseased."

Ibid, page 177.

> " ... Frolich has reported eight characteristics which he considers helpful. These are dystrophy, anorexia, anemia, occasional slight edema, cessation in gain of weight or loss of weight, susceptibility to infection, intestinal disturbances and now and then more pronounced symptoms such as hematuria ... "

Berglund, Medes, Huber, Longcope and Richards, *The Kidney in Health and Disease*, page 150, 1935.

> "In scorbutic (vitamin C deficient) guinea pigs, Bessesen described a progressive increase in renal weight, amounting to 58 per cent at death from scurvy ... "

Wiggers, *Physiology in Health and Disease*, page 967, 1934.

> " ... Recent knowledge as to the character of the vitamin makes it probable that it also acts by virtue of its unique reducing properties to promote oxidative and respiratory functions of tissues."

Ibid, page 968.

> "Another group of symptoms (of vitamin C deficiency) appears to be more related to oxidative disturbances of more highly differentiated cells. This is particularly true of certain manifestations referable to the nervous system, e. g., the tachycardia and rapid respirations, sensory paresthesias, pains, hyperalgesia, patchy anesthetic areas and loss of the knee jerk ... "

Petter, Vitamin C and Tuberculosis, *The Journal-Lancet*, 57:221, May, 1937.

> "Guinea pigs on vitamin C deficient diets show decreased resistance to tuberculosis infection and disease ...
>
> "Clinically, vitamin C deficiency is definitely demonstrable in all forms of tuberculosis, most marked in the febrile and destructive forms of the disease ...
>
> " ... Grant has shown that the addition of vitamin C to an adequate diet increases the resistance to tuberculosis, while — interestingly — the addition of vitamin D to a C deficient diet lowers the resistance ... "

Osol, Treatment of Pneumonia with Vitamin C, *American Druggist,* 95, 5:55, 138, May 1937.

> "Vitamin C does not find its only use in the treatment of scurvy and prescorbutic conditions. Already it has been used with good results in the treatment of cataract of the eye; in increasing capillary resistance and preventing capillary bleeding due to vitamin C deficiency; and in treating certain types of anemias.
>
> "The latest report on another therapeutic application of vitamin C promises an even greater field of usefulness for this important factor. In a recent issue of the Munchener medizinische Wochenschrift, Drs. J. Gander and W. Niederberger report the results of treatment of fifteen cases of pneumonia with the vitamin. Four case histories are described in detail."

Sherman, *Chemistry of Food and Nutrition*, Fifth Edition, page 441, 1937.

> "There are now a number of observations on record which indicate that vitamin C helps to protect the body from, or defer the intensification of, such changes as are characteristic of the aging process ...
>
> "Liberality of intake of vitamin C protects against capillary fragility which is a part of the aging process in most people, even those who escape disease; and under stress of combating a toxin, the body may or may not develop arteriosclerosis according to the liberality with which vitamin C is supplied. In view of such findings, and those which indicate that different passably healthy people may have very different concentrations of vitamin C in their tissues, it would seem to be well for us to keep ourselves well 'saturated' with vitamin C by taking a liberal portion of our needed food

calories in the form of fruits and vegetables."

*Chicago Herald and Examiner*, Vitamin C in Natural Form Foe to Paralysis, October 9, 1937. (Dr. C. W. Jungeblut)

"First, vitamin C from natural food sources, such as oranges, lemons and animal glands, is far more effective in treating and preventing infantile paralysis than synthetic vitamin C, called ascorbic acid, cevitamic acid and so on.

"Second, when there is more vitamin C in the body, there is less danger of having infantile paralysis.

"Third, certain persons make use of the vitamin C that they eat better than others. They are more resistant to disease."

Booth and Hansen, The Present Day Status of the Vitamins, *The Journal-Lancet*, 57, 12:538-539, December 1937.

"Chief Symptoms of Avitaminosis C

"In Man and Animals (guinea pig):

1. Scurvy — increasing pallor, irritability, spongy and bleeding gums, loosened teeth, sore and swollen joints, petechiac and large superficial hemorrhages, epistaxis, sore mouth, dyspnea, loss of energy, anorexia, loss of weight, anemia, edema, fragility of bones and pseudo-paralysis.

2. Less extreme deficiency
   a. Hemorrhagic tendencies.
   b. Dental caries, pyorrhea.
   c. Vague aches and pains.
   d. Fatigue, pallor, anemia.
   e. Abnormal cutaneous pigmentation.
   f. Increased susceptibility to infection in general, and to specific cases of diphtheria, poliomyelitis, and tuberculosis.
   g. Joint disease strikingly similar to rheumatic fever.
   h. Vague nerve disturbance; increased pulse and respiration.
   i. Sensory nerve disorders (paresthesias).
   j. Increased capillary fragility.

**Edited by Royal Lee**

VITAMIN NEWS

VITAMIN PRODUCTS CO. • MILWAUKEE, WISCONSIN

October 15, 1937 VOL. 5

## BIBLIOGRAPHY FOR VITAMIN CHART

## (VITAMIN D)

1. Becker, J. E., *Journal of the American Dietetic Association*, 10:391, 1935.
— Eddy, W. H. and Dalldorf, G., *The Avitaminoses*, page 269, The Williams and Wilkins Co., Baltimore, 1937.
— Harris, L. J., *Lancet*, No. 222, 1031, 1932.
— Harris, L. J., *Vitamins in Theory and Practice*, pages 122, 140-141, Cambridge University Press, London, 1935.
— Howell, William H., *Textbook of Physiology*, Twelfth Edition, Revised, page 972, W. B. Saunders Co., Philadelphia, 1933.
— Kay, H. D. and Guyatt, B. L., *Nature*, 131:468, 1933.
— Macleod, J. J. R., *Physiology in Modern Medicine*, Seventh Edition, page 734, C. V. Mosby Company, St. Louis, 1935.
— Mathews, Albert P., *Principles of Biochemistry*, page 417,439-440, William Wood and Co., Baltimore, 1936.
— McCollum, E. V., *Safeguarding the Growing Child*, No. 5.
— McGowan, J. P., *Journal of Biological Chemistry*, 26:1138, 1933.
— Medical Research Council, *The Influence of Diet on Caries on Children's Teeth*, pages 129-130, 132, London, 1936.
— Medical Research Council, *Vitamins: A Survey of Present Knowledge*, pages 48, 93, 100, 242, London, 1932.
— Orr, W. J., Holt, L. E., Jr., Wilkins, L. and Boone, F. G., The Calcium and Phosphorus Metabolism in Rickets, with special reference to ultraviolet ray therapy, *American Journal of Diseases of Children,* 26:362, 1923.
— Orr, W. J., Holt, L. E., Jr., Wilkins, L. and Boone, F. G., The Calcium and Phosphorus in the Diet to the Absorption of These Elements from the Intestine, *American Journal of Diseases of Children*, 28:574, 1924.
— Quigley, D. T., *Notes on Vitamins and Diets*, pages 19-20, 127, Consolidated Book Publishers, Inc., Chicago, 1933.
— Schabad, *J. A., Arch. F. Kinderh.*, 52:68, 1910.
— Schloss, E., Ergebn. *Inn. Med. Kinderh.*, 15:55, 1917.
— Sherman, H. C. and Smith, S. L., *The Vitamins*, Second Edition, Monograph Series, No. 6, pages 298-299, The Chemical Catalog Co., Inc., New York, 1931.
— Stearns, G. and Jeans, P. C., *Proceedings of the American Society of Biological Chemistry*, 114, c, 1936.
— Stepp, W., Kuhnau, J. and Schroeder, H., *The Vitamins and Their Clinical Application*, Ferdinand Enke, Stuttgart, Germany, 1936.
— Sure, Barnett, *Vitamins in Health and Disease*, page 114, The Williams and Wilkins Co., Baltimore, 1933.
— Telfer, S. V., Studies on Calcium and Phosphate Metabolism, Part I: The Excretion of Calcium and Phosphorous, *Quarterly Journal of Medicine,* 16:45, 1922-1923.
— Telfer, S. V., Studies on Calcium and Phosphate Metabolism, Part II: The Metabolism of Calcium and Phosphorous in Rickets, *Quarterly Journal of Medicine*, 16:63, 1922-1923.
— Telfer, S. V., Studies on Calcium and Phosphate Metabolism, Part III: The Absorption of Calcium and Phosphorous and Their Function in the Skeleton, *Quarterly Journal of Medicine,* 17:245, 1924.

— Wiggers, C. J., *Physiology in Health and Disease*, pages 967, 971, 1031, Lea & Febiger, Philadelphia, 1934.

2. Harris, L. J., *Vitamins in Theory and Practice*, page 122, Cambridge University Press, London, 1935.
— Medical Research Council, *Vitamins: A Survey of Present Knowledge*, pages 242, 269, London, 1932.
— Wiggers, C. J., *Physiology in Health and Disease*, page 969, Lea & Febiger, Philadelphia, 1934.

3. Richardson, G. C., *Illinois Medical Journal*, 65:367, 1934.

4. Gunn, F. D., *Proceedings of Society of Experimental Biology and Medicine*, 24:120, 1926.
— Laurens, H. and Soon, J. W., *Proceedings of the Society of Experimental Biology and Medicine*, 22:114, 1924.
— Sanford, H. N. Gastever, R. H. and Wyatt, L., *American Journal of Diseases of Children*, 43:566, 1922.

5. Gunn, F. D., *Proceedings of the Society of Experimental Biology and Medicine*, 24:120, 1926.
— McNealy, R. W., Shapiro, P. F., and Milnick, P., *Surgery, Gynecology and Obstetrics*, 60:785, 1935.
— Phillips, R. A., Robertson, D. F., Corson, W. C., and Irwin, G. F., *Annals of Internal Medicine*, 4:1134, 1934.
— Richardson, G. C., *Illinois Medical Journal*, 65:367, 1934.
— Stanford, H. N. Gastever, R. H. and Wyat, L., *American Journal of Diseases of Children*, 43:566, 1922.
— Stepp, W., Kuhnau, J. and Schroeder, H., *The Vitamins and Their Clinical Application*, Ferdinand Enke, Stuttgart, Germany, 1936.

6. Jeans, P. C. and Stearns, G., *Proceedings of the Society of Experimental Biology and Medicine*, 31:1159, 1934.
— Jeans, P. C. and Stearns, G., *Proceedings of the Society of Experimental Biology and Medicine*, 32:1464, 1935.
— Medical Research Council, *Vitamins: A Survey of Present Knowledge*, page 48, London, 1932.
— Quigley, D. T., *Notes on Vitamins and Diets*, page 21, Consolidated Book Publishers, Inc., Chicago, 1933.
— Sherman, H. C. and Smith, S. L., *The Vitamins*, Second Edition, Monograph Series, No. 6, page 320, The Chemical Catalog Co., Inc., New York, 1931.
— Stearns, G., Jeans, P. C. and Vandecar, V., *Journal of Pediatrics*, 9:1, 1936.
— Stearns, G. and Jeans, P. C., Proceedings of the American Society of Biological Chemistry, 114, c, 1936.
— Stepp, W., Kuhnau, J. and Schroeder, H., *The Vitamins and Their Clinical Application*, Ferdinand Enke, Stuttgart, Germany, 1936.
— Wiggers, C. J., *Physiology in Health and Disease*, page 969, Lea & Febiger, Philadelphia, 1934.

7. Richardson, G. C., *Illinois Medical Journal*, 65:367, 1934.

8. *Vitamin D Milk*, 3, 7:27, October, 1936.

9. Harrow, B. and Sherwin, C. P., *The Chemistry of the Hormones*, pages 31-32, The Williams and Wilkins Co., Baltimore, 1934.
— Medical Research Council, *The Influence of Diet on Caries in Children's Teeth*, pages 129-130, London, 1936.
— Stepp, W., Kuhnau, J. and Schroeder, H., *The Vitamins and Their Clinical Application*, Ferdinand Enke, Stuttgart, Germany, 1936.
— Wolf, William, *Endocrinology in Modern Practice*, page 367, W. B. Saunders Co., Philadelphia, 1936.

10. Eddy, W. H. and Dalldorf, G., *The Avitaminoses*, page 269, The Williams and Wilkins Co., Baltimore, 1937.
— Quigley, D. T., *Notes on Vitamins and Diets*, pages 20, 43-44, 88, 127, Consolidated Book Publishers, Inc., Chicago, 1933.

— Sure, Barnett, *Vitamins in Health and Disease*, page 188, The Williams and Wilkins Co., Baltimore, 1933.

11. Mathews, Albert P., *Principles of Biochemistry*, page 442, William Wood & Co., Baltimore, 1936.
— Presnell, A. K., The Relation of Vitamin D to Skin Respiration, *Journal of Biological Chemistry,* 121, 1:5-8, October, 1937.

12. Barborka, C. J., Diet and Preventive Dentistry, *Journal of the American Dental Association,* 23, 6:977-985, 1936.
— Cantarow, A., *Calcium Metabolism and Calcium Therapy*, Lea & Febiger, Philadelphia, 1931.
— Eddy, W. H. and Dalldorf, G., *The Avitaminoses*, pages 218-219, The Williams and Wilkins Co., Baltimore, 1937.
— Harris, L. J., *Vitamins in Theory and Practice*, Footnote page 127, Cambridge University Press, London, 1935.
— Mathews, Albert P., *Principles of Biochemistry*, pages 439-440, William Wood & Co., Baltimore, 1936.
— Medical Research Council, *Vitamins: A Survey of Present Knowledge*, pages 48-49, 73, 239, London, 1932.
— Quigley, D. T., *Notes on Vitamins and Diets*, page 43, Consolidated Book Publishers, Inc., Chicago, 1933.
— Stepp, W., Kuhnau, J. and Schroeder, H., *The Vitamins and Their Clinical Application*, Ferdinand Enke, Stuttgart, Germany, 1936.
— Wiggers, C. J., *Physiology in Health and Disease*, pages 971, 987, Lea & Febiger, Philadelphia, 1934.

13. Macleod, J. J. R., *Physiology in Modern Medicine*, Seventh Edition, page 734, C. V. Mosby Co., St. Louis, 1935.
— Mathews, Albert P., *Principles of Biochemistry*, page 439, William Wood & Co., Baltimore, 1936.
— Stearns, G., Jeans, P. C. and Vandecar, V., *Journal of Pediatrics*, 9:1, 1936.
— Stepp, W., Kuhnau, J. and Schroeder, H., *The Vitamins and Their Clinical Application*, Ferdinand Enke, Stuttgart, Germany, 1936.

14. Berglund, Medes, Huber, Longcope and Richards, *The Kidney in Health and Disease*, page 151, Lea & Febiger, Philadelphia, 1935.
— Mathews, Albert P., *Principles of Biochemistry*, page 439, William Wood & Co., Baltimore, 1936.

15. Barborka, C. J., Diet and Preventive Dentistry, *Journal of the American Dental Association,* 23, 6:977-985, 1936.
— Quigley, D. T., *Notes on Vitamins and Diets*, page 89, Consolidated Book Publishers, Inc., Chicago, 1933.
— Rhinehart, B. A., *Radiology*, 24:1, 1933.

16. Eddy, W. H. and Dalldorf, G., *The Avitaminoses*, page 269, The Williams and Wilkins Co., Baltimore, 1937.
— Medical Research Council, *Vitamins: A Survey of Present Knowledge*, page 54, London, 1932.
— Quigley, D. T., *Notes on Vitamins and Diets*, pages 20, 43-44, 88, 98, 127, Consolidated Book Publishers, Inc., Chicago, 1933.
— Sherman, H. C. and Smith, S. L., *The Vitamins*, Second Edition, Monograph Series, No. 6, page 388, The Chemical Catalog Co., Inc., New York, 1931.
— Stepp, W., Kuhnau, J. and Schroeder, H., *The Vitamins and Their Clinical Application*, Ferdinand Enke, Stuttgart, Germany, 1936.

17. Barborka, C. J., Diet and Preventive Dentistry, *Journal of the American Dental Association,* 23, 6:977-985, June, 1936.
— Harris, R. S. and Bunker, J. W. M., *American Journal of Roentgenology and Radium Therapy,* 33:25-30, 1935.

18. Barborka, C. J., Diet and Preventive Dentistry, *Journal of the American Dental Association,* 23, 6:977-985, June, 1936.
— East, Bion R., Vitamin D Milk: Its Significance to the Public Health and the Milk Industry, *Journal of Medicine*, pages 418-423, October, 1934.
— Eddy, W. H. and Dalldorf, G., *The Avitaminoses*, page 269, The Williams and Wilkins Co., Baltimore, 1937.
— Macleod, J. J. R., *Physiology in Modern Medicine*, Seventh Edition, pages 734, 749-750, C. V. Mosby Co., St. Louis, 1935.
— Mathews, Albert P., *Principles of Biochemistry*, page 439, William Wood & Co., Baltimore, 1936.
— McCollum, E. V., Relationship Between Diet and Dental Caries, *Journal of Dental Research.*
— Quigley, D. T., *Notes on Vitamins and Diets*, page 19, Consolidated Book Publishers, Inc., Chicago, 1933.
— Sure, B., *Vitamins in Health and Disease*, page 109, The Williams and Wilkins Co., Baltimore, 1933.
— *Vitamin D Milk*, 2, 1:2, January, 1935.

19. Hamilton, B. and Schwartz, C. J., *Journal of Clinical Investigation*, 11:817, 1932.
— Trumper and Cantarow, *Biochemistry in Internal Medicine*, page 150, W. B. Saunders Co., Philadelphia, 1933.
— *Vitamin D Milk*, Parathyroid Enlargement as Related to Sunshine and Vitamin D, 3, 4:16, April, 1936.

20. Dworzak, H., *Med. Klinik.*, January, 1936.
— East, Bion R., Vitamin D Milk: Its Significance to the Public Health and the Milk Industry, *Journal of Medicine,* page 419, October, 1934.

21. Eddy, W. H. and Dalldorf, G., *The Avitaminoses*, page 220, The Williams and Wilkins Co., Baltimore, 1937.
— Macleod, J. J. R., *Physiology in Modern Medicine*, Seventh Edition, page 734, C. V. Mosby Co., St. Louis, 1935.
— Macleod, J. J. R., *Physiology in Modern Medicine*, Seventh Edition, page 734, C. V. Mosby Co., St. Louis, 1935.

22. Macleod, J. J. R., *Physiology in Modern Medicine*, Seventh Edition, page 734, C. V. Mosby Co., St. Louis, 1935.

Booth and Hansen, The Present Day Status of the Vitamins, *The Journal-Lancet,* 57, 12:530-544, December, 1937.

> "In rickets, calcium salts are incompletely deposited, or even not at all, both in the maturing proliferative cartilage and in bone which is in process of formation. This failure in lime-salt deposition is the most striking feature in the pathology of rickets and is the essential cause of the gross changes in the skeleton. The only change outside the skeleton is hypertrophy of the parathyroid glands..."

"Chief Symptoms of Avitaminosis D:

> 1. Rickets: irritability, craniotaoes, prominent frontal bosses, delayed closing of fontanelles, pigeon breast, rachitic rosary, flaring ribs, epiphysseal enlargement at wrists and elbows, marked perspiration, delayed eruption of teeth, muscular weakness, protruding abdomen and bowing of legs.
> 2. Spasmophilia or infantile tetany: carpopedal spasm, laryngospasm and convulsions, and spasticity.
> 3. Osteomalacia: extreme softening of bones, especially in pregnancy.
> 4. Osteoporosis: failure of normal deposition of calcium phosphate leading to impaired calcification of bone.
> 5. Cessation of growth.
> 6. Abnormal ratio of calcium and phosphorus in the blood.

7. Dental malformation and caries..."

"Clinical Application of Vitamin D:

1. Prevention and cure of infantile rickets and tetany.
2. Prevention and cure of osteomalacia.
3. Formation and maintenance of normal tooth structure.
4. In defective calcium and phosphorus metabolism.
5. Routinely during infancy and periods of rapid growth, in pregnancy and lactation.
An adequate intake of calcium and phosphorus is also necessary in all cases."

Bills, *Journal of the American Medical Association*, 108:13-15, January 2, 1937.

"Thus, we distinguish eight forms of vitamin D, and it seems possible that others can be produced...

"Summary...Eight forms of vitamin D have been artificially prepared. At least two forms occur in fish oils, which may or may not be identical with certain of those made in vitro."

Norris, Seven Kinds of Nutritional Leg Weakness: Why Chicks Go Down and What to Do, *Poultry Tribune*, pages 14, 29, April 1937.

"In chicks with rickets (the leg weakness resulting from a lack of vitamin D), the bones rather than the nervous tissues are affected. Rickets results either from a failure of the bones to harden or calcify properly, or from the removal of calcium and phosphorus by a stiff-legged, stilted gait, accompanied by difficulty in balancing the body over the legs. When rickets becomes very severe, the legs of the chicks are unable to sustain the weight of the body and the chick can no longer stand..."

Medical Research Council, *The Influence of Diet on Caries in Children's Teeth*, page 132, London, 1936.

"...prove conclusively that a high vitamin D intake before the full eruption of the permanent teeth is of significant value in diminishing the incidence of caries in such teeth after eruption..."

Eddy and Dalldorf, *The Avitaminoses*, page 236, William and Wilkins, 1937.

"The requirements of pregnancy and of normal tooth structure are related since rachitic lesions in the milk teeth occur before birth. For a time it was believed that the fetus was immune to rickets. This seems a rather surprising point of view since osteomalacia is commonly related to pregnancy and the combined requirements of mother and fetus are naturally greater than those of the mother alone. At any rate undeniable evidence of rickets during intrauterine life now exists, including rachitic disease of the teeth."

Ibid, page 240

"Many cases of malnutrition appear to benefit from vitamin D, particularly disorders in which calcium is excreted excessively, and tetany, in which the blood calcium is reduced in amount. Improvement has followed the use of vitamin D in some cases of osteogenesis imperfects and celiac disease (Schultz)."

**Edited by Royal Lee**

CATALYN NATURES SOURCE OF VITALITY MADE IN U.S.A.

# VITAMIN NEWS

CATALYN NATURES SOURCE OF VITALITY MADE IN U.S.A.

VITAMIN PRODUCTS CO. • MILWAUKEE, WISCONSIN

November 15, 1937 VOL. 5

## BIBLIOGRAPHY FOR VITAMIN CHART

## (VITAMIN E)

1. Dryerre, H., Vitamins and the Prevention of Abortion in Sheep, *Nature*, 132:751, 1933
— Eddy, W. H. and Dalldorf, G., *The Avitaminoses*, pages 248, 250, The Williams and Wilkins Co., Baltimore, 1937
— Evans, H. M., *Journal of the American Medical Association*, 99:469-474, 1932.
— Howell, W. H., *A Textbook of Physiology*, Twelfth Edition, Revised, page 974, W. B. Saunders Co., Philadelphia, 1933.
— Mathews, A. P., *Principles of Biochemistry*, pages 443-445, William Wood & Co., Baltimore, 1936.
— Matitill, H. A. and Clayton, M. M., Vitamin E and Reproduction on Synthetic and Milk Diets, *Journal of Biological Chemistry*, 68:665-685, 1926.
— Medical Research Council, *Vitamins: A Survey of Present Knowledge*, page 117, London, 1932.
— Pacini, A. J., *Wheat Germ Oil — Vitamin E*, pages 23-24, The American Physician, Inc., New York, 1935.

2. Eddy, W. H. and Dalldorf, G., *The Avitaminoses*, page 248, The Williams and Wilkins Co., Baltimore, 1937.
— Pacini, A. J., *Wheat Germ Oil — Vitamin E*, pages 17-18, The American Physician, Inc., New York, 1935
— Pacini A.J., Why We Need Vitamin E, *Health Culture Magazine,* January, 1936.

3. Blumberg, H. A., A Growth Deficiency Disease Curable by Wheat Germ Oil, *Journal of Biological Chemistry,* 108, 1:227-238, January, 1935.
— Eddy W. H., and Dalldorf, G., *The Avitaminoses*, page 248, The Williams and Wilkins Co., Baltimore, 1937.
— Pacini, A. J., *Wheat Germ Oil — Vitamin E*, pages12-13, The American Physician, Inc., New York, 1935.
— Sure, B., *The Vitamins in Health and Disease*, page 123, The Williams and Wilkins Co., Baltimore, 1933.

4. Davidson, J. R., An Attempt to Inhibit the Development of Tar Carcinoma in Mice, *Canadian Medical Association Journal,* 32:364-366, 1935.
— Eddy, W. H. and Dalldorf, G., *The Avitaminoses*, page 248, 254-255, The Williams and Wilkins Co., Baltimore, 1937.
— Mathews, A. P., *Principles of Biochemistry*, page 445, William Wood & Co., Baltimore 1936.
— Pacini, A. J., *Wheat Germ Oil — Vitamin E*, pages 10, 39, The American Physician, Inc., New York, 1935.

5. Pacini, A. J., *Wheat Germ Oil — Vitamin E*, page 15, The American Physician, Inc., New York, 1935.

6. Olcott, H. S., Paralysis in the Young of Vitamin E Deficient Female Rats, *Journal Of Biological Chemistry,* Scientific Proceedings of the American Society of Biological Chemists, 119, 1:1xxiv, June 1937.
— Pacini, A. J., *Wheat Germ Oil — Vitamin E*, pages 15, 16, The American Physician, Inc., New York, 1935.

7. McGonigle, G. C. M., *Illinois Medical Journal,* page 212, March 1935 (Health Department, Stockton-on-Tees, England).

8. Blumenfeld, C. M., Weight Changes in the Suprarenal Glands of Albino Rats on Vitamin E Deficient and Fat Deficient Diets, *Endocrinology* 18:367-381, 1934.
— Eddy, W. H. and Dalldorf, G., *The Avitaminoses*, page 248, 250, The Williams and Wilkins Co., Baltimore, 1937.
— Gierhake, Experimental Studies on Vitamin E, *Arch. F. Gynekol.* 156:348-350, 1933.
— Mathews, A. P., *Principles of Biochemistry*, page 445, William Wood & Co., Baltimore 1936.
— McQueen-Williams, M., Increased Gonadotropic Content of Anterior Hypophysis from Vitamin E Deficient Female Rats, *Anatomical Record,* 58, No. 4, Suppl. 77, 1934.
— Medical Research Council, *Vitamins: A Survey of Present Knowledge*, page 109, London, 1932.
— Nelson, W. O., Studies on the Anterior Hypophysis, III; The Anterior Hypophysis in Vitamin E Deficient Rats, *Anatomical Record*, 56:241-253, 1933.
— Pacini, A. J., *Wheat Germ Oil — Vitamin E*, page 20, The American Physician, Inc., New York, 1935.
— Verzar, F., The Action of Vitamin E, *Magyar Orvosi, Arch.*, 32:273-292, 1931.
— Verzar, F., Hypertrophy of the Uterus and Vitamin E. Internal Secretion and Avitaminoses, *Pflugers Arch.*, 227:491-510,1931.
— Verzar, F., *Arch. Ges. Physiol. Mensch u. Tiere*, The Actions of Vitamin E on the Hypertrophy of the Uterus, 227, 4:499-510, 1931.
— Verzar, F., The Anti-Sterility or Fertility Vitamin, *Ztschr. F. vitaminforsch,* 1:116-134, 1932.
— Verzar, F., Vitamin and Internal Secretions, *Schweiz. Med. Wochenschr.*, 62:57-60, 1932.
— Verzar, F., Arvay, A. and Kokas, E. von, Basal Metabolism of Vitamin E Deficient Rats and the Correction of the Vitamin E Deficiency by Means of the Anterior Pituitary Hormone, Internal Secretions and Avitaminosis, *Biochem. Ztschr.*, 240:19-27, 1931.
— Verzar, F. and Kokas, E. von, The Action of Vitamin E Deficiency on the Hair Growth of Rats, *Pflugers Arch. Ges. Physiol.*, 227, 4:511-516, 1931.

9. Blumberg, H. A., A Growth Deficiency Disease Curable by Wheat Germ Oil, *Journal of Biological Chemistry,* 108, 1:227-238, January, 1935.
— Medical Research Council, *Vitamins: A Survey of Present Knowledge*, pages 107-108, London, 1932.
— Pacini, A. J., *Wheat Germ Oil — Vitamin E*, page 10, The American Physician, Inc., New York, 1935.
— Sure B., *The Vitamins in Health and Disease*, page 123, The Williams and Wilkins Co., Baltimore, 1935.

10. Evans, H. M. and Burr, G. O., *Journal of Biological Chemistry*, 76:273-297, 1928.
— Medical Research Council, *Vitamins: A Survey of Present Knowledge*, page 107, London, 1932.
— Pacini, A. J., *Wheat Germ Oil — Vitamin E*, page 15, The American Physician, Inc., New York, 1935.

11. Evans, H. M. and Burr, G. O., *Journal of Biological Chemistry*, 76:273-297, 1928.
— Pacini, A. J., *Wheat Germ Oil — Vitamin E*, page 15, The American Physician, Inc., New York, 1935.

12. Adamstone, F. B. and Card, L. E., The Effects of Vitamin E Deficiency on the Testis of the Male Fowl, *Journal of Morphology,* 56:339-359, 1934.
— Eddy, W. H. and Dalldorf, G., *The Avitaminoses*, pages 247, 250-251, The Williams and Wilkins Co., Baltimore, 1937.
— Evans, H. M., Vitamin E, *Journal of the American Medical Association*, 99:469-474, 1932, 99:469-474, 1932.
— Evans, H. M. and Burr, G. O., The Anti-Sterility Vitamin Fat-Soluble E, *Proceedings of the National Acad-*

*emy of Science,* 11:334-341, 1925.
— Evans, H. M. and Burr, G. O., *Journal of Biological Chemistry*, 76:273-297, 1928.
— Macleod J. J. R., *Physiology in Modern Medicine*, page 742, C. V. Mosby Co., St. Louis, 1935.
— McCollum, E. V. and Simmonds, N., *The Newer Knowledge of Nutrition*, Fourth Edition, pages 368-369, The Macmillan Co., New York, 1929.
— Medical Research Council, *Vitamins: A Survey of Present Knowledge*, page 112, London, 1932.
— Pacini, A. J., *Wheat Germ Oil — Vitamin E*, pages 19, 23, 25, 38, The American Physician, Inc., New York, 1935.
— Stepp, W., Kuhnau, J. and Schroeder, H., *The Vitamins and Their Clinical Application*, Ferdinand Enke, Stuttgart, Germany, 1936.

13. Ringsted, A., *A Preliminary Note on the Appearance of Paresis in Adult Rats Suffering from Chronic Avitaminosis E*, Biochemical Journal, 29:788, 1936.
— Sherman, H. C. and Smith, S. L., *The Vitamins*, Second Edition, Monograph Series, No. 6, page 344, The Chemical Catalog Co., Inc., New York, 1931.
— Stepp, W., Kuhnau, J. and Schroeder, H., *The Vitamins and Their Clinical Application*, Ferdinand Enke, Stuttgart, Germany, 1936.
— Sure, B., *The Vitamins in Health and Disease*, page 123, The Williams and Wilkins Co., Baltimore, 1933.

14. Eddy, W. H. and Dalldorf, G., *The Avitaminoses*, pages 241, 250-251, The Williams and Wilkins Co., Baltimore, 1937.
— Evans, H. M. and Burr, G. O., The Anti-Sterility Vitamin Fat-Soluble E, *Proceedings of the National Academy of Science,* 11:334-341, 1925.
— Ewing, P. V., *The Hog Breeder,* 10, 3, 1935.
— Gass, H. and Schmidt, C. L. A., Calcium and Phosphorus Metabolism in Rats During Pregnancy and Lactation and the Influence of the Reaction of the Diet Thereon, *Journ. of Biological Chemistry*, 86, 1:417, 1930.
— Harris, L. J., *Vitamins in Theory and Practice*, page 179, Cambridge University Press, 1935.
— Howell, W. H., *A Textbook of Physiology*, Twelfth Edition, Revised, page 973, W. B. Saunders Co., Philadelphia, 1933.
— Juhasz-Schaffer, Vitamin E. VI, Sterility in Female Rats in Avitaminoses E., *Virchow's Arch.*, 282:662-679, 1931.
— Macleod, J. J. R., *Physiology in Modern Medicine*, pages 742, 974, C. V. Mosby Co., St. Louis, 1935.
— Marchesi, F., Vitamin E and Reproductive Function in Albino Rats, *Sperimentale,* 89:119-165, 1935.
— Mason, K. E., Differences in Testis Injury and Repair After Vitamin A Deficiency, Vitamin E Deficiency and Inanition, *American Journal of Anatomy,* 52:153-240, 1933.
— Mathews, A. P., *Principles of Biochemistry*, pages 443-445, William Wood & Co., Baltimore 1936.
— McCollum, E. V. and Simmonds, N., *The Newer Knowledge of Nutrition*, Fourth Edition, pages 368-369, The Macmillan Co., New York, 1929.
— Medical Research Council, *Vitamins: A Survey of Present Knowledge*, pages104-105, 106,107, 112, London, 1932.
— Pacini, A. J., *Wheat Germ Oil — Vitamin E*, pages 10, 23, The American Physician, Inc., New York, 1935.
— Stepp, W., Kuhnau, J. and Schroeder, H., *The Vitamins and Their Clinical Application*, Ferdinand Enke, Stuttgart, Germany, 1936.

15. Pacini, A. J., *Wheat Germ Oil — Vitamin E*, page 10, The American Physician, Inc., New York, 1935.
– Ringsted, A., A Preliminary Note on the Appearance of Paresis in Adult Rats Suffering from Chronic Avitaminosis E., *Biochemical Journal,* 29:788, 1933.
– Sure, B., *The Vitamins in Health and Disease*, page 123, The Williams and Wilkins Co., Baltimore, 1933.

– Verzar, F., The Action of Vitamin E, *Magyar Orvosi, Arch.*, 32:273-292, 1931.
– Verzar, F. and Kokas, E. von, The Action of Vitamin E, Deficiency on the Hair Growth of Rats, *Pflugers Arch. Ges. Physiol.*, 227, 4:511-516, 1931.

16. Medical Research Council, *Vitamins: A Survey of Present Knowledge*, page 108, London, 1932.
— Pacini, A. J., *Wheat Germ Oil — Vitamin E*, page 10, The American Physician, Inc., New York, 1935.
— Stepp, W., Kuhnau, J. and Schroeder, H., *The Vitamins and Their Clinical Application*, Ferdinand Enke, Stuttgart, Germany, 1936.

Booth and Hansen, Present Day Status of Vitamins, *Journal Lancet*, 57, 12:542, December 1937.

"Chief Symptoms of Avitaminosis E

A. In Man
1. Habitual and threatened abortion.
2. Uterine hypoplasia, amenhorrhea, sterility.

B. In Animals (rat and chicken).
1. Failure of reproduction.
(a) Female — resorption of young during gestation.
(b) Male — sterility with irreversible, incurable lesions in the testes which do not respond to a high Vitamin E diet.
(1) Loss of fertilizing power.
(2) Absence of motility of spermatozoa.
(3) Loss of sperm.
(4) Loss of sex interest.
2. Paresis in young rats from maternal deficiency.
3. Muscular weakness, atrophy of voluntary muscles in young animals.

"Clinical Applications of Vitamin E.

1. Treatment of sterility, habitual, and spontaneous abortion in man. Vogt-Moller successfully treated seventeen out of twenty cases of habitual abortion with wheat germ oil, after noting favorable results in sheep and cows.
2. Possibly in hypoplasia and hypofunction of the gonads.

*Medical Times,* Chemical Nature of Vitamin E Established, 65, 8:xxvi, August 1937. (Abstracted from *American Professional Pharmacist,* July 1937) (Fernholz).

"…. The lack of this vitamin in the diet of rats leads to progressive disturbance in the nutrition of fetal placenta and a maceration and resorption of the fetuses in the uterus without affecting estrus and the faculty of fertilization. The administration of vitamin E in the form of wheat germ oil or suitable concentrates during the earliest stages of pregnancy is capable of anticipating and preventing this fetal destruction. Considerable evidence has been presented in the recent literature as to the efficacy of wheat germ oil in habitual abortion and stillbirth in women."

Pacini, Wheat *Germ Oil — Vitamin E,* page 15, American Physician, Inc., 1935.

"A day or so before weaning, rats born from others deficient in vitamin E develop a strikingly severe paralysis involving the hind legs and the musculature of the body. There is no relation, it seems, between the appearance of the paralysis and growth. It arises in animals that have grown normally and that show the usual vigor.

"Thus, where there is little vitamin E in the milk, there is great susceptibility to infantile paralysis infection; and where there is considerable vitamin E in the milk, there is less susceptibility to infection."

Oncken, Physiological Effects of Vitamin Deficiencies, *Illinois Medical Journal,* December 1934.

"Certainly a vitamin demanded imperatively for the control of sex and sex functions in so many lower animals, as is vitamin E, must play a definite counterpart in the human economy.

"As to the offspring themselves, the young from vitamin E surfeited mothers are more intelligent and keen than are those from mothers deprived of vitamin E to the point where the young are just born. In this respect vitamin E exerts an action rivaling that of vitamin B."

Eddy and Dalldorf, *The Avitaminoses,* page 248, Williams and Wilkins, 1937.

"Others have been less conservative. The following functions of wheat germ oil in the human dietary have been postulated.

1. Increased vigor.
2. Increased mental acumen as evidenced by the relative learning capacity of rats on Vitamin E rich and poor diets.
3. Aphrodisiac values
4. Some influence on the endocrines, e.g., on the pituitary by Verzar.
5. Possible prevention of anemia though hematopoietic value denied by Nelson, Mattill and Evans.
6. Anti-abortion value based on observation of Vogt-Moller.
7. Possible action on cell multiplication and perhaps thereby cancer prevention based on fact that rats on high E show greater resistance to the induction of tar cancers.

"The evaluation of such claims obviously awaits further clinical evidence. Sure expresses his views of the matter as follows:

'Since vitamin E is abundantly distributed in nature it has been doubted whether any human sterilities can be attributed to its deficiency. Obstetricians, however, state that at least 6 to 8 per cent of sterilities cannot be accounted for by diseased conditions in either father or mother. The diet of many people in the country is derived mainly from degerminated cereals, from which vitamin E has been removed by milling. Furthermore that diet is not supplemented sufficiently by eggs and vegetables. It remains therefore, to be demonstrated clinically that such cases will not respond to vitamin E administration. In Europe, Poulsson (1927) and Vogt Moller (1931) have cured a few cases of habitual abortion in women by the ingestion of vitamin B during pregnancy.'"

# NOTES

VITAMIN NEWS

VITAMIN PRODUCTS CO. • MILWAUKEE, WISCONSIN

December 15, 1937 VOL. 5

## BIBLIOGRAPHY FOR VITAMIN CHART

### (VITAMIN F)

1. Boyd, Eldon M. and Connell, W. Ford, Essential Unsaturated Fatty Acids in the Relief of the Common Cold, *Canadian Medical Association Journal*, 37:38, July, 1937.

2. Evans, H. M. and Burr, G. O., New Dietary Deficiency with Highly Purified Diets; the Biological Effect of Fat in the Diet, *Proceedings of the Society of Experimental Biology and Medicine,* 35:390-397, 1927.

3. Hinsberg, K. and Holland, G., The Iodine Absorption Value of the Blood Fats in Normal and Pathological Conditions, *Klinische Wochenschrift*, 12:1601-1602, 1933.

4. Burr, G. O. and Beber, A. F., Metabolism Studies with Rats Suffering from Fat Deficiency, *Proceedings of the Society of Experimental Biology and Medicine,* 31:911-912, 1934.
— Haven, F. L., Effect of Dietary Fats on Growth and Composition of Tumors, *Proceedings of the Society of Experimental Biology and Medicine*, 32:743-747, 1935.

5. Pacini, August J. and Avis, H. Wentworth, *Vitamin F in Cosmetics, Soap, Perfumery and Cosmetics*, September, 1936.

6. Mathews, Albert O., *Physiological Chemistry*, page 609, William Wood & Co., Baltimore, 1925.

7. Burr, G. O. and Burr, M. M., A New Deficiency Disease Produced by the Rigid Exclusion of Fat from the Diet, *Journal of Biological Chemistry,* 82:345-367, 1929.
— Burr, G. O. and Burr, M. M., On the Nature and Role of the Fatty Acids Essential in Nutrition, *Journal of Biological Chemistry,* 86:587-621, 1930.
— Cornbleet, T., Use of Maize Oil (Unsaturated Fatty Acids in the Treatment of Eczema), *Archives of Dermatology and Syphilology,* 31:224-226, 1931.
— Graham, C. E. and Griffith, A. H., Observations on the Nutritive Value of Certain Fats, *Proceedings of the Society of Experimental Biology and Medicine*, 28:756-761, 1931.
— Hansen, A. E., Serum Lipid Changes and Therapeutic Effects of Various Oils in Infantile Eczema, *Proceedings of the Society of Experimental Biology and Medicine,* 31:160-161, 1933.
— Hansen, A. E., Study of Iodine Number of Serum Fatty Acids in Infantile Eczema, *Proceedings of the Society of Experimental Biology and Medicine,* 300:1198-1199, 1933.
— Pacini, August J., Are Allergies a Vitamin Deficiency Symptom, *Health Culture,* 42, 3:18-19, 60-62, March, 1936.
— Pacini, August J., Vitamin F (Unsaturates), *American Perfumer,* December, 1936.
— Roche, A. and Roche J., Cutaneous Eruptions Attributed to Deficiency of Lipid in the Rat, *Comptes Rendus*

*de la Societe Biologique*, 109:463-464, 1932.
— Shepherd, M. I., *Survey of Vitamin F in Cosmetics*, pages 3-5, Pharmaceutical Specialties Co., Chicago, 1936.
— Shepherd, M I., Vitamin F in Skin Creams, *Drug & Cosmetic Industry*, March, 1936.
— Shepherd, M. I. and Linn, D. R., Evaluation of Vitamin F, *Drug & Cosmetic Industry*, page 629, May, 1936.
— Sinclair, R. G., Some Observations on the Growth of Rats on Fat-Free and Fat-Containing Diets, *Proceedings of the Society of Experimental Biology and Medicine,* 27:1059-1062, 1930.
— Tanze, U., The Effects of Fatty Acids on Nutrition, *Scientific Papers from the Institute for Physical and Chemical Research, Tokyo,* 22:13-28, 1932.
— Tanze, U., The Effects of Fatty Acids on Nutrition, *Scientific Papers from the Institute for Physical and Chemical Research, Tokyo*, 22:1-14,1933.
— Weinstein, M. L. and Glennon, K., Vitamin F Ointments, *Illinois Medical Journal,* June, 1937.

8. Shepherd, M. I., Survey of Vitamin F in Cosmetics, *Pharmaceutical Specialties Co*., page 5, 1937.

9. Burr, G. O. and Burr, M. M., A New Dietary Disease Produced by the Rigid Exclusion of Fat from the Diet, *Journal of Biological Chemistry,* 82:345-367, 1929.
— Burr, G. O. and Burr, M. M., On the Nature and Role of the Fatty Acids Essential in Nutrition, *Journal of Biological Chemistry,* 86:587-621, 1930.
— Burr, G. O. and Burr, M. M. and Miller, E. S., *Journal of Biological Chemistry*, 91:1, 1932.
— Evans, H. M. and Lepkovsky, S. C., *Journal of Biological Chemistry, 96:143-157, 1932.*
— Funk, C., Casper, S. and Casper, H., *Proceedings of the Society of Experimental Biology and Medicine*, 28:816, 1931.
— Graham, C. E. and Griffith, W. H., *Proceedings of the Society of Experimental Biology and Medicine*, 28:756-761, 1931.
— Hawk P. B. and Gergeim, O., *Practical Physiological Chemistry*, P. Blakinston's Son and Company, Philadelphia, 1931.
— Hume, E. M. and Smith, H. H., *Journal of Biochemistry*, 25:300, 1931.
— Shepherd, M I., *Vitamin F in Skin Creams*, Drug & Cosmetic Industry, March, 1936.
— Sinclair, R. G., *Proceedings of the Society of Experimental Biology and Medicine*, 27:1059, 1930.
— Weinstein, M. L. and Glennon, Kathryn, Vitamin F Ointments, *Illinois Medical Journal,* June, 1937.

10. Burr, G. O. and Brown, W. R., On the Fatty Acids Essential in Nutrition, *Proceedings of the Society of Experimental Biology and Medicine*, 30:1349-1352, 1933.
— Burr, G. O. and Burr, M. M., A New Deficiency Disease Produced by the Rigid Exclusion of Fat from the Diet, *Journal of Biological Chemistry,* 82:345-367, 1929.
— Burr, G. O. and Burr, M. M., On the Nature and Role of the Fatty Acids Essential in Nutrition, *Journal of Biological Chemistry,* 86:587-621, 1930.
— Pacini, August J., Vitamin F (Unsaturates), *American Perfumer,* December, 1936
— Shepherd, M I., Vitamin F in Skin Creams, *Drug & Cosmetic Industry,* March, 1936.
— Shepherd, M. I. And Linn, D. R., Evaluation of Vitamin F, *Drug & Cosmetic Industry,* page 629, May, 1936.

11. Pacini, August J., Are Allergies a Vitamin Deficiency Symptom, *Health Culture,* 42, 3:18-19, 60-62, March, 1936.

12. Graham, C. E. and Griffith, A. H., Observations on the Nutritive Value of Certain Fats, *Proceedings of the Society of Experimental Biology and Medicine,* 28:756-761, 1931.

13. Evans, H. M., Lepkovsky, S. and Murphy, E. A., Vitamin Need of the Body for Certain Unsaturated Fatty Acids: A Digest of Three Communications, *Journal of Biological Chemistry,* 106:431, 441, 445, 1934.

14. Planotov, G., The Influence of Unsaturated Fatty Acids on the Virulence of Tubercle Bacilli, *American Review of Tuberculosis*, 21:362-369, 1930.

15. Burr, G. O. and Brown, W. R., On the Fatty Acids Essential in Nutrition, *Proceedings of the Society of Experimental Biology and Medicine*, 30:1349-1352, 1933.
— Burr, G. O. and Burr, M. M., A New Deficiency Disease Produced by the Rigid Exclusion of Fat from the Diet, *Journal of Biological Chemistry*, 82:345-367, 1929.
— Evans, H. M. and Burr, G. O., New Dietary Deficiency with Highly Purified Diets, *Proceedings of the Society of Experimental Biology and Medicine,* 25:41-48, 1927.
— Shepherd, M I., Vitamin F in Skin Creams, *Drug & Cosmetic Industry,* March, 1936.
— Sinclair, R. G., Evidence of the Synthesis of Essential Unsaturated Fatty Acids by the Rat, *Journal of Biological Chemistry,* 114:94, 1936.
— Tanze, U., The Effects of Fatty Acids on Nutrition, *Scientific Papers from the Institute for Physical and Chemical* Research, *Tokyo,* 22:13-28, 1932.
— Tanze, U., The Effects of Fatty Acids on Nutrition, *Scientific Papers from the Institute for Physical and Chemical Research, Tokyo,* 22:1-14, 1933.
— Weinstein, M. L. and Glennon, Kathryn, Vitamin F Ointments, *Illinois Medical Journal*, June, 1937.

16. Shepherd, M. I. And Linn, D. R., Evaluation of Vitamin F, *Drug & Cosmetic Industry,* page 629, May, 1936.
— Weinstein, M. L. and Glennon, Kathryn, Vitamin F Ointments, *Illinois Medical Journal*, June, 1937.

17. Burr, G. O. and Burr, M. M., On the Nature and Role of the Fatty Acids Essential in Nutrition, *Journal of Biological Chemistry*, 86:587-621, 1930.
— Evans, H. M. and Burr, G. O., New Dietary Deficiency with Highly Purified Diets, *Proceedings of the Society of Experimental Biology and Medicine*, 25:41-48, 1927.
— Evans, H. M. and Burr, G. O., New Dietary Deficiency with Highly Purified Diets, *Proceedings of the Society of Experimental Biology and Medicine*, 25:390-397, 1927.
— Evans, H. M., Lepkovsky, S. and Murphy, E. A., Vitamin Need of the Body for Certain Unsaturated Fatty Acids: A Digest of Three Communications, *Journal of Biological Chemistry,* 106:431, 441, 445, 1934.
— Shephard, M. I., Vitamin F in Skin Creams, *Drug & Cosmetic Industry,* March 1936.
— Weinstein, M. L. and Glennon, Kathryn, Vitamin F Ointments, *Illinois Medical Journal*, June, 1937.

Pacini, Vitamin F (Unsaturates), *American Perfumer*, December 1936 (abstracted by Pacini).

> "Symptoms suggesting vitamin F deficiency are apparently more prevalent among humans than symptoms suggesting deficiencies due to all other vitamins combined. Dry skin, brittle, lustreless and falling hair, dandruff, brittle fingernails and eczema, and kidney diseases are exaggerately numerous and ubiquitously distributed … "

Boyd and Connell, Essential Unsaturated Fatty Acids in the Relief of the Common Cold, *Canadian Medical Association Journal,* 37:38, July 1937.

"In the present investigation a systematic study was made to determine if these unsaturated fatty acids had any real value in the prevention and treatment of the common cold.

> "Following a control period of seven weeks, beginning January 1, 1937, during which colds were recorded, 15 minims of purified linoleic and linolenic acids ('vitamin F') were given daily to 41 medical students for a further seven weeks, and 65 others served as controls. Vitamin F reduced the average incidence of colds by 64 per cent and the average duration by 78 per cent, there being at the same time little appreciable difference in the incidence and duration of the untreated group. Of the treated group, 71 per cent responded favorably and 20 per cent showed no relief. Unpleasant reactions occurred in one-third of the treated cases, diarrhea, nausea and vomiting being the chief side effects, but most of these were temporary and disappeared on taking the substance with, rather than between, meals."

Booth and Hansen, The Present Day Status of the Vitamins, *The Journal Lancet,* pages 542-543, December 1937.

> "Vitamin F has become of practical importance because of the great amount of propaganda in cosmetic literature dealing with dermatological conditions. There has been considerable question among investigators as to whether the expression vitamin F should actually be used in this connection.

> "In 1927, Burr working with Evans on vitamin E found that animals reared on highly purified low-fat diets still failed to attain normal development and nutrition. Subsequent investigations by Burr and Burr revealed that rats on fat deficient diets have early cessation of growth, scaliness of feet and hands, scaliness of the tail so marked that the tip frequently becomes necrotic and falls off, hematuria, and early death. McAmis, Mendel and Anderson reported somewhat similar findings in animals on fat-free regimen. Burr and Burr were the first to find that fats of high degree of unsaturation given in relatively small amounts caused complete disappearance of symptoms. Later, they definitely established that esters of linoleic and linolenic acids were essential for the normal nutrition of the rat hence, the expression, 'the essential unsaturated fatty acids.' There has been much controversy as to whether this type of deficiency should be considered a type of avitaminosis. Most reports in the literature term this disorder a fat deficiency disease. Evans and his co-workers as well as others have been referring to this essential factor as vitamin F.

> "The lack of these unsaturated fatty acids has been known to cause disturbances in gestation and lactation. As regards the human subject little is known. Relatively recently at the University of Minnesota, one of the workers in this field maintained himself on a strictly fat-free diet for a period of over six months — resulting in some rather interesting but not entirely conclusive findings (Brown, et al). In infants maintained on a diet otherwise complete but strictly devoid of fat, it has been shown that eczema developed. Several investigators have found that certain infants suffering from outspoken eczema of long duration have been found to be benefited by internal administration of oils rich in unsaturated fatty acids over a variable length of time (Hansen; Cornbleet)."

Pacini, Are Allergies A Vitamin Deficiency Symptom, *Health Culture*, 42,3:18-19, 60-62, March 1936.

> " ... The most probable answer at present is that allergic people are those who are not vitamin F protected, or more simply, those who have been eating the wrong kind of fats or have been fat-sparing in their diets.

"BRONCHIAL ASTHMA AND ECZEMA. Probably the closest link in support of the vitamin F deficiency concept of allergy is the recent work of Cornbleet and Pace, appearing in one of the American Medical Association publications. These men treated more than eighty cases of allergic eczema with an oil containing some linoleic acid. They reported very satisfactory results in these selected cases of allergic eczema … "

" … and a person who is vitamin F deficient is very likely it now seems to be allergic."

Shepherd, *Survey of Vitamin F in Cosmetics*, page 3, Chicago, 1936.

"It is now definitely established that the complete removal of certain indispensable unsaturated fatty acids from the diet result in the appearance of 'deficiency' symptoms which involve:

(1) skin and epidermal damage;
(2) the endocrine glands;
(3) certain of the viscera, in particular the kidneys;
(4) the general state of nutrition;
(5) and possibly the constitutional physiology that permits allergic susceptibility to take place.

"There are several classical epidermal symptoms of vitamin F deficiency. They include:

(1) in the skin, a thickening, a dryness, a roughness, a tendency to pigment, a proneness to develop sores and an ultimate eczema;
(2) in the hair, a distinct brittleness, a thinning and finally an alopecia;
(3) in the nails, distinct brittleness, tendency to ridged and roughened disfigurements eventuating in eczema."

Ibid, page 4.

" … Physicians have observed eczema intensify when the afflicted parts were exposed to sunlight, providing the eczema were of the so-called allergic type — the only type produced by vitamin F deficiency …

"Frequently, the first and very distinctive sign of vitamin F deficiency is brittleness of the finger nails. More rarely a true eczema of the finger nails may occur … "

Tanze, The Effects of Fatty Acids on Nutrition, *Scientific Papers of the Institute for Physical and Chemical Research, Tokyo*, 22:1-14, 1993 (Abstract).

"Fat-starved rats developed a definite nutritional disorder characterized by a loss of hair, later on inflammation, then dermatitis … There was a retarded growth. Immediately upon restoring linoleic acid to the diet, a soft, fine coating of hair appeared in the denuded areas, growth was normally resumed and the animals became normal. The hair developed a lustrous sheen and the eyes became extremely bright and clear. Oleic acid was ineffective and linolenic acid was neither constant nor at any time as effective as linoleic acid. No sparing action of linoleic acid or linolenic acid for vitamin B was found …The fatty acids from cod liver oil were not effective."

# NOTES

**VITAMIN NEWS**

VITAMIN PRODUCTS CO. • MILWAUKEE, WISCONSIN

January 15, 1938 VOL. 6

## BIBLIOGRAPHY FOR VITAMIN CHART

## (VITAMIN G)

1. Eddy, W. H. and Dalldorf, G., *The Avitaminoses*, page 121, The Williams and Wilkins Co., Baltimore, 1937
— Harris, L. J., *Vitamins in Theory and Practice*, page 76, Cambridge University Press, London, 1935.
— Mathews, Albert P., *Principles of Biochemistry*, page 425, William Wood & Co., Baltimore, 1936.
— Sherman, H. C. and Ellis, L. N., Necessary Versus Optimal Intake of Vitamin G (B.), *Journal of Biochemistry,* 104:91-97, 1934.
Sherman, H. C. and Smith, S. L., *The Vitamins*, Second Edition, Monograph Series, No. 6, page 146, The Chemical Catalog Co., Inc., New York, 1931.
— Wiggers, Carl J., *Physiology in Health and Disease*, page 962, Lea & Febiger Co., Philadelphia, 1934.

2. Mathews, Albert P., *Principles of Biochemistry*, page 429, William Wood & Co., Baltimore, 1936.
— Stepp, W., Kuhnau, J. and Schroeder, H., *The Vitamins and Their Clinical Application*, Ferdinand Enke, Stuttgart, Germany, 1936.

3. Sherman, H. C. and Smith, S. L., *The Vitamins*, Second Edition, Monograph Series, No. 6, page 146, The Chemical Catalog Co., Inc., New York, 1931.
— Wiggers, Carl J., *Physiology in Health and Disease*, page 962, Lea & Febiger Co., Philadelphia, 1934.

4. Stepp, W., Kuhnau, J. and Schroeder, H., *The Vitamins and Their Clinical Application*, Ferdinand Enke, Stuttgart, Germany, 1936.

5. Adams, Philip D., The Oxygen Uptake and Composition of the Skin of Rats in Vitamin G Deficiency, *Journal of Biological Chemistry,* 116, 2:641-651, December, 1936.
— Harris, L. J., *Vitamins in Theory and practice*, pages 76-77, Cambridge University Press, London, 1935.
— Macleod, J. J. R., *Physiology in Modern Medicine*, Seventh Edition, page 746, C. V. Mosby Co., St. Louis, 1935.
— Medical Research Council, *Vitamins: A Survey of Present Knowledge*, page 151, London, 1932.
— Sherman, H. C. and Smith, S. L., *The Vitamins*, Second Edition, Monograph Series, No. 6, pages 142-143, 146, The Chemical Catalog Co., Inc., New York, 1931.
— Sure, B., *The Vitamins in Health and Disease*, page 136, The Williams and Wilkins Co., Baltimore, 1933.
— Wiggers, Carl J., *Physiology in Health and Disease*, page 962, Lea & Febiger Co., Philadelphia, 1934.

6. Sherman, H. C. and Smith, S. L., *The Vitamins*, Second Edition, Monograph Series, No. 6, page 146, The Chemical Catalog Co., Inc., New York, 1931.
— Sure, B., *The Vitamins in Health and Disease*, pages 143-144, The Williams and Wilkins Co., Baltimore, 1933.

7. Barborka, C. J., Diet and Preventive Dentistry, *Journal of the American Dental Association,* 23, 6:977-985,

June, 1936.
— Harris, L. J., *Vitamins in Theory and Practice*, page 71, 74, Cambridge University Press, London, 1935.
— McCollum, E. V. and Simmonds, N., *The Newer Knowledge of Nutrition*, Fourth Edition, Chapter XXIII, pages 374-392, The Macmillan Co., New York, 1929.
— Medical Research Council, *Vitamins: A Survey of Present Knowledge*, pages 150-151, London, 1932.
— Schuler, R., Chemistry and Physiology of Vitamin B, *Drug & Cosmetic Industry,* 39, 2:179-181, August, 1936.
— Stepp, W., Kuhnau, J. and Schroeder, H., *The Vitamins and Their Clinical Application*, Ferdinand Enke, Stuttgart, Germany, 1936.
— Wolbach, *Journal of the American Medical Association,* 108:7-120, January 2, 1937.

8. Eddy, W. H. and Dalldorf, G., *The Avitaminoses*, page 134, The Williams and Wilkins Co., Baltimore, 1937.
— Mathews, Albert P., *Principles of Biochemistry*, page 430, William Wood & Co., Baltimore, 1936.
— Medical Research Council, *Vitamins: A Survey of Present Knowledge*, page 253, London, 1932.
— Remp, D. G. and Bing, F. C., Inanition as a Factor in Vitamin G Deficiency, *Journal of Nutrition,* 8:457-462, 1934.
— Sure, B., *The Vitamins in Health and Disease*, page 144, The Williams and Wilkins Co., Baltimore, 1933.
— Wiggers, Carl J., *Physiology in Health and Disease*, page 317, Lea & Febiger Co., Philadelphia, 1934.

9. Adams, Philip D., The Oxygen Uptake and Composition of the Skin of Rats in Vitamin G Deficiency, *Journal of Biological Chemistry*, 116, 2:641-651, December, 1936.
— Berglund, Medes, Huber, Longcope and Richards, *The Kidney in Health and Disease*, page 256, Lea & Febiger, Philadelphia, 1935.
— Eddy, W. H. and Dalldorf, G., *The Avitaminoses*, pages 131, 137-138, 140, 144, The Williams and Wilkins Co., Baltimore, 1937.
— Harris, L. J., *Vitamins in Theory and Practice*, page 75, Cambridge University Press, London, 1935.
— Macleod, J. J. R., *Physiology in Modern Medicine*, Seventh Edition, page 746, C. V. Mosby Co., St. Louis, 1935.
— McCollum, E. V. and Simmonds, N., *The Newer Knowledge of Nutrition*, Fourth Edition, page 374, The Macmillan Co., New York, 1929.
— Medical Research Council, *Vitamins: A Survey of Present Knowledge*, pages 150-151, London, 1932.
— Schuler R., *Drug & Cosmetic Industry*, 39, 2:179-181, 186, August, 1936.
— Sherman, H. C. and Smith, S. L., *The Vitamins*, Second Edition, Monograph Series, No. 6, pages 142-143, The Chemical Catalog Co., Inc., New York, 1931.
— Stepp, W., Kuhnau, J. and Schroeder, H., *The Vitamins and Their Clinical Application*, Ferdinand Enke, Stuttgart, Germany, 1936.
— Sure, B., *The Vitamins in Health and Disease*, pages 126, 137, The Williams and Wilkins Co., Baltimore, 1933.
— Wolbach, *Journal of the American Medical Association,* 108:7-120, January 2, 1937.

10. Eddy, W. H. and Dalldorf, G., *The Avitaminoses*, pages 134, 136-137, The Williams and Wilkins Co., Baltimore, 1937.
— Macleod, J J. R., *Physiology in Modern Medicine*, Seventh Edition, page 746, C. V. Mosby Co., St. Louis, 1935.
— McCollum, E. V. and Simmonds, N., *The Newer Knowledge of Nutrition*, Fourth Edition, page 374, The Macmillan Co., New York, 1929.
— Medical Research Council, *Vitamins: A Survey of Present Knowledge*, pages 150-151, London, 1932.
— Schuler R., *Drug & Cosmetic Industry*, 39, 179-181, 186, August, 1936.
— Sherman, H. C. and Smith, S. L., *The Vitamins*, Second Edition, Monograph Series, No. 6, pages 142-143, The

Chemical Catalog Co., Inc., New York, 1931.
— Stepp, W., Kuhnau, J. and Schroeder, H., *The Vitamins and Their Clinical Application*, Ferdinand Enke, Stuttgart, Germany, 1936.

11. Eddy, W. H. and Dalldorf, G., *The Avitaminoses*, page 144, The Williams and Wilkins Co., Baltimore, 1937.
— Lepkovsky, S. and Krause, M. E., The Tripartite Nature of Vitamin G, *Proceedings of the American Institute of Nutrition,* Abstracted in *Journal of Nutrition,* 13, 6, Suppl., page 12, June 10, 1937.
— Sherman, H. C. and Smith, S. L., *The Vitamins*, Second Edition, Monograph Series, No. 6, pages 121, 142-143, The Chemical Catalog Co., Inc., New York, 1931.
— Sure, B., *The Vitamins in Health and Disease*, pages 136-137, The Williams and Wilkins Co., Baltimore, 1933.

12. Fitzmorris, C. S., *Cincinnati Journal of Medicine*, 16:585, 1936.
— Mathews, Albert P., *Principles of Biochemistry*, pages 430-432, William Wood & Co., Baltimore, 1936.
— Rhoads and Miller, *Journal of the American Medical Association*, 103, 387, 1934.

13. Adams, Philip D., The Oxygen Uptake and Composition of the Skin of Rats in Vitamin G Deficiency, *Journal of Biological Chemistry,* 116, 2:641-651, December, 1936.

14. Eddy, W. H. and Dalldorf, G., *The Avitaminoses*, pages 131-132, 134, 136-137, The Williams and Wilkins Co., Baltimore, 1937.
— Macleod, J. J. R., *Physiology in Modern Medicine*, Seventh Edition, page 746, C. V. Mosby Co., St. Louis, 1935.
— Mathews, Albert P., *Principles of Biochemistry*, page 430, William Wood & Co., Baltimore, 1936.
— McCollum, E. V. and Simmonds, N., *The Newer Knowledge of Nutrition*, Fourth Edition, page 374, The Macmillan Co., New York, 1929.
— Medical Research Council, *Vitamins: A Survey of Present Knowledge*, pages 150-151, London, 1932.
— Schuler R., *Drug & Cosmetic Industry*, 39, 2:179-181, 186, August, 1936.
— Sherman, H. C. and Smith, S. L., *The Vitamins*, Second Edition, Monograph Series, No. 6, pages 121, 142-143, The Chemical Catalog Co., Inc., New York, 1931.
— Stepp, W., Kuhnau, J. and Schroeder, H., *The Vitamins and Their Clinical Application*, Ferdinand Enke, Stuttgart, Germany, 1936.
— Sure, B., *The Vitamins in Health and Disease*, pages 126-127, 137, The Williams and Wilkins Co., Baltimore, 1933.

15. Sherman, H. C. and Smith, S. L., *The Vitamins*, Second Edition, Monograph Series, No. 6, page 143, The Chemical Catalog Co., Inc., New York, 1931.

16. Berglund, Medes, Huber, Longcope and Richards, *The Kidney in Health and Disease*, pages 149-150, 256, Lea & Febiger, Philadelphia, 1935.
— Medical Research Council, *Vitamins: A Survey of Present Knowledge*, page 151, London, 1932.
— Sherman, H. C. and Smith, S. L., *The Vitamins*, Second Edition, Monograph Series, No. 6, page 143, The Chemical Catalog Co., Inc., New York, 1931.

17. Eddy, W. H. and Dalldorf, G., *The Avitaminoses*, page 132, The Williams and Wilkins Co., Baltimore, 1937.
— Medical Research Council, *Vitamins: A Survey of Present Knowledge*, page 151, London, 1932.
— Stepp, W., Kuhnau, J. and Schroeder, H., *The Vitamins and Their Clinical Application*, Ferdinand Enke, Stuttgart, Germany, 1936.

18. Macleod, J. J. R., *Physiology in Modern Medicine*, Seventh Edition, page 746, C. V. Mosby Co., St. Louis, 1935.
— Medical Research Council, *Vitamins: A Survey of Present Knowledge*, page 151, London, 1932.
— Stepp, W., Kuhnau, J. and Schroeder, H., *The Vitamins and Their Clinical Application*, Ferdinand Enke, Stuttgart, Germany, 1936.
— Sure, B., *The Vitamins in Health and Disease*, page 136, The Williams and Wilkins Co., Baltimore, 1933.

19. Clapp, C. A., *Cataract: Its Etiology and Treatment*, pages 76-77, Lea & Febiger, Philadelphia, 1934.
— Eddy, W. H. and Dalldorf, G., *The Avitaminoses*, page 147, The Williams and Wilkins Co., Baltimore, 1937.
— Medical Research Council, *Vitamins: A Survey of Present Knowledge*, page 151, London, 1932.
— Oncken, Mildred, Physiological Effects of Vitamin Deficiencies as Summarized Briefly from Recent and Authenticated Research Experiments, *Illinois Medical Journal,* December 1934.
— Sure, B., *The Vitamins in Health and Disease*, pages 136, 143-144, The Williams and Wilkins Co., Baltimore, 1933.

20. Medical Research Council, *Vitamins: A Survey of Present Knowledge*, pages 151-151, London, 1932.
— McClendon, J. F., *A Manual of Biochemistry*, page 6, John Wiley & Sons, Inc., New York, 1934.
— Stepp, W., Kuhnau, J. and Schroeder, H., *The Vitamins and Their Clinical Application*, Ferdinand Enke, Stuttgart, Germany, 1936.
— Wolbach, *Journal of the American Medical Association,* 108:7-120, January 2, 1937.

21. Eddy, W. H. and Dalldorf, G., *The Avitaminoses*, pages 133-134, The Williams and Wilkins Co., Baltimore, 1937.
— Mathews, Albert P., *Principles of Biochemistry*, page 427, William Wood & Co., Baltimore, 1936.
— McCollum, E. V. and Simmonds, N., *The Newer Knowledge of Nutrition*, Fourth Edition, page 374, The Macmillan Co., New York, 1929.
— Medical Research Council, *Vitamins: A Survey of Present Knowledge*, pages151-151, London, 1932.
— Schuler R., *Drug & Cosmetic Industry*, 39, 2:179-181, 186, August, 1936.
— Sure, B., *The Vitamins in Health and Disease*, page 128, The Williams and Wilkins Co., Baltimore, 1933.

22. Sherman, H. C. and Smith, S. L., *The Vitamins*, Second Edition, Monograph Series, No. 6, pages 142-143, The Chemical Catalog Co., Inc., New York, 1931.

Abstract from *Journal of Nutrition*, 13, 6, Supplement page 12-13, June 10, 1937 of "Vitamin B Deficiencies as Influenced by Dietary Carbohydrates," by Morgan, Cook and Davison, speech delivered at the Fourth Annual Meeting of the American Institute of Nutrition, April 1937.

> "Lactose, sucrose and cornstarch were used as 54 to 70% of the basal diets fed to young rats deprived of one or more of the vitamin B factors. Growth, dermatitis, cataract formation, blood and urine sugar and calcium were determined on animals kept in individual screen-floored cages on these regimens for 8 to 16 weeks.
>
> "Three factors of the vitamin B complex were used, a wheat germ preparation of vitamin $B_6$, a rice-bran preparation of the filtrate factor and crystalline lactoflavin. Crystalline vitamin $B_1$ (Merck) was given in ample amount to all the rats. The three vitamin $B_2$ preparations were given each alone, all combinations of two together as well as all three together.
>
> "The lactose diet with no vitamin $B_2$ factors produced as good conditions as with $B_6$ and flavin. The

filtrate factor, however, improved growth. The cornstarch diet was but little improved by addition of filtrate factor but much improved by both B and flavin. The sucrose diet gave better growth than the others when supplemented by all the factors but apparently supplied none of them spontaneously.

"Thus the intestinal flora supported by lactose produces flavin and $B_6$, cornstarch carries the filtrate factor or favors its intestinal formation, and sucrose neither carries nor allows the intestinal production of any of these factors."

McCollum, *Recent Advances in Nutritional Research*, pages 25-26, Bruce Publishing Company, St. Paul, 1937.

"There is unanimity of opinion among investigators that pellagra is due to some dietary deficiency, which has been called vitamin $B_2$, P-P factor, and vitamin G. For some years it was generally believed that a form of dermatitis in the rat which is caused by inadequate diet was the analog of human pellagra. This is now known to be a mistaken view. Maize, which has generally been abundant in the diet of the human pellagrin, prevents or cures the rat dermatitis. The factor necessary for the prevention of the rat dermatitis is now called vitamin $B_6$. The nature of the substance or substances, a deficiency of which causes human pellagra, is entirely unknown. The administration of liver, yeast or wheat germ, produces cures, the former, often dramatic changes in the patient. Some studies with liver fractions seem to indicate that pellagra is due to double deficiency of unknown substances. The experimental status of our knowledge in this field does not warrant further discussion here."

Booth and Hansen, Present Day Status of the Vitamins, *Journal Lancet,* 57, 12:536, December 1937.

"Chief Symptoms of Avitaminoses $B_2$ (G) Complex.

A. In man.

1. Pellagra — due probably to avitaminosis P. P. of the vitamin $B_2$ complex.
2. Acrodynia believed by some to be caused by the lack of one or more of the factors in vitamin B complex. Because of its cutaneous manifestations, acrodynia is often mentioned in connection with vitamin $B_2$ complex.
3. Little is known of lactoflavin deficiency in the human subject."

"Clinical Applications of Vitamin B .

1. Prevention and cure of pellagra.
2. Promotion of growth and well-being (due to lactoflavin).
3. Possible prevention of cataract formation.
4. Increase of vitamin $B_2$ content of milk in lactation.
5. Cure of stomatitis and glossitis of chronic alcoholism and of alcoholic pellagra — by early treatment with a high caloric diet and 75 grams of yeast or of liver extract daily. (Blankenhorn and Spies)
6. Treatment of acrodynia."

**Edited by Royal Lee**

# NOTES

# VITAMIN NEWS

VITAMIN PRODUCTS CO. • MILWAUKEE, WISCONSIN

February 15, 1938 VOL. 6

## CAN VITAMINS BE STANDARDIZED AS TO UNIT CONTENT?

Pharmacologists have attempted to find scientific short cuts for determining the merit of vitamins by means of their effect upon animals and to establish units of potency based on these results.

Where the chemical identity of a vitamin was thought to be established, the vitamin became subject to standardization in quantitative measurement.

Both methods were intended to remove from the user of the product (patient or physician) the necessity of depending upon their own means of appraisal (the clinical test), which in any case, must be the final arbiter of quality. Vitamin concentrates used for therapeutic purposes are far less in need of standardization than those used for food fortification, for their continued acceptance by a physician must of necessity be accompanied by tangible results, but the user of a food product containing added vitamins has less opportunity to be able to judge its merit by the less obvious effect of the small quantities present.

In our efforts to be scientific, however, it is important that we defer the job of establishing units for measurement before a foundation of fact has been built. It appears that in this case, in our efforts to be more scientific, premature assumptions have caused most of our vitamin technologists to be a great deal less scientific.

As in all new sciences, a little knowledge is dangerous. The proponents of the scheme to test vitamins by animal experiment overlooked one vital matter that is the basic principle of animal nutrition — that each species has a biochemistry peculiar to itself, and each has its own preferential food substances. The caloric value of hay, for example, determined by its effect on cows and horses, is no criterion of its nutritional merit as a food for humans.

Biological standardization of vitamins (C, D, and G especially), according to most recent findings, has failed to be a success because of this principle, and chemically pure "vitamin C" (ascorbic acid) is of no benefit whatsoever to some species and according to its discoverer, Szent-Gyorgyi, fails to have its expected effects in treating some of the outstanding and characteristic symptoms of scurvy in the human.[1]

The first forms of synthetic vitamin D were loaded with toxic materials that were not detected in the rat experiments [2] and only recent research by German chemists have made possible a pure and non-toxic synthetic product through the use of monochromatic ultraviolet light in its synthesis by irradiation. The rat, unhappily for us, responded to the toxic product as well as to the "human" form of the vitamin without showing ill effects. Naturally, the manufacturers of such abortions do not advertise their mistakes and the substitution of biological tests for clinical experience delayed the development of true vitamin D for a considerable time. The real truth came out only by the discovery that the "rat" vitamin was useless as a "chick" vitamin, the chicken requiring the same form of vitamin D (in metabolizing egg shell calcium) as is effective for maintaining the health of the human race.

In the case of vitamin G, a separate chemical form has been found for each of the three species so far studied.[3].

Further work promises to greatly extend this principle of "species specificity." Since the present concept of vitamins involves whole "chemically related families," in the case of each vitamin, as we have preached for some years, this picture appears reasonable. No animal feeder in a zoo tries to maintain all the different species of animals on the same forms of fats, carbohydrates and proteins, nor on the same proportions. Some species cannot even survive unless they are supplied with certain special foods that are peculiar to their native location. There are 200 different sugars in Nature, more starches in all probability, a great diversity of fats (some fatty acids are unique in having only one source), and proteins are different for each species of animal. Why not a diversity of vitamin molecules with species preference? If there were not such a variety we would have an exception to the general rule.

Now as to the possibility of isolating chemically a "vitamin principle," we might as well try to isolate a "carbohydrate," a "protein" or a "fat," and say it was chemically pure and supplied all the carbohydrate, protein or fat requirements of a species. Even though we realize that cellulose is a favorable nutritive medium to supply carbohydrate to the horse, that is no reason to assume that the horse will not thrive best on an assortment of carbohydrates. The group most acceptable to the horse will not fall in the same spot on the list of all possible carbohydrates as will the group best adapted to the human, but it can overlap.

The now obsolete idea that "caloric" measurement determined the nutritional values of food materials has been abandoned on identically the same grounds that we argue here — that it failed to distinguish between the "species preference" that caused a great variation in the assimilation and use of the food material in question.

The calorie has been discarded as a unit of food value since the discovery of the importance of these new food factors that the calorie did not measure.

In our slight present knowledge of vitamin chemistry, we have so far found four forms of vitamin A, six forms of vitamin B, three forms of vitamin C, twelve forms of vitamin D, etc.

The naïve assumption that vitamin A can be measured as milligrams of carotene now is obviously a premature jump at a conclusion. A patient can be shown to have a deficiency of vitamin A even though his skin is yellow with unassimilated carotene. It has been shown that carotene may not be converted into vitamin A in certain diseases in the human, and the liver normally has this function.[4] It is apparent here that the chemical identification of a "vitamin," after too limited experimentation, followed by a pharmacopeial standard of "so and so" many milligrams of the compound so identified, can be a grievous error. The well-known tendency of political bodies and quasi-politicians to refuse to admit their mistakes is well exemplified in these cases of the promotion and acceptance of both carotene and toxisterol as vitamins A and D respectively.

Ascorbic acid has proven quite useless in controlling a condition of bleeding gums, loose teeth and "black and blue spots" (pseudo bruises) that indicate a definite scurvy condition.

Crystalline vitamin B has no such reputation for treating heart conditions as has the concentrate of vitamin B complex.

And so on down the line of vitamin D, vitamin E, vitamin F and vitamin G.

"Seals of Acceptance" are merely an endorsement of the exploded "biological unit" and "chemically purified" theories. The granters of "Seals of Acceptance" refuse to accept clinical evidence of merit, and even go so far as to condemn products that they have admittedly failed to test or investigate in any way. How can such unreliable purveyors of swivel-chair opinions command any respect among thinking people?

We can say then that it is not practical to rate a vitamin in quantitative units depending upon its assumed identity as a certain chemically known molecule. Such an assumption has resulted in errors that probably have cost us years of progress in the vitamin field and has caused embarrassment for those who accepted the principle as fact and attempted to put it into practice.

We can say that animal tests are of value only to the extent of offering evidence as to the kind of deficiency symptoms to associate with a particular vitamin, but the chemical nature of the factor that has the same effect in the human may be quite different but closely related and probably associated in foods. The term "vitamin complex" recognized this association of "closely related families" that the recent experiments with the "molecular still," as developed at the Eastman Kodak Laboratories, has shown. To chemically separate or crystallize out the special factor that is best for some test animal may mean (and usually does) the elimination of the special factor that is best for the human.

Concentrates made by determining the physical properties and solubilities with consequent extraction with proper solvents obtains the whole group of related factors. To use them as a group is just as sensible as to use a variety of su gars and starches as Nature provided them in a diet, instead of preferring refined cane sugar or glucose as a sole source of carbohydrate.

It is evident when we see the true picture as it is unfolding, that vitamin units as previously established are just as wide of the mark in measuring vitamin merit. This is not an argument against real measuring units, but against false and misleading ones.

Men mined and sold coal for warming their habitations long before scientists discovered how to measure its worth for the purpose in heat units. Vitamin concentrates will be sold and will produce results without being tested for unit content for years before the real and correct means will be developed for measuring its effect other than "the rule of thumb."

Until better ways of determining facts are available, the only safe guide in ascertaining the merit of any commodity is to inquire into the reputation of the product *among those qualified to know — its experienced users.*

[1] *Los Angeles Times*, New Lemon Vitamin Cure for Bleeding, March 14, 1937 (*Abstract of Nature,* Volume 138, pages 27 and 798, July 4 and November 7, 1936 respectively).

[2] Sherman, H. C., *Chemistry of Food and Nutrition*, Fifth Edition, pages 455-456, The Macmillan Company, N. Y., 1937.

[3] Lepkovsky, S. and Krause, M E., Tripartite Nature of Vitamin G. (Abstract from *Journal of Nutrition*, 13, 6, Supplement page 12, June 10, 1037).

[4] Schneider, R. and Widmann, E., The Hepato-hormonal Direction of Vitamin A Metabolism and the Etiology of Paget's Disease, *Klin. Wchnschr.*, 14:1786, 1935 (Abstract by Endocrinology, 20, 3:451, May 1936).

**Edited by Royal Lee**

# NOTES

# VITAMIN NEWS

VITAMIN PRODUCTS CO. • MILWAUKEE, WISCONSIN

March 15, 1938 VOL. 6

## THE MINERAL ELEMENTS OF NUTRITION

Of all the nutritional materials necessary to health, the minerals have received the least attention by the investigators of science. It has required the study of vitamins to bring this fact into prominence. Vitamins as a class probably should be considered as factors of mineral metabolism and promoters of mineral assimilation, as each of the vitamins are now known to be involved in the normal control of the metabolism of the most important of the nutritional elements — calcium.

We have to admit in the beginning that there is no background of any kind of systematic research to look to for information on this subject. Our information today is wholly dependent upon occasional discoveries here and there, and mainly in the study of animal nutrition. These results of animal tests may be, we believe, applied to the human with considerably more parallelism than in the case of animal tests with vitamin concentrates, for we are dealing with less highly organized and complex chemical entities, in which the variations in the physiological chemistry of the different species may be of less moment. (In the case of the vitamins, such differences in physiological chemistry may result in complete ineffectiveness of a vitamin when used for a different species. The chicken, for instance, requires a fat-soluble vitamin C that is quite different chemically from the water-soluble vitamin C required by the human, and vitamin D as developed for the rat is useless for the hen).

The form in which mineral elements are required may be one or more of four general classifications — organic or inorganic, colloidal or crystalloidal.

An organic mineral may be defined from a nutritional viewpoint as a mineral element in some chemical combination that is peculiar to the reactions of a living cell. Such a combined mineral may be either crystalloidal or colloidal. Example: phytin of bran or the lecithin of wheat germ, both carrying organic phosphorus, and the phytin — magnesium, too.

An inorganic mineral is a mineral substance in the form in which it occurs before it has been acted upon by living cells. Plants absorb minerals in this form, and they are changed after absorption into organic forms, but that is not to say that the original inorganic forms are not also essential parts of the economy of living cells, both plant and animal.

A colloidal mineral is one that has been so altered that it will no longer pass through cell walls or other organic membranes. This colloidal mineral may still be either organic or inorganic in certain cases, although as a general rule, it is necessary for the mineral to become changed into the organic form in order to get it into a colloidal form.

The crystalloidal form of a mineral or salt is the form in which it will form crystals. As a general rule, colloids will not form crystals. (Outstanding exception is blood hemoglobin.)

The crystalloidal form is the pure mineral substance. To form the colloidal form, some greater or less amount of other materials must be present. (This is true only of minerals; there are many pure colloids, gelatine, for instance, of non-mineral nature.) Pure sodium silicate, for instance, is crystalloid, but the presence of small amounts of sodium chloride changes it to a colloid. The difference is simply in its molecular makeup, the colloid molecule being composed of a group of about 50,000 of the crystalloid molecules. That is why it will not pass through a cell wall. A snowflake is a water crystal, but built up of a vast number of water molecules. It will not go through an opening that would pass a smaller crystal, but under certain conditions, the water in the air takes the form of flakes of relatively similar type. That is just what occurs when a crystalloid, through some apparently slight influence, changes spontaneously to a colloid. In adding the salt to the sodium silicate solution, the electrostatic balances are altered by reason of the water becoming conductive (pure water is not, and salt is one of the best ionizers to make it conductive), and possibly the sodium silicate molecules become attracted together in groups electrostatically.

It is obvious that a cell must be able to convert crystalloids to colloids to prevent the loss of its essential elements by diffusion out again. Glucose is a crystalloid; glycogen a colloid. Insulin is believed to make the conversion. Blood sugar, as glucose, passes into the muscle cell, and without insulin, it cannot be retained.

The great class of colloids in living cells are the proteins. In the plant, the retention of minerals is accomplished by attaching the mineral molecules to proteins. These proteins are probably the simplest of all proteins, and may have been evolved for the special purpose.

Plant juices, therefore, contain both mineral forms, as absorbed as well as in the colloidal form. Milk contains a colloidal form of a calcium compound that is of a protein nature. Proteins are destroyed by heat, and that explains the loss of assimilable calcium in milk when it is pasteurized.

Cooking also destroys the plant minerals that are in the colloidal form. An attempt was made to preserve fruit juices without cooking by filtering through porcelain to remove the organisms, but the product was found to have lost nutritional values. The reason here is apparent — the colloids also were held back.

Potassium is probably the most important of the mineral elements that must be supplied in the organic form. Plant juices are high in potassium, but our intake of raw juices is never very high. Potassium is an antagonist of phosphorus; too much causes a sensitization of the nervous system (particularly the parasympathetic), which may be excessive if phosphorus deficiency is present. Horses on a high green grass diet become jittery and nervous; bran with its phosphorus content prevents and cures the condition. Phosphoric acid has been used, added to the drinking water, with the same effect. The phosphorus then need not be in the organic form. In fact, it has been shown that the phytin of bran is split by an intestinal enzyme into phosphoric acid and its other components. Few of us escape some of the effects of phosphorus deficiency, for our use of refined cereals greatly limits our intake of this element.

Calcium is put to work in the body in numerous forms, and it is a reflection upon our modern institutions of research that so little is known about just what forms are required, how they are made, and what their functions are. We do know that the form of organic calcium in raw milk is of exceptional value to the child in supplying the material for tooth and bone development, and that in the adult as well as in the child, a calcium deficiency results in susceptibility to infectious disease. From a viewpoint of nutritional therapy, the best form of calcium is still a matter of argument. Dicalcium phosphate has been much promoted commercially, but its assimilation is admittedly difficult by reason of the low solubility. Calcium gluconate has high solubility, but its effects are not outstanding, even where acute deficiency exists. The lactate does often produce spectacular results in some symptoms of calcium deficiency such as fever blisters, canker sores in the mouth, cold sores, etc., but again may fail in another apparently identical case. Probably the differences are due to differences in vitamin reserves, as vitamins A, C, D and F in particular regulate the calcium balances between the blood, lymph and intracellular fluids.

The blood contains calcium in, at least, half a dozen forms, the main divisions being a distinction between the diffusible and non-diffusible, and between serum, plasma and corpuscle calcium. Passing an electric current through blood serum drives a form of both diffusible and non-diffusible to each electrode, distinguishing four kinds of serum calcium besides the plasma and corpuscle calcium.

Vitamin D and the parathyroid hormone both act to increase the diffusible calcium of blood serum. The presence of vitamin A is necessary to prevent the serum calcium from precipitating in such forms as kidney stones, and a deficiency of phosphates aids this precipitation.[1] In Paget's disease, it has been shown that the liver has lost its ability to convert carotene into vitamin A,[2] and the bone degeneration characteristic of this disease is the consequence. We see that the maintenance of bone, therefore, depends upon vitamins A, C and D, at least. (In vitamin C deficiency, the bones become decalcified, the outstanding reaction is scurvy.)

Calcium metabolism also depends upon the presence of minute amounts of other more rare elements, of which manganese and fluorine have recently come to the front. These will be discussed under these respective headings.

It is a common experience for the physician to prescribe remedies for obvious deficiencies, observe a certain degree of encouraging improvement, and then have the patient come to a standstill before complete recovery. This is clearly a case where the replacement therapy has been incomplete. Suppose vitamin C is supplied for a case of incipient scurvy, characterized by decalcification of the supporting tissues of the teeth, with resultant looseness of these important organs. A certain degree of improvement occurs, then the case drags along without complete recovery. Calcium deficiency obviously could be the reason, and vitamin D, too, is necessary and may not be present (the vitamin D puts the calcium into the blood stream; the vitamin C unloads it where it is required), and all these activities may possibly be hindered by fluorine and manganese deficiency. The complexity of the problem is discouraging, but the remarkable results produced give us the stimulus to keep on the trail of an explanation of the failures, for such is the price of progress.

## REFERENCES

[1] Bliss, A. R., Jr., Livermore, G. R., and Prather, E. O., Jr., The Relation of Vitamin A and Vitamin D to Urinary Calculus Formation, *The Journal of Urology,* 30, 6:642, December 1933.

[2] Schneider, E. and Widmann, E., The Hepatohormonal Direction of Vitamin A Metabolism and the Etiology of Paget's Disease, *Klin. Wchnschr.*, 14:1786, 1935.

**Edited by Royal Lee**

# NOTES

VITAMIN NEWS

VITAMIN PRODUCTS CO. • MILWAUKEE, WISCONSIN

March 15, 1938 VOL. 6

## WHY NOT BE HONEST ABOUT IT ?

In these pages, we have at various times called attention to some of the obvious basic principles underlying the use and preparation of vitamin concentrates.

Today, these principles, to be set forth again below, are becoming more and more obvious as new facts are established. They show that the methods in use to rate vitamin concentrates in terms of the "units" commonly used are fallacious and misleading and that the physician or layman who depends upon such statements of "unit" content is being imposed upon by the manufacturers of such materials.

Why not be honest about the matter and admit the facts? Here they are:

1. The vitamins are all now known to exist as complexes, groups or families of related and similar organic principles.

To rate any vitamin complex in terms of any one of its fractions is just as illogical as to set up as a standard for the carbohydrate component of a diet, a specified quantity of pure cane sugar. (It is just as criminal to purify vitamins as food components as to denature carbohydrates; they cease to be natural foods (1a) and become drugs, the effects of which may be quite at variance with that of the original complex, and of a narrower original range of action.) (1b) (1c) (1d) (1e)

2. The different factors of a complex have quite a different value in serving as the vitamin for different species.

To set up as a standard unit a given quantity of a pure vitamin, therefore, can be as deceiving as to specify for the carbohydrate component of a diet a given quantity of pure cellulose. (Cellulose is carbohydrate only for such species of test animals as goats, cows and horses. Its value is zero in human nutrition.)

Do not be fooled. These statements are not idle arguments, but are basic laws of nutrition. You can ignore them only at your own risk, for it will be yourself and those who depend upon your opinions who will suffer from the consequences of ignorance.

The fetish of "scientific standardization" has been the downfall of many makers of vitamin concentrates.

Vitamin A was said to be standardizable in terms of carotene. Now we find that many patients show an A deficiency because they cannot convert carotene to vitamin A. (2a) (2b) (2c)

Vitamin A was said to be standardizable in rat units. Now we find that in equal amounts according to rat units, Vitamin A from spinach is *10 times* as effective in the human as the vitamin A from fish oil. (3)

Vitamin B was said to be standardizable in terms of pure "thiamin." Now we know that the vitamin B complex contains 14 known components besides thiamin. (4)

Vitamin C was said to be standardizable in terms of "Ascorbic Acid." After its discoverer received the Nobel Prize for his work, he found that it lacks the antihemorrhagic factor, the deficiency of which is the real cause of scurvy. (5a) (5b) (5c) (5d)

Vitamin D was standardized in terms of rat units, with the later finding that the rat vitamin was not vitamin D at all, and that all the irradiated materials sold up to that point contained a new substance having toxic properties (toxisterol). (6a) (6b) (6c) (6d)

Vitamin E was not recognized as necessary for the human until of late, but it is now known to be essential, and in purified forms loses its potency, being most effective if the "complex" is not taken apart. (7a) (7b)

Vitamin G investigations have brought to light a chemically different vitamin G for each species tested in one series of experiments (8a) (8b) (8c)

Do the promoters of these abortions and fake products (though made in the good faith of ignorance) tell you about their mistakes? *No*. A thousand times *no*.

You must be canny enough to apply the old common sense test. Use only products of known clinical value. Ask the man who has used them or make your own tests. It is not the physician anyway who has supported the business of the makers of phoney products. It is the layman who bought them "over the counter" without a prescription nine times out of ten, thinking that the "old reliable firm" back of the product knew what it was doing.

---

(1a) "Man commits a crime against nature when he eats the starch from the seed and throws away the mechanism necessary for the metabolism of that starch." (*Time*, $B_1$, 32,2:39, July 11, 1938, quoting Dr. R. R. Williams)

(1b) "It would seem that we are not justified in considering rat units of vitamin D in irradiated ergosterol as being equivalent to the same number of rat units of vitamin D in cod liver oil as a curative or prophylactic remedy for rickets." (Barnes, D. J., Brady, M. J. and James, E. W., Comparative Value of Irradiated Ergosterol and Cod Liver Oil as a Prophylactic Antirachitic Agent When Given in Equivalent Dosage According to the Rat Unit of Vitamin D, *American Journal of Diseases of Children,* 39:45, 1930)

(1c) Irradiated vitamin D is a different substance from cod liver oil D. (Abstract of Steenbock, H. Kletzein, S. N. F., and Halpin, J. G., The Reaction of the Chicken to Irradiated Ergosterol and Irradiated Yeast as Contrasted with the Natural Vitamin D of Fish Liver Oil, *Journal of Biological Chemistry,* 97:249, 1932)

(1d) "Deprecating the promiscuous use of viosterol, Brehm points out 'It is important in treating a patient not to produce by overtreatment a more serious condition than that originally treated. Natural vitamins, when indicated, seem preferable to synthetic vitamins.'" (*Modern Medicine*, Viosterol During Pregnancy, page 62, October, 1937)

(1e) Vitamin D factor in viosterol and cod liver oil are not identical. Ten times as many vitamin D units in viosterol do not give as much protection as plain cod liver oil. (Abstract of DeSanctis, Rudolph and Craig, J. D., A Five-Year Clinical Study of the Prophylactic Value of Antirachitic Agents, *New York State Journal of Medicine* 34:16, 712-714, 1934)

(2a) " ... In several cases of Paget's disease, the carotene content was normal, but the vitamin A content was markedly subnormal. From this, it is inferred that in this disease, there is some liver disturbance which interferes with the conversion of carotene to the vitamin." (*Endocrinology,* 20, 3:451, May 1936 abstracting Schneider and Widmann, The Hepato-hormonal Direction of Vitamin A Metabolism and the Etiology of Paget's Disease, *Klin. Wchnschr.*, 14:1786, 1935)

(2b) Greaves and Schmidt found that carotene was much less assimilable and effective than vitamin A itself and that the conversion of carotene to vitamin A was accomplished only in the presence of normal amount of bile. (Abstract of Greaves and Schmidt, *American Journal of Physiology,* 111:492-502, April 1935)

(2c) Palmer points out that the conversion of carotene to vitamin A occurs in the liver probably through the medium of an enzyme and that the ability to make this conversion is necessary to the effective utilization of carotene as vitamin A. (Abstract of Palmer, L.S., *Journal of American Medical Association*, 110, 21:1751, May 21, 1938)

(3) Friderichsen and Edmund point out that the vitamin A factor from spinach is 10 times as effective, unit for unit, in clinical tests, as the vitamin A from fish liver oils, besides producing a more prolonged action. (Abstract of Frederichsen, C. and Edmund, Carsten, Studies of Hypovitaminosis A: II. A New Method of Testing and Resorption of Vitamin A from Medicaments, *American Journal of Diseases of Children*, 53:89-109, January 1937; III. Clinical Experiments in the Vitamin A Balance in Children after Various Diets, ibid, 533:1179-1201. March 1937)

(4) Williams, Robert R. and Spies, Tom D., *Vitamin $B_1$ and Its Use in Medicine*, pages 133-134, Macmillan Co., New York, 1938)

(5a) Elmby and Warburg have cured scorbutic patients by the use of lemon juice in cases that were not amenable to treatment with ascorbic acid. (Abstract of Elmby, A., and Warburg, E., *Lancet,* 233, 1363, 1937)

(5b) "Dr. Szent-Gyorgyi later found, along with vitamin C in fruit juices and adrenals, a 'permeability factor' which he calls vitamin P, not present in synthesized C ... " (*Time,* Paprika Prize, page 55, November 8, 1937)

(5c) "Because the isolated vitamin C lacks something that the true vitamin as found in juices retains, the synthetic product is not proving a substitute for orange and tomato juices in preventing borderline cases of scurvy, and other less tangible but real childhood ills, Dr. Henry G. Poncher of Chicago told 70 members of the Texas and Dallas Pediatrics Society here recently at a meeting held by the organization." (*Drug Trade News*, M. D. Holds Synthetic Vitamin D Not Complete, 12, 23:46, December 6, 1937)

(5d) "So Szent-Gyorgyi had to depend upon an occasional human. These were sufficient, however. In repeated tests he found that his citrin, or vitamin P from lemons or red pepper, in 14 days would clear up a hemorrhagic condition when pure vitamin C from some other source was useless." (*Los Angeles Times,* New Lemon Vitamin Cure for Bleeding: Scientist Working Here to Separate 'Citrin' from its 'Twin,' Vitamin C, March 14, 1937)

(6a) " ... Moderate over-irradiation under some conditions produces a substance ('toxisterol' or 'substance 248') which has a marked tendency to cause pathological calcification of the soft tissue of the body while being relatively ineffective in curing rickets ... Some of the early reported toxic manifestations following high dosage with irradiated ergosterol were doubtless due to the presence of considerable amounts of toxisterol, perhaps as the result of technical defects in the irradiation procedure." (Sherman, H. C., *Chemistry of Food and Nutrition,* Fifth Edition, pages 455-456, The Macmillan Company, New York, 1937)

(6b) See reference 1c.

(6c) See reference 1e.

(6d) "Previous studies showed (a) that the liver oils of different species of fish contain forms of vitamin D which react differently, per rat unit, on chickens ... " (Bills, C. E., Massengale, O. N., Hickman, K. D. C. and Gray, E. LeB., A New Vitamin D in Cod Liver Oil, Abstract from Proceedings of the American Society of Biological Chemists, *Journal of Biological Chemistry,* 123, 3:x-xi, May 1938)

(7a) Evans and the Emersons isolated three different related principles in the vitamin E complex and found that the complex was more effective than any of the single factors. They ask "is a mixture more effective than any of its separate constituents and what is pure vitamin E?" Evans and his associates express the opinion that probably several closely related factors each provide the vitamin E function in different degrees. (Abstract of Evans, H. M., Emerson, O. H., and Emerson, Gladys A., The Isolation from Wheat Germ Oil of an Alcohol-Tocopherol, Having the Properties of Vitamin C, *Jour. Biol. Chem.*, 113:319, Feb. 1936)

(7b) "A caution, of course, is necessary. There should be no confusion between crystalline Vitamin E and wheat germ oil. The one, like viosterol, is a single component of a natural product (synthetic in the case of viosterol); the natural product contains the natural vitamin in an environment most favorable to its best work. There is as much difference in the usefulness of crystalline vitamin E and wheat germ oil as there is between viosterol and cod liver oil. The two, in either case, are not identical substitutes." (New York Physician, November 1935 as quoted by Pacini, August J., in his Wheat Germ Oil: Vitamin E, page 41, *The American Physician* , Inc., New York)

(8a) The experiments demonstrated that an extract of rice bran may be separated into two fractions by means of treatment with fullers' earth. The unabsorbed fraction was the antidermatitic factor for the chick and the absorbed portion served as the same factor for the rat. (Abstract of Lepkovsky, S. and Jukes, T. H., The Effect of Some Reagents on the 'Filtrate Factor' [A Water-Soluble Vitamin Belonging to the Vitamin B Complex and Preventing a Dietary Dermatitis in Chicks], *Journal of Biological Chemistry*, 114, 1:109-116 [114], May 1936.)

(8b) The filtrate factor which is potent for the chick is found, in all probability, to be a different factor than a human pellagra-preventive principle. (Abstract of Jukes, T. H. and Lepkovsky, S., The Distribution of the "Filtrate Factor" [A Water-Soluble Vitamin Belonging to the Vitamin B Complex and Preventing a Dietary Dermatitis in Chicks] in Certain Feeding-Stuffs, *Journal of Biological Chemistry,* 114, 1:117-121 [121], May 1936.

(8c) The fact is pointed out that pellagra in the human is caused by deficiency of a different factor than either rat pellagra or chicken pellagra. (Abstract of von Euler, The Water-Soluble Vitamins, *Annual Review of Chemistry,* 5:364, 1936)

**Edited by Royal Lee**

VITAMIN NEWS

VITAMIN PRODUCTS CO. • MILWAUKEE, WISCONSIN

VOL. 6

## NUTRITIONAL FACTORS AFFECTING THE HEART

Those who have had occasion to make many heart examinations by means of diagnostic apparatus, such as the electrocardiograph, sphygmograph, cardiophone, etc., concur in the comment that a functionally sound or normal heart is as uncommon as a perfect set of teeth.

Perfection in either case is dependent upon adequate nutritive factors. We know now that it is the great exception to find an individual without definite physical marks of deficiency, and the heart is no more immune to such deficiencies than are the teeth or the endocrine system.

The nervous control of the heart is affected by means of a balance of power of the two divisions of the autonomic nervous system — a resultant of the opposing stimuli received from the sympathetic and vagus (or parasympathetic) innervation.

The sympathetic tends to speed up and increase the circulation of blood in response to physiological demands; the vagus inhibits according to similar demands. (The former is the accelerator; the latter the brake.)

Exercise, anger and emotions initiate stimuli to the sympathetic. Deficiency of the organic potassium (found in green leaf vegetables) can paralyze the vagus, allowing these stimuli to the sympathetic division to have too great and too prolonged an effect. The result is "sympatheticotonia," with tendency to:

- tachycardia
- hypertension
- rapid respiration
- dry mouth
- paralysis of muscles and of accommodation
- exophthalmos
- low gastric acidity (hypochlorhydria)
- gastrointestinal hypotonicity
- spastic sphincter
- leukopenia
- constipation[1]
- dehydration

"V-P" Organic Mineral tablets are a convenient and rapid means for supplying organic potassium.

Worry, shock, bad news, fright, etc. initiate stimuli to the vagus, and deficiency of the phosphoric radical[2] paralyzes the sympathetics, permitting too great and too prolonged an effect from these causes that initiate vagal stimuli.

The result is "vagotonia," with tendency to:

- bradycardia
- angina pectoris
- hypotension
- irregular respiration
- excessive salivation
- spasm of muscles of accommodation
- enophthalmos
- leukocytosis
- gastric and duodenal ulcers
- hyperchlorhydria
- nervous indigestion
- gastrointestinal hypermotility
- relaxed sphincter
- spastic gastrointestinal musculature
- diarrhea
- hydration

It is evident now why heart symptoms and digestive disorders are usually concomitant.

Where the vagus is not opposed and becomes dominant, by reason of partial paralysis of the sympathetic system, the common cause is phosphorus and phosphate deficiency. "V-P Phosphade" is a quick and convenient means for restoring balance in that case.

Let us here consider the patient having a heart that is somewhat impaired functionally or organically, so that it is unable to respond to demands for reserve effort. Suppose a deficiency of potassium develops, with consequent over-stimulation by the sympathetics by reason of the impaired vagus inhibition. The heart will be found to be laboring as if under the demands of exercise — an engine without a governor. Nutritional deficiency here aggravates a situation that would not otherwise be serious.

With vitamin deficiency to starve the endocrines, and mineral deficiency to paralyze either or both divisions of the autonomic system, any combination of the two lists of consequences of autonomic unbalance is possible.

Vitamin B deficiency alone can so impair the muscular and nervous functions as to cause extreme embarrassment of the heart.

On the next page is shown a graph of an interesting case. Patient, female, age 30. In graph No. 1 (10;45 A.M.), we see three feeble pulsations, followed periodically by three barely distinguishable attempts at contraction. Six tablets of "V-P" Vitamin B Complex were administered and at 11:00 A.M., 15 minutes later, graph No. 2 was made. A normal pulse was found with a rise in systolic blood pressure of 17 mm. nearer normal (83 mm. to 100 mm).

[1] Robertson and Doyle, Intestinal Stasis in Low Mineral Diets, *Journal of Nutrition*, 9, 5:553-569, May 10, 1935, point out this potassium deficiency as a probable common cause of constipation.

[2] Action is by reason of loss of calcium from the nerve cell through its reversion to carbonate from phosphate, the carbonate being inert physiologically.

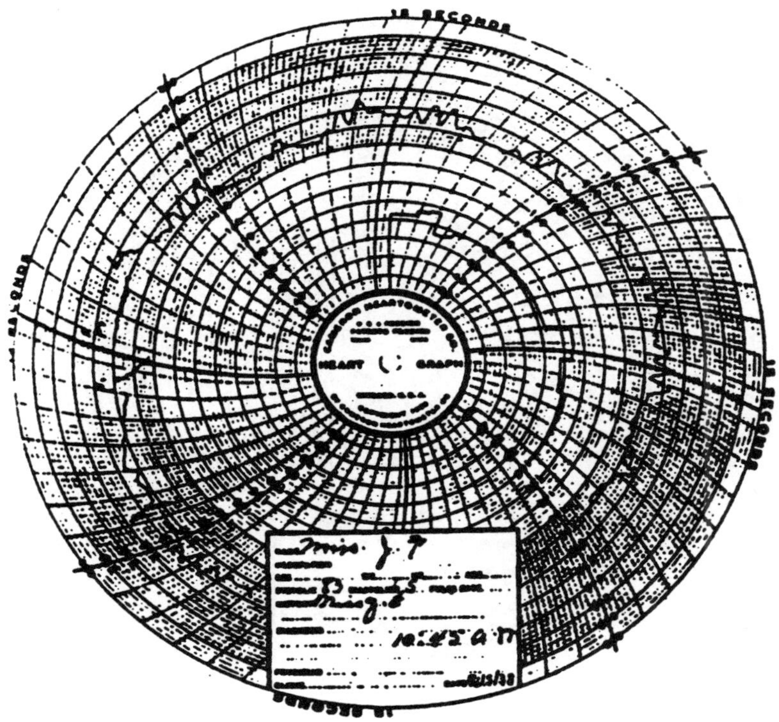

10:45 A.M.
How would you diagnose this case?
(Acute deficiency of Vitamin B Complex)

In hyperthyroidism we find a result of vitamin deficiency (aggravated by iodine and organic potassium paucity), in which the oversecretion of thyroid hormone brings about an excessive elimination of calcium and phosphates. The end result is a specific form of autonomic unbalance modified by the presence of thyrotoxicosis.

That explains the phenomenal relief in hyperthyroidism that usually follows the use of "Catalyn" with "V-P Phosphade" and "V-P" Organic Minerals which is frequently successful even where occurrences have necessitated successive thyroidectomies. It is obvious that surgery cannot cure a dietary deficiency, but can only remove consequences.

The older books on materia medica highly recommended metaphosphoric acid as a remedy for nervous indigestion and nervous instabilities. The more recent authorities have thrown out such recommendations with the statement that "hydrochloric acid should be preferred," naively assuming that the indigestion was due to a lack of this component of gastric juice. The phosphoric radical, on the other hand, is really the natural remedy to stop the excessive secretion of hydrochloric acid present in nervous indigestion and allied conditions.

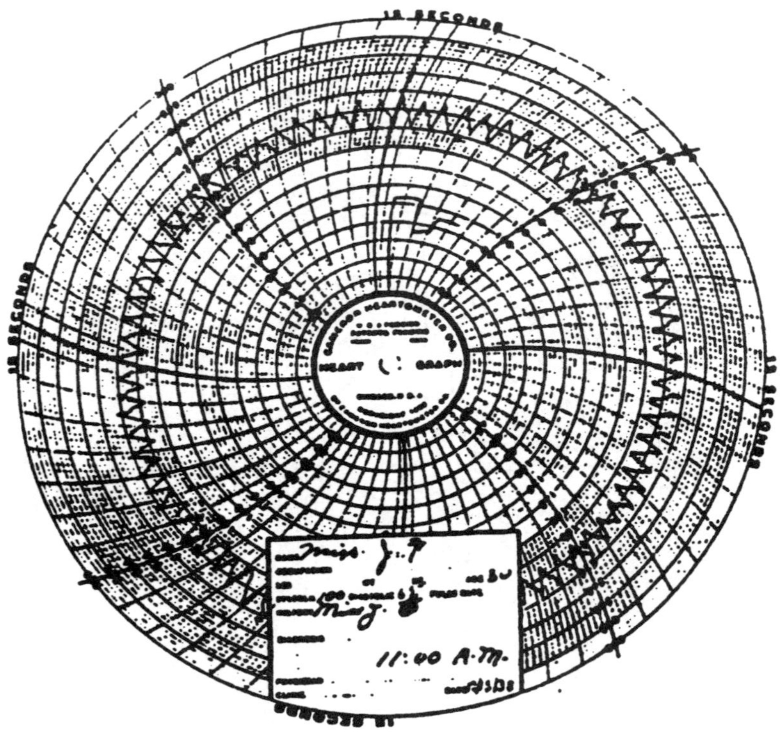

11:00 A.M.
Same day, same patient
(A nearly normal graph)

Often where both potassium and the phosphoric radical are lacking, we may need both "V-P Phosphade" and "V-P" Organic Minerals in the same case.

The old-time veterinarians prescribed metaphosphoric acid for horses that were "skittish" and nervous from too much green grass and oats (containing organic potassium in abundance and no phosphoric radical, wheat being the only cereal carrying it in substantial amounts).

We recall that cod liver oil was also described once by the authorities as being "no better than so much butter." Effective prescriptions including linseed oil for application to the skin, were changed to call for "sweet oil," under the mistaken assumption that "oil was oil," with resultant total loss of effect, the original effectiveness having been due to the Vitamin F content of the linseed.

These items of history are brought to your attention to emphasize the fact that you are accountable for results only, and your patients depend upon your judgement based upon your experience. The longer a physician has practiced, the more he depends upon his own observations and the less he depends upon those of others.

**Edited by Royal Lee**

VITAMIN NEWS

VITAMIN PRODUCTS CO. • MILWAUKEE, WISCONSIN

VOL. 7

# VITAMIN B COMPLEX THERAPY AND CARDIAC PATHOLOGIES

by

**William A. Hanson**

One of the first noticed and most important effects of vitamin B avitaminosis is the bradycardia so prevalent among beriberi sufferers. Harris[1] claims that this cardiac effect is due to an excess of lactic acid, which is not iodized in the absence of vitamin B.

The lowered respiratory quotient described by Stepp, Kuhnau, and Schroeder[2] in avitaminosis B is not due to the lactic acid factor, but to the lack of another $B_1$ fraction which effects the catalysis of pyroracemic acid. This clearly indicates the complex nature of the vitamin B heart factors.

Sherman and Smith[3] suggest that the vitamin B factor concerned with the removal of lactic acid (which factor Harris holds responsible in avitaminosis B for bradycardia) is entirely different from the factor which in avitaminosis causes heart block and further different from the factor which in conjunction with torulin regulates water distribution in the body.

Carter[4] has shown that pigeon heart block can be cured by administration of whole wheat but not by administration of vitamins $B_1$, $B_2$, or the fat-soluble concentrates. In a latter communication,[5] he carries his experiments further and concludes that a wheat germ constituent different from vitamin $B_1$ leads to a complete restoration of cardiac function in case of pigeon heart block.

It should be evident that a complex vitamin concentrate is the only scientific one to use in cardiac conditions because of the innumerable various factors, all necessary, which are present in the vitamin B complex. Stepp, Kuhnau, and Schroeder[6] recognize this fact when they say, "— in cases of vitamin $B_1$ deficiency not responding upon administration of highly purified vitamin $B_1$ preparations in a manner expected, it is recommended, therefore, to prescribe yeast (Brewer's or dry) which contains all the factors of the vitamin B group — "

"V-P" Vitamin B Complex concentrate contains these vitamins and associated food principles of the vitamin B group and is in a much more concentrated form than yeast preparations.

In such pathologies, therefore, it would seem beneficent to employ complex vitamin concentrates. Remarkable results from administration of our own "V-P" Vitamin B complex concentrate are indicated on the charts on pages 90, 100 and 124 of *Vitamin News*. These results will be demonstrated in your own office on our Endocardiograph should you desire. Clinical results show no such rapid and complete effects upon administration of crystalline vitamin B.

"V-P" Vitamin B complex concentrate was developed over a ten year period of clinical tests on human subjects. It is a food concentrate obtained by physical means in order to insure the presence of all the vitamins in the B group and the associated food principles necessary to produce completely satisfactory results from Vitamin B therapy.

## BIBLIOGRAPHY

[1] Harris, *Vitamins in Theory and Practice,* Cambridge University Press, England, 1935, pp. 64-67.
[2] Stepp, Kuhnau, and Schroeder, *The Vitamins and Clinical Application,* English translation, Vitamin Products Co., Milwaukee, 1938, p. 24.[3]. Sherman and Smith, *The Vitamins,* Chemical Catalog Company, New York, second edition, 1931, p. 81.
[4] Carter, *Biochemical Jol.* 24:1811, 1930.
[5] Carter, Maintenance Nutrition in the Pigeon and Its Relation to Heart Block, *Biochemistry,* 28:933-939, 1934.
[6] Stepp, Kuhnau, and Schroeder, *The Vitamins and Clinical Application,* English translation, Vitamin Products Co., Milwaukee, 1938, p. 64.

The effect of vitamin B in five-minute period in a 32-year-old patient, J. B. of San Diego, California

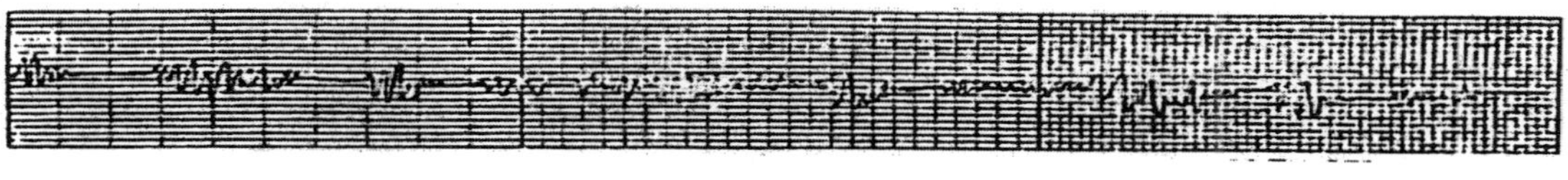

10TH SEC. 25TH SEC. 50TH SEC.

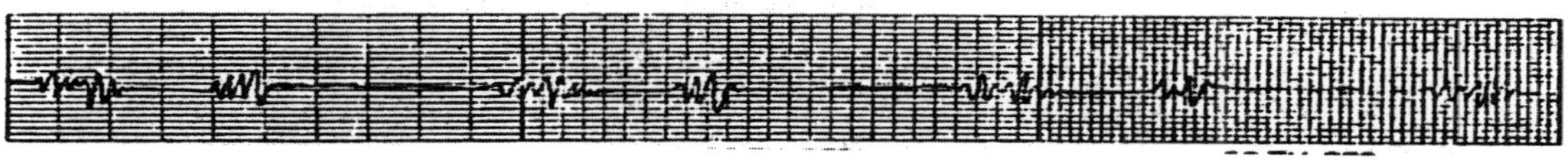

10TH SEC. 25TH SEC. 50TH SEC.

Graphs by permission of Endocardiograph Co., Milwaukee, Wisconsin

Pulse rate, 55 before administration of vitamin B, and pulse rate, 70 afterwards.

The first graph shows very short rest periods and considerable fibrillation.

Second graph shows well-defined rest periods and a great reduction in fibrillation. This is due to the restoration of the function of nerve tissue and is illustrative of the rapid action of the vitamin B fraction that is required by the heart. This fraction is not identical with crystalline vitamin $B_1$, but is part of the vitamin B complex as found in wheat germ.

The response of heart block in the human to treatment with "V-P" Vitamin B Complex

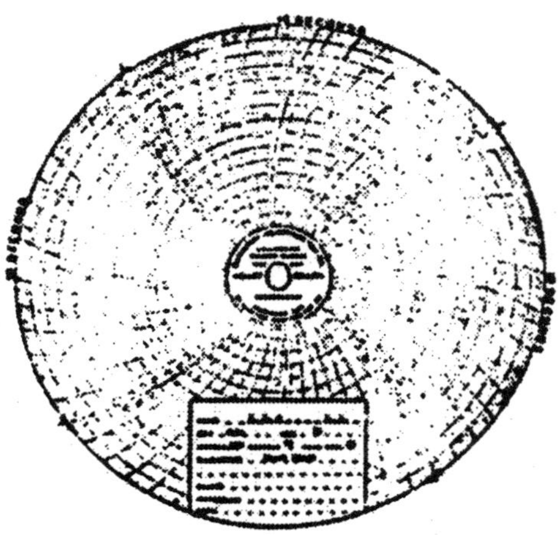

Before Taking Vitamin B

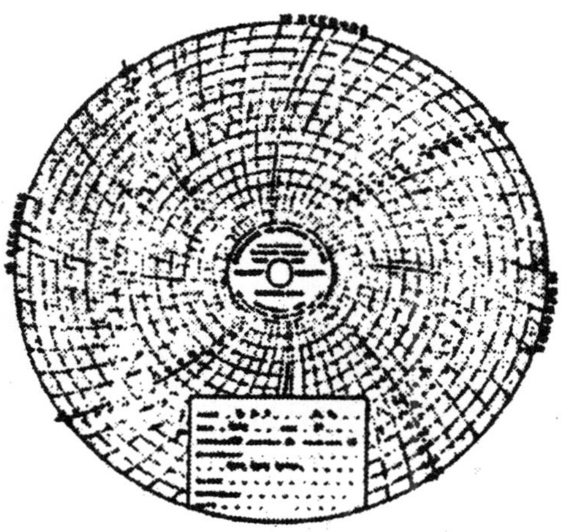

After 4 Days' Treatment

"The writer has had a personal experience with 'complete heart block' that after eight weeks' duration, subsided in four days on your vitamin B complex. The pulse of 28 stepped up to the normal 72, and the character and amplitude of the graph changed from a typical 'block' graph to one that was normal.

"On several occasions since then on the least indication of a possible return, he has resorted to vitamin B of other makes, and he is convinced they are not as efficacious as your 'B complex.' Your tablet seems to take hold and give instantaneous results."

*(signed) W. D. D., M. D.*

# NOTES

VITAMIN NEWS

VITAMIN PRODUCTS CO. • MILWAUKEE, WISCONSIN

## ABSTRACTS ON RELATION OF VITAMIN DEFICIENCIES TO HEART DISORDERS

"In rats, a Vitamin $B_1$-free ration produces a distinct bradycardia, which disappears on addition of the vitamin (as yeast) to the ration. In underfeeding, bradycardia develops as a result of the inanition and is not relieved by administration of the vitamin."

Parade, Vitamin B Researches, I. Relation Between Deficiency of Vitamin $B_1$ and Bradycardia, Z. *Vitaminforsch.* 6:327-334, 1937, as Abstracted by *Chemical Abstracts*, 32, 7:2577, April 10, 1938.

"CARDIOVASCULAR MANIFESTATIONS OF VITAMIN $B_1$ DEFICIENCY: The cardiovascular manifestation of beriberi most commonly encountered are dyspnea and palpitation on exertion, tachycardia and edema. The heart is generally enlarged both to the right and to the left. Systolic murmurs are common. Basilar pulmonary rates are frequent. The arterial blood pressure is usually normal or low, frequently with an increased blood pressure. On palpation, a bounding quality is noted in the larger arteries and 'pistol shot' sounds may be heard on auscultation. The venous pressure is generally increased but may be normal. The skin is usually warm and of normal color. Cyanosis is rare; edema may be mild and only in dependent parts, or diffuse and extreme. Electrocardiograms generally show alterations, chiefly in the T waves. Circulatory failure may be predominately right sided or left sided. Sudden circulatory collapse (shock) has been observed, as well as syncope due to hypersensitivity of the cartoid sinus.

"It is thus apparent that the cardiovascular manifestations of vitamin $B_1$ deficiency do not, at least in the present state of our knowledge, comprise a rigid and easily recognized clinical syndrome. Furthermore, not infrequently, rheumatic, arteriosclerotic, or syphilitic heart disease may have superimposed injury due to vitamin $B_1$ deficiency.

"However, there are technical measurements of the circulation which may prove to be of significant value in the differentiation of beriberi from other types of cardiovascular disorders. The circulatory minute volume and circulation time are both increased in the cardiovascular complications of beriberi whereas other causes of congestive failure, except hyperthyroidism, result in conspicuous slowing of the circulation. The important points in establishing the diagnosis of cardiovascular disease dependent on deficiency of vitamin $B_1$ are, in addition to those points already presented, the presence of other manifestations of vitamin $B_1$ deficiency, such as polyneuritis, or of deficiencies of other portions of the B complex, such as glossitis and pellagrous skin changes. Indeed, it is rare to observe 'beriberi heart' without at least minimal signs of polyneuritis; the history of dietary inadequacy or of conditioning factors which lead to vitamin $B_1$ deficiency in spite of an apparently normal diet; the disappearance of signs and symptoms following adequate $B_1$ therapy."

Strauss, Therapeutic Use of Vitamin $B_1$ in Polyneuritis and Cardiovascular Conditions; *Clinical Indications, Journal of the American Medical Association*, 110, 13:953-956, (955), March 26, 1938.

"Nutritional disorders may affect the heart along with other tissues, sometimes seriously. Beriberi, a disease which is primarily the consequence of vitamin B deficiency (tropical avitaminosis), has been shown to cause hydropic degeneration (intracellular edema) of the myocardium, particularly of the right ventricle, with cardiac dilation and failure. Relief is obtained neither by digitalis nor by diuretics but by the administration of antineuritic vitamin B."

White, *Heart Disease*, Page 437, MacMillan Co., 1936.

"Evans found that vitamin C increased the urinary output in each of 8 cases of cardiac failure and in another with considerable edema of the lower extremities of unknown etiology. In 2 cases, the increase was slight; in 4, it was either moderate or considerable and in 3 cases, it was great. When a quantitative estimate was made of the excess of urinary output over fluid intake in the 9 cases over a period of 173 days, it was found that vitamin C induced greater diuresis than digitalis, but less than theobromine, theobromine with sodium salicylate, and ammonium chloride. In each of 3 patients in whom cardiac failure had occurred with auricular fibrillation, vitamin C induced diuresis actually in excess of that produced by digitalis, although never with the same degree of clinical improvement nor with reduction of the ventricular rate. These results direct attention to the need of providing an adequate supply of vitamin C for all patients with cardiac failure. To ensure a constant state of vitamin C saturation in heart failure, it is probably enough to include in the patient's diminished fluid intake an adequate proportion of lemon and orange juice.

Evans, Vitamin C in Heart Failure, *Lancet* London, 1:308, February 5, 1938, as Abstracted by *Journal of the American Medical Association*, 110, 18:1526, April 30, 1938.

" ... Sudden death from heart disease in relatively young or middle-aged persons is caused, in a measure, by blood vessel and heart disease resulting from a lack of sufficient foods containing vitamin C ... "

Quigley, *Notes on Vitamins and Diets*, Page 126, Consolidated Book Publishers, Inc., Chicago, 1933.

"An analysis was made of the cardiac rate, electrocardiographic complexes and the response to drugs of rats in the non-deficient state and in repeatedly induced vitamin $B_1$ deficiency. The heart rate fell slowly during feeding on a deficient diet, but returned to normal within a few hours after an adequate dose of vitamin $B_1$. In most cases of deficiency, changes occurred in the electrocardiographic complexes. Exercise did not produce more rapid heart changes in the deficiency. The cardiac responses of deficient and normal rats to adrenaline were the same. Atropine and section of the vagus nerve did not abolish the changes caused by deficiency. Deficient rats were more sensitive to the toxic effects of strophanthin."

Weiss, Haynes and Zoll, Electrocardiographic Manifestations and the Cardiac Effect of Drugs in Vitamin $B_1$ Deficiency in Rats, *American Heart Journal,* 15:206-220, 1938, as abstracted by *Chemical Abstracts*, 32, 22:9202, November 20, 1938.

"The cardiac disturbance is of great diagnostic importance in distinguishing beriberi from other unrelated forms of neuritis and is the most serious threat to life in the patient not already endangered by infectious disease. Cardiac symptoms come and go but are always present at some stage of beriberi. They consist of shortness of breath, precordial pain, boring in nature, which may be as severe as that in angina pectoris.

"The heart is enlarged and the liver swollen and tender. The veins of the neck are engorged. The pulse is weak. The cardiac symptoms, when severe, cause intense suffering and discomfort. The patients toss about in bed unable to compose themselves. They may die suddenly in such attacks. Respiration is so laborious it resembles that of respiratory obstruction."

Eddy and Dalldorf, *The Avitaminoses*, The Chemical, Clinical and Pathological Aspects of the Vitamin Deficiency Diseases, pages 92-93, The Williams and Wilkins Company, Baltimore, 1937.

"The symptoms of acute cardiac beriberi closely resemble those of infantile beriberi. Patients with predominating cardiac symptoms usually die suddenly, and often without a history of prodromal symptoms. At any time during the course of the disease, and often without warning to the physician, symptoms of acute cardiac failure may suddenly appear. This cardiac failure is characterized by paroxysmal onset of precordial pain, dyspnea, cyanosis, increased venous pressure, tachycardia, murmurs, and a small, thready pulse. Transient elevation of the systolic and diastolic blood pressure and electrocardiograph changes are frequently described. Examination of the heart shows striking enlargement, especially to the right, associated with pulmonary congestion, cyanosis, and vasomotor collapse ... "

Williams and Spies, Vitamin $B_1$ and Its Use in Medicine, *The Macmillan Medical Monographs*, Page 21, The Macmillan Company, New York, 1938.

"THE HEART. The most common cause of sudden death from vitamin $B_1$ deficiency is acute cardiac failure. The classical picture of postmortem is a dilated and hypertrophied heart. The right auricle and right ventricle are conspicuously enlarged; the chambers are filled with blood and the valves are normal. At times, when the enlargement of the right auricle and ventricle is pronounced, the left heart may be small. In such instances, the walls are 'paper thin' as a result of the dilation of the right auricle and conus arteriosus. Chronic passive congestion of the liver, spleen, kidneys, and intestines are nearly always present, and pulmonary edema occurs in at least 50% of the cases."

Ibid Page 62.

"THE MECHANISM OF CARDIOVASCULAR FAILURE IN VITAMIN $B_1$ DEFICIENCY. The beriberi heart results from failure to utilize sufficient quantities of vitamin $B_1$. It is characterized by two outstanding features: 1, the predominance of cardiac enlargement on the right side; 2, diminished contractile power. Lack of satisfactory anatomical or physiological explanations for these findings has led to the following hypotheses as explanations of the mechanism of the heart failure.

"1. Degeneration of the vagus nerve ...

"2. Respiratory paralysis ...

"3. Water retention or edema hypothesis ... "

Ibid Pages 64 and 65.

"NUTRITIONAL HEART DISEASE IN CHILDREN. Waring presents thirteen cases of cardiac disturbances of nutritional origin. The diagnosis of nutritional cardiac disease was made on the basis of the following observations: cardiac enlargement, shown by percussion and by roentgen examination, without accompanying murmur; negative results of urinalyses; absence of sluggishness of reflexes; a history of deficient diet, and a more or less rapid response to rest and sufficient food. Dietetic histories in most cases were vague, but malnutrition was generally evident. Twelve of the thirteen patients were Negro children aged from 14 to 48 months. The cause of cardiac enlargement does not appear in these cases. Whether deficiency of vitamin $B_1$, deficiency of protein or general dietetic deficiency is the fundamental cause is still a matter of some disagreement. All the patients improved on adequate diets strengthened with materials rich in vitamin $B_1$. It appears that the cardiac changes are not entirely due to a lack of $B_1$ but to a rather more general deficiency of dietary materials and that a satisfactory response to dietetic treatment may be expected in cases in which the illness is not too far advanced."

Waring, Nutritional Heart Disease in Children, *American Journal of Diseases of Children,* 55:750, April 1938, as Abstracted by *Journal of the American Medical Association*, 110, 24:2033-2034, June 11, 1938.

" ... The heart beat is affected in both pigeons and rats. There is bradycardia and heart block which clear up promptly when the vitamin (B) is given."

Macleod, *Physiology in Modern Medicine,* Page 475, The C. V. Mosby Company, St. Louis, 1935.

"A few years ago, Dr. Drury and I discovered that the hearts of rats suffering from lack of vitamin $B_1$ beat only half as fast as those of normal rats — i.e. they had what clinicians would call bradycardia.

"The interesting point I am leading up to is this, that further investigations in my laboratory have shown that the low heart-rate has to do with the excess of lactic acid, which in the absence of vitamin $B_1$ cannot be got rid of. The lactic acid seems to poison the heart muscle and prevent it functioning at full rate. Give vitamin $B_1$, the lactic acid can be disposed of, and the heart is soon beating at its normal rate again."

Harris, *Vitamins in Theory and Practice*, Pages 65-67, The Macmillan Company, New York, 1935.

"A most interesting finding recently made in England is that a deficiency of vitamin B produces abnormal slowness of the heart beat. It was proved that this was produced by the specific effect of vitamin B deficiency, not by insufficient food intake. Since heart failure in mankind is a common cause of death, and frequently occurs in persons apparently in excellent health, the application of such experimental results to human ailments may very well be expected."

Sure, *The Vitamins in Health and Disease,* Page 41, The Williams and Wilkins Co., Baltimore, 1933.

"Experimentally it has been demonstrated that vitamin B deficiency produces an abnormal rhythm of the heart, known as 'bradycardia.' In this disease the heart rate in the rat is reduced from a normality of 500-550 beats per minute to 300-350. Since the American diet is often low in vitamin B, is it not possible that some forms of cardiac disease are due to cumulative effects of vitamin B deficiency? No clinical evidence is available, however. A statistical investigation of the dietary history of men dying of cardiac diseases would be of medical interest.

Ibid Page 191

Tohoku states that vitamin B deficiency is also known to cause heart enlargement.

Tohoku, *Journal of Experimental Medicine,* Page 184, 1935.

" ... Bradycardia is common (in vitamin B deficiency)."

Wiggers, *Physiology in Health and Disease,* Page 960, Lea and Febiger, Philadelphia, 1934.

"Vitamin $B_1$ deficiency in rats caused bradycardia, not of vagus origin, and depression of the T wave and the ST segment of the electrocardiogram. It is not clear whether or not the bradycardia is due to certain metabolites produced in excess in this condition (lactic and pyruvic acids and alpha-ketoglutamic acid). Synthetic vitamin administration in normal dogs is reported to produce, on the other hand, a marked and sustained bradycardia. The addition of vitamin C to the perfusion solution of the isolated frog's heart increases the extent of contraction, especially when added after perfusion has been carried out for some time. Acute vitamin C deficiency in the guinea pig is reported to be associated with proliferative lesions along the margins of the heart valves. No changes in the electrocardiograms of normal children receiving therapeutic doses of vitamin D over a long period of time occur, contrary to the results of previous workers."

Eyster, Heart, *Annual Review of Physiology,* 1:317-344, 1939.

# NOTES

VITAMIN NEWS

VITAMIN PRODUCTS CO. • MILWAUKEE, WISCONSIN

VOL. 7

# FOOD FACTS OR THEORIES — WHICH TO FOLLOW?

## The Wrong Path Leads to An Untimely Death

Most of us possess sufficient common sense to follow the course indicated by established facts rather than to follow a theoretical hypothesis when the two conflict. However, often we are overpowered by the publicity spread by the promoters of theories who profit by such theories, when the facts are of so little profit to anyone that they are not so well publicized.

The facts regarding nutritional matters represent a very outstanding example of such a situation. The exploiters of denatured and synthetic foods that annually destroy more human life than the most bloody war imaginable are not interested in facts. If they can promote a theory that will help sales, such theories are published widely without regard for the real truth. This is not only true about the manufacturers of such denatured foods as white flour and white sugar, but also is true of the manufacturers of synthetic and chemically pure vitamins.

It has been our pleasure to recently read a new book, *Nutrition and Physical Degeneration* by Weston A. Price, published by Paul B. Hoeber, Inc., New York, 1939. Dr. Price proceeds to delineate some facts, ascertained by himself after traveling to all parts of the globe to get them himself first-hand.

He says that tuberculosis, heart disease, physical deformities, dental disease, and lowered resistance in general were uniform and inevitable consequences in every race or tribe of people where a change from native foods to modern commercial foods took place. To illustrate, in French Equatorial Africa the native population in 1911 was twenty million; today two and a half million. Innumerable photographs and detailed examples from all parts of the world are offered as irrefutable evidence for his statements. In high valleys in Switzerland where no commercial foods were brought in, the incidence of tuberculosis was zero, the incidence of dental caries in school children was 0.3 cavities per individual. (Three children had to be examined to find one defective tooth.) This is one twenty-fifth the incidence of caries found elsewhere in Switzerland.

In Australia, after examining skulls of the native race of various periods in museums at Canberra and Sydney, he states that if a scale were extended a mile long and the decades were indicated by inches, it is apparent that there has been more degeneration in the last few inches than in the preceding mile. Dr. Price observes, "This gives some idea of the virulence of the blight contributed by our modern civilization."

Among the natives of the Torres Straits Islands, the same picture was found. The government physician in charge of the group stated that in thirteen years, he had seen only one case of suspected malignancy among four thousand islanders. In the same time he had operated several dozen malignancies in the three hundred of the white population.

The significant statement is made that dental caries is arrested in those native individuals whose diet was changed back to their original form after being on refined foods for a period. The open cavities ceased to be active.

An interesting case at home is described by Dr. Price of a five-year-old boy with rheumatic fever, arthritis, and an acute heart involvement who had been hospitalized for two and one-half years. The mother had been told there was no chance of recovery. Severe tooth decay was a part of the picture. (The American Heart Association has reported that 75% of heart disease begins before ten years of age.) Dr. Price changed the white flour part of the diet to whole wheat (fresh), oatmeal, whole milk and high-vitamin butter with extra natural vitamin D complex (from cod liver). The boy was badly crippled with arthritis, swollen knees, wrists, rigid spine, cried by the hour (bedfast). Rapid improvement occurred under the new diet, and six years later is reported normal except for being taller and heavier than average.

Dr. Price also relates the failure of the synthetic form of vitamin D (he refers to the "so-called vitamin D") known as Viosterol, which produced marked pathological calcification of the kidney in obstetrical cases (tests on a group of 540), which, of course, did not occur in those groups where the natural vitamin D complex was used (as cod-liver oil).[1,2]

We think that Dr. Price's book is a history-making step forward that will stand out among the mass of theory that has flooded the medical world, and which has so misled the public that the word "Viosterol" has almost become synonymous with "vitamin D."

The purveyors of such frauds as Viosterol are as criminally negligent as the miller of white flour who bleaches it to remove the last traces of vitamin, so it will not by any possible chance support life, to keep off insects that otherwise would consider it as food. We have nothing but respect for Steenbock, the inventor of the process for making Viosterol, for he was also the original discoverer of the fact that it was not vitamin D, and he published his findings for any interested person to see.[3,4] But by that time the commercial interests had taken possession of his process, and he was powerless to retrieve it.

It has since made many millions of dollars for its owners, but at what a price![2,5,6]

We have called attention before in these pages to the dangers of viosterol. (*Vitamin News,* page 51). We have been astonished that a food and drug administration could overlook such a product that is so widely circulated as a nutritional factor for infants and children, that is in reality a death-dealing poison. At the same time, we can recall the successful prosecution of a natural food product admittedly harmless where purchasers as well as prescribing physicians testified under oath as to the beneficial and indispensable nature of the article in question. Is it possible that politics enter into the matter of enforcement of the food and drug laws? If that is true, there is no choice left for Patrick Henry's immortal "Give me liberty or give me death." It is just "Death" — Death to be dealt out by the highest bidder.

The criminally asinine negligence of the Food and Drug Administration in this case is only equaled by the performance of the War Department in the Civil War and the Indian Wars following. The Winchester repeater was manufactured and available before the Civil War, but the War Department was asleep at the switch. Even as late as Custer's Last Stand, the soldiers were slaughtered merely because they had to use the pitiful single-shot, antiquated army muskets while the Indians were well equipped with Winchester repeaters that all the trading posts had been selling for years in exchange for furs.

It seems to be the history of civilization for the people of a democratic government to be "sold down the river" by dishonest, ignorant or indifferent public servants. No other argument is needed for a wholesale review of laws intended to protect the people, but which work out to betray them, by taking away their personal liberty to choose what food they must have to live, under the pretense of regulating the sale of drugs.

What is the remedy? Publicity and more publicity. Doctor, if you would like extra copies of this issue to pass out to your patients, drop us a post card stating how many you need. And a letter to your Congressman or Senator would not be out of order, asking him why we have laws that list all foods that cure deficiency diseases as drugs, and which prohibit their sales until the "consensus of opinion" of "experts" has accepted the facts regarding their value. Is this not putting theory ahead of facts? Is not the old principle of law requiring truthful statements as to uses and effects a sufficient protection for the purchaser? And ask him why the laws are not enforced against synthetic poisons masquerading as "foods," where the facts are so perfectly established? Is it because of the political power and influence of the owners of the Viosterol patents, the Alumni Research Foundation of the University of Wisconsin?

I fear that too many people have been taking for granted the philanthropic motives of that institution. A thousand dollars a day in royalties would put a lot of pressure on anybody's conscience.

That is why we need a food and drug law. But the really big offenders always get away, and one of their prize tricks is to make it appear by hook or crook that those who see the rotten picture and call public attention to it are themselves law violators. What better way to dynamite criticism? (We have some very interesting facts in our possession for anyone who would like to study this picture further.)

These tactics would be for more difficult of accomplishment if we all insisted on accepting only facts that we could prove ourselves, and no facts are easier to prove than the truth about nutritional products. They either consistently do their work or they do not.

Here is a case where "V-P" concentrates did their work. Can you figure what the mathematical probabilities are of this result being a coincidence? Or would you be inclined to agree with us that it just is a natural result of a more complete nutrition?

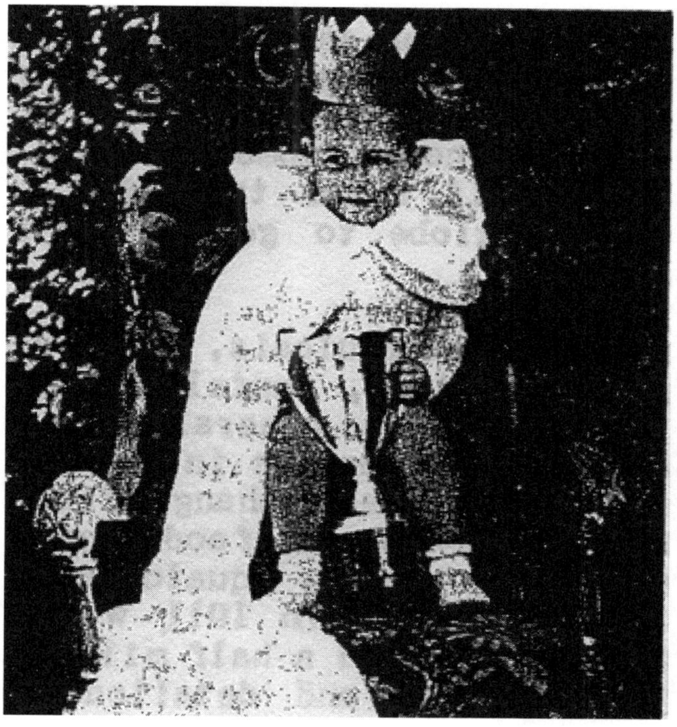

This sunny young man of 22 months was prema--turely born, an incubator baby, and the attending physician doubted his ability to survive. His father, a chemist, realizing that the only hope for aid was in nutritional support, started the addition of a daily ration of "V-P" vitamins to the milk within a week after birth. At the age of 22 months, our young friend won first prize in a baby contest over 465 other contenders, with the phenomenal score of 100.

[1] Price, W. A., *Nutrition and Physical Degeneration*, Page 411, Paul B. Hoeber, Inc., New York, 1939.
[2] Brehm, Potential Dangers of Viosterol During Pregnancy with Observations of Calcification of Placentae, *Ohio Surgical and Medical Journal*, 33:990, 1937.
[3] Steenbock, Keltzein and Halpin, The Reactions

of the Chicken to Irradiated Ergosterol and Irradiated Yeast as Contrasted with the Natural Oils, *Journal of Biological Chemistry,* 97:249, July 1932.

[4] Haman and Steenbock, the Antirachtic Effectiveness of Vitamin D from Various Sources, *Journal of Biological Chemistry,* 114, 222:505-514, June 1936.

[5] Bills, Massengale, McDonald and Wirick, The Action of Activated Ergosterol in the Chicken, *Journal of Biological Chemistry*, 108, 222:323-330, February 1935.

[6] Spies, *Archives of Internal Medicine*, page 433, September 1932.

VITAMIN NEWS

VITAMIN PRODUCTS CO. • MILWAUKEE, WISCONSIN

VOL. 7

# WHY V-P VITAMIN PRODUCTS ARE NOT OFFERED FOR COUNCIL ACCEPTANCE

This question is often asked us. There are several reasons why we do not want to obtain this endorsement.

The first is that we do not want to be under the restriction that requires that any therapeutic claims be in accordance with the consensus of medical opinion. We insist on our right to publicly state the facts about the uses of our products now, and not twenty years from the date of their discovery, for it takes that long for the "consensus" to accept new things that are revolutionary in nature.

For example, we pioneered in telling the profession about the value of vitamins in treating heart conditions. The consensus of medical opinion even at this late day, for example, is that "there is no connection between vitamins and heart disease, and no vitamin product is of any value in treating heart conditions." That is the statement made by the best experts the Food and Drug Department was able to assemble to aid in the prosecution of the manufacturer of a vitamin product in a recent case.

Pages 126 (a) and 126 (b) of *Vitamin News* herewith attached indicate how far wrong these so-called "experts" were.

Pasteur was ridiculed for twenty years because his ideas were so revolutionary. The truth means nothing to the "expert." He will believe nothing, and accept nothing that does not carry an explanation that fits his preconceived theories. We have facts to offer that need no apologies. We offer them for consideration by any physician who is sufficiently open-minded to want to make his own tests. If they do not fit past theories, thta is no reason for us to hesitate in passing them on after they have been proven beyond doubt. These facts mean life or death to the patient with heart disease.

The "experts" called in the above case were the best medical and vitamin men obtainable from the faculties of the University of Wisconsin and Marquette University. To make the statement these men did, in this year of 1939, is illustrative of the same peculiar antipathy to new ideas that was shown by the opponents of Pasteur. Such men have to die off and be replaced by men educated in the "new school" before progress can take place.

For us to operate in accordance with the A. M. A. Council is to permit such antiquarians to dictate our business policies.

Our business is founded, rather, upon the endorsement of the physicians, who have given our products the real test of clinical use. The following unsolicited comment from a California physician is typical.

"I believe you and others will be interested in Mrs. F., who was suffering from hypertension since last January. She had been under intensive treatment by another physician from January to October 1 without any improvement.

During this time, she had suffered two mild strokes and was so debilitated that at times she was so weak that she had to be fed. I started her on one-half Catalyn twice a day on October 1. In five days, I had reduced her pressure from 240, where it had been for ten months, to 220. I increased to one tablet night and morning and in the next five days, the pressure was reduced another twenty points. I increased to one tablet t.i.d. and the pressure was down to 180 at the end of two weeks. Her two sons returned at this time and the excitement and additional guests caused her pressure to go up to 220 again. I then added organic mineral tablets one a day. Prior to this time, I had allowed her up for short intervals, but put her back in bed and have kept her there for the past month. Her reading yesterday was 162 over 86. She is again being allowed up for short intervals and expects to have her feet under the table at tomorrow's dinner." (December 25, 1937)

"Another interesting fact relative to her treatment — on October 11, her pulse was very intermittent, missing every second or third beat. By December 1, it had become almost steady. On that date, I counted one hundred beats without a miss.

"Needless to say, I am a rabid enthusiast over Catalyn products. I make no hesitancy in saying frequently that I believe vitamin therapy is the biggest thing in medicine yet developed, and I am heartily in accord with your idea of multiple vitamin therapy. It seems to me the only logical view to take of vitamin deficiency. Also, your vitamin products are exclusively prescribed by myself and are the only ones recommended to my compeers."

Sincerely yours,

........, M.D.

Another unwarranted position taken by the Council is the acceptance of synthetic vitamins as equivalent to the natural product. It has accepted Viosterol as vitamin D whereas it is known to be actually a chemically different substance from real vitamin D. It has not yet revoked the acceptance, even though there is no doubt as to the fact that Viosterol is a dangerous artificial substance for the real thing.

Neither does the Council properly recognize the difference between vitamin complexes and the pure products. All wholesome food materials are complexes; we have no means of exhaustively specifying what they contain.

The difference between complexes and pure vitamins is very well indicated by their value in supplying nutrition to yeast. The yeast plant requires vitamins of the B and G groups to live. It takes up these vitamins from the media it lives in, and concentrates them to some extent thereby. We offer graphic charts to show the great difference in the life-giving properties of our "V-P" Complexes as compared to the chemically pure substitutes, unit for unit.

There is much the same variation in results in the use of these vitamin products in treating human vitamin deficiencies. That is why the unit offers no reasonable basis for comparing the nutritive value of different vitamin products, or their therapeutic values either.

When the A.M.A. Council is willing to be guided by facts alone, and ceases to follow unfounded and dangerous theories, we will seek its endorsement. That endorsement will then mean something. As long as it denies facts in order to justify a position founded on theory, it is on dangerous ground, and we see no prestige for us in having such endorsement.

"What the rank and file of the medical profession ten or fifteen years ago did not know about nutrition fills many books today.

"Prof. E. V. McCallum, one of the distinguished nutrition authorities, declared in 1935 that 'deficiency of vitamin $B_1$ constitutes one of the major health problems of the world.' Opposed to this is a dictum of obscure origin, but one frequently and forcibly uttered by medical gentlemen who seem to substantiate one another, assuring the bewildered laity that people in this country get plenty of vitamins in their ordinary diet.

"Intuition is all very well as far as it goes, but it becomes ridiculous when doctors cling to it long after the accumulating weight of new knowledge shows that the old idea was wrong."

Brady, Intuition and Nutrition, *Milwaukee Sentinel*, Nov. 4, 1939

Effect of "V-P" Vitamin B Complex on Yeast Growth

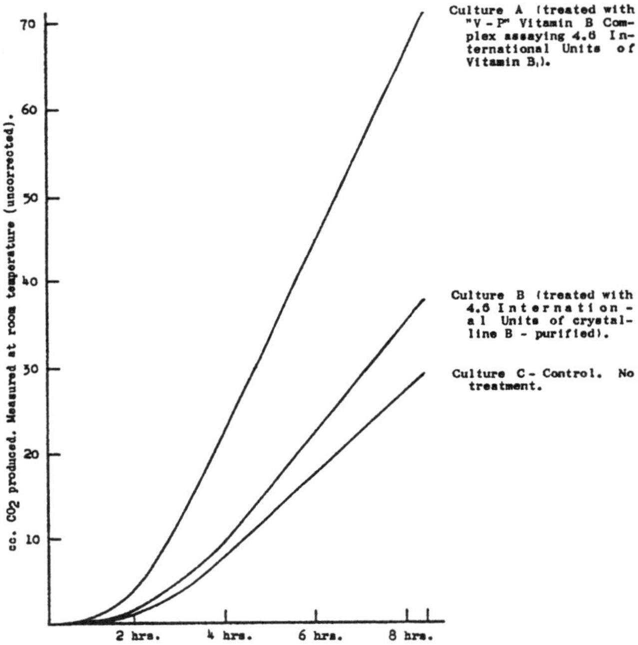


Graph 1

Effect of "V-P" Vitamin G Complex on Yeast Growth

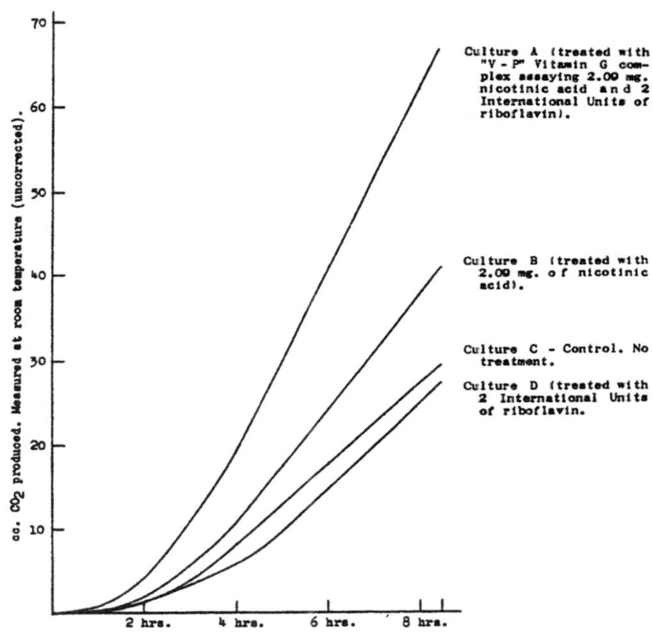


Graph 2

"There is a principle which is a bar against all information, which is proof against all argument, and which cannot fail to keep a man in everlasting ignorance. That principle is condemnation before investigation."

— Herbert Spencer

"The supreme misfortune that can befall any man is for him to embrace a theory in preference to a fact."

— Leonardo da Vinci

"Receiving thankfully all that physiology or chemistry or any other science can give us, let us still hold that that alone is truth which is proved clinically, and that which is clinically proved needs no further evidence."

— Sir James Paget

**Edited by Royal Lee**

# NOTES

VITAMIN NEWS

VITAMIN PRODUCTS CO. • MILWAUKEE, WISCONSIN

VOL. 8

## THE RELATIONSHIP BETWEEN VITAMIN D AND VITAMIN F

To begin by a review of the primary facts, we recall that vitamin D maintains the carrying capacity of the blood serum for calcium and phosphorus. In case of vitamin D deficiency, the blood stream fails to take on calcium and phosphorus from the alimentary system. The administration of vitamin D in such a situation will immediately raise the blood content of both calcium and phosphorus.

Vitamin F is, on the other hand, a depressor of the blood calcium. It, however, cooperates with vitamin D in insuring an adequate assimilation of calcium, since the lowering of blood calcium is accomplished by its diffusion into the tissues. The two vitamins, therefore, while obviously antagonistic, if one limits his observations to the blood-calcium levels, are partners in the basic function of assimilating calcium, and transferring supplies of that element from the alimentary system to the bone, the interruption of which sets up that syndrome known as rickets.

It is, no doubt, this cooperative function of vitamin F that is responsible for the reversal of effect of vitamin D when it is administered in quantities beyond the "threshold of tolerance" of the subject. Then the flow of calcium is reversed, from the tissues into the blood serum. This reversal of action accounts for the observed fact that a deficiency or excess of vitamin D may be similar in effect.[1] It indicates that the reserves of vitamin F are exhausted temporarily.

> "Duguid stated that vitamin D with acid sodium phosphate produced severe tubular nephritis but with alkaline phosphate there was more extensive calcification. Randall has called attention to the occurrence of renal calculi in vitamin D deficiency. This observation again emphasizes the similarity of the effects of deficiency and excess of vitamin D."[1]

It also indicates the unquestionably low "buffer" supply of vitamin F in such cases, and explains why the reversal may occur in one patient under a given dosage and not in another.

Recent researches have shown that the natural sources of vitamin D, such as cod-liver oil, butter and yeast also contain potent forms of vitamin F.[2] It is this vitamin F of cod-liver oil that, no doubt, is responsible for the vast difference between the clinical performance of the cod-liver oil and purified or synthetic vitamin D (such as Viosterol), that is so well known today. The latter products apparently owe their toxicity to the lack of vitamin F, which is necessary to complete the delivery of the calcium to its destination, and without which the blood-calcium levels may reach toxic figures.

The probable presence in cod-liver oil of vitamin F was predicted in these pages[3] with the comment that "this would account for the great difference in the toxicity of cod-liver oil D as compared to irradiated ergosterol." Predictions based upon clinical performance are usually sound.

Recent researches have pointed out the presence in cod-liver oil of a factor other than the vitamin D that is specifically destructive to the bacillus tuberculosis.[4] The older books on materia medica lauded cod-liver oil as a most useful remedy to combat tuberculosis. Later, cod-liver oil was branded as a quack remedy by the "smarter" young generation, who said that the value previously observed was merely due to its fat content, and that butter or lard would be more acceptable substitutes. Billings[5] cautiously stated in 1914 as to its use in tuberculosis, "cod-liver oil is still highly recommended though it is doubtful whether it is of greater value than other easily digested fats." Boissevain[6] has found that vitamin F complex caused an attenuation of virulence of tubercle bacilli. Platonov[7] cited the fact that tuberculosis increased during the World War when fats were scarce (causing a low vitamin F intake). He experimentally demonstrated that guinea pigs were immune to lethal doses of tubercle bacilli that had been treated with the vitamin F complex, and suggested that the natural immunity of the horse to tuberculosis was probably due to the high content of the vitamin F complex in its blood. (Is that why the horse thrives best on oats, the highest carrier of vitamin F among the common grains?) Archard et al[8] found that the serum content of vitamin F complex was lowered in the acute stage of infectious disease, rising to normal with recovery. They concluded that the resistance of the patient was proportional to the serum content of vitamin F complex. (Vitamin F complex throughout this discussion is intended to mean the unsaturated fatty-acid component, of which the biologically active fraction is yet to be identified.)

It is tragic that such vitally valuable facts have so long been overshadowed by theory. The report of the University of Wisconsin investigators stated that tuberculosis of the skin (lupus) was particularly amenable to the application of cod-liver oil, but not to vitamin D alone. Stille[9] in 1868 stated in his *Materia Medica* that lupus was more easily cured by the use of cod-liver oil than by any other remedy. He also quoted Dr. Walshe on the use of cod-liver oil for tuberculosis (Pulmonary) as follows:

> "It more rapidly and effectually induces improvement in the general and local symptoms than any other known agent."

But the careful observations of the practicing physician are ignored and ridiculed by the professors who compile the text books, unless a plausible theory is attached.

I am stressing this point to emphasize to every physician who reads this the vital importance of carefully investigating the reliability of all his sources of information, for the responsibility is his alone if he is misled by false prophets and permits his patients to fail to regain their health thereby.

Stille also stated in 1868 that cod-liver oil was occasionally an effective remedy for diabetes. We have had many reports that our vitamin F concentrate was useful in controlling the blood sugar in diabetes. Now we have more evidence:

> " ... The administration of linoleic acid by mouth lowered the blood sugar in diabetics sometimes as much as 100 per cent in from three to four hours."[10]

It has been said, too, that oatmeal was assimilable by the diabetic without the appearance of any of its starch as urinary sugar (first observed by Von Noorden). Not all diabetics react favorably, but the students of diabetes have been baffled to this day for an explanation. Some have even called the "oatmeal treatment" the "carbohydrate treatment."

Now these facts all fall into their proper place. Oatmeal, as stated on page 31 of this publication, was first observed to be a source of vitamin F long ago. Some diabetics respond to the vitamin B treatment, some to the vitamin F treatment. It is certainly worthwhile (for the patient) to make a test of a few days on the first one and then on the other, one tablet with each meal, to see if his pancreas has yet arrived at the state where it is totally unresponsive to kindness.

Diabetes should be called the "white-sugar disease." Keep in mind the South American Honey Bear referred to in this publication which developed diabetes on a diet of corn syrup. Natural carbohydrates, such as cereals, all have both vitamin B and vitamin F in their germinal cells, and as Dr. Spies of vitamin B fame says, it is A crime to sell cereal products without the vitamins in them to insure their metabolism.

In discussing cereal products, we must not forget the old poisoner — bleached flour. Heart disease in general should be designated bleached-flour disease. We cannot pick up a paper without reading of the sudden death from "bleached-flour disease" of some prominent man in the prime of life.

Why is bleached flour on the market? Why, simply because flour is perishable unless it is devitaminized by bleaching. It becomes a permanent commodity when bleached; it will not support the life of a gnat or weevil, and the uninformed human creatures who are fed the stuff fail to get their allotment of vitamins. What results? Lacking the vitamin B complex, the nervous system degenerates. (First "nervous indigestion for ten years or so, then heart symptoms, arrhythmias in the beginning, fibrillation in the end.) The heart may speed up, or slow down, sometimes to half speed like an automobile motor with half of its ignition system out of commission. (Heart block appears to be a specific reaction to the degenerative effect of vitamin-B-complex deficiency.) Then, again, the deficiency of vitamin F may cause a calcification of the coronary arteries with attendant angina pectoris. On the slightest exertion, the victim is seized with the most excruciating pains in the chest. It is no coincidence that vitamin F has proven the most valuable vitamin remedy for this condition. (Vitamin C is also useful.)

Yes, half of us are starving to death and without the slightest suspicion of malnutrition, either on the part of the patient or of the doctor.

In fact, the doctor often has less suspicion of the true state of affairs than many laymen. Someday the designation "doctor of medicine" will become of less importance than "doctor of nutrition." The past definition of "medicine" is that it is something of no reference to health, of no interest to the well person.

The "doctor of nutrition" will be consulted less by the sick than by the well. There are more men employed today in watching the factors that affect the performance of our automobiles — checking the air in our tires, checking the oil levels, checking the freezing point in our radiator solutions and checking the fuel tank, than there are making repairs. But the doctor of medicine is a doctor of repairs. Is there not something wrong with our method or with our philosophy? Is it the doctor's fault, or isn't it, that we let ourselves break down before seeking counsel?

[1] Reed, Struck and Steck, *Vitamin D*, page 173, University of Chicago Press, 1939.
[2] *Annual Review of Biochemistry,* Vol. VII, pages 82, 86 and 87. 1938; Ibid, Vol. VIII, page 130, 1939.
[3] *Vitamin News*, published by Vitamin Products Company, page 38, October 15, 1934.
[4] *Badger Quarterly*, U. W. Finds that "Vitamin Fraction" Cures Skin TB, 1, 1:6, January 1939.
[5] Billings, *Forchhelmer's Therapeutic of Internal Diseases,* Vol. III, page 507, D. Appleton & Co., 1914.
[6] Boisbovian, The Action of Unsaturated Fatty Acids on Tubercle Bacilli, *American Review of Tuberculosis*, 13:84-89. 1926.
[7] Platonov, The Influence of Unsaturated Fatty Acids on the Virulence of Tubercle Bacilli, *American Review of Tuberculosis,* 21:362-369, 1930.
[8] Archard, Grigaut, LeBlanc and David, The Lipoid Equilibrium of the Blood Serum in Acute Diseases, *Journal de*

*Physiologie at de Pathologie Generale*, 26:415, 1928.
[9] Stille, *Therapeutics and Materia Medica*, Third Edition, Revised, Vol. II, page 810, Henry C. Lea, 1868.
[10] Hinsberg and Holland, The Iodine Absorption Value of the Blood Fats in Normal and Pathological Conditions, *Klin. Wchnschr.*, 12:1601-1602, 1933.

**Edited by Royal Lee** **3/30/40**

VITAMIN NEWS

VITAMIN PRODUCTS CO. • MILWAUKEE, WISCONSIN

VOL. 8

# SYNTHETIC VS. NATURAL VITAMINS

When a chemist begins the study of any material, he has as his chief objective the mapping of the molecular structure, and he feels that his work is unfinished until he succeeds in synthetically duplicating its construction.

Previous to the days of vitamin investigation, no chemist had the temerity to suggest the synthetic production of foodstuffs from non-food sources. The obvious lack of accessory food factors in such products made their commercial exploitation out of the question, regardless of the fact that it has long been possible to make sugar from calcium carbide (via acetylene) or from wood pulp.

In the vitamin field, however, no such practical knowledge of the dangers of consuming synthetic materials has existed in the public mind to protect the layman from exploitation by unscrupulous or ignorant purveyors of nutritional products, who on every hand are barking their wares in health food, grocery, and drug stores.

Each year sees new advertising campaigns break all sales records with new products of assembled synthetic conglomerations of so-called "Vitamins." The buyers are looking for sustenance. Proof that they fail to find it in these mushroom proportions is unmistakable in the short life of each of these trade names in the mind of the public. Here today and gone tomorrow. Every druggist can show a "morgue" of dead products that sold as leaders while the advertising pressure was applied, and were not called for again after the first crop of customers had hopefully laid its money on the counter for the privilege of testing the new and scientifically advertised "Elixir of Life." A product that cannot create its own repeat business is unquestionably worthless, regardless of the so-called "biological units" it may contain.

We reiterate the principle: "Animal tests are indispensable to determine the symptoms of vitamin deficiency, but are worthless to determine what will cure those symptoms when observed in the human species."

The natural vitamin complexes contain the various closely related principles that are normally found together in foods. The more we study those complexes, the more complex they appear. That is why synthetic and chemically purified "vitamins" are really not vitamins at all. They are only fragments of vitamins, just as the vegetable fiber in hay is a fragment of the carbohydrate complex. Goats, rabbits, and guinea pigs can thrive if fed this single fragment of the carbohydrate group (as it naturally occurs *unpurified)*, but we cannot. Hay is not a carbohydrate for the human, but we get some benefit from the associated minerals and vitamins it contains.

The unparalleled results produced by "V-P" Vitamin Complexes are due to the presence of these associated synergists which make up each complex.

That is why "V-P" Vitamin A Complex will so effectively relieve those frequent cases of hypertension, cystitis, and sinusitis that develop because of vitamin A deficiency.

> That is why "V-P" Vitamin B Complex so effectively cooperates with liver extract in anemia and corrects the heart arrhythmias found in almost a third of the adults over fifty, which are common specific reactions to Vitamin B deficiency.
>
> That is why "V-P" Vitamin C Complex so promptly brings down the temperature in infectious diseases where the deficiency has paralyzed the phagocytic activity.
>
> That is why "V-P" Vitamin E Complex so promptly relieves the eczematous conditions that often result from a deficiency of the fat-soluble vegetable group.
>
> That is why "V-P" Vitamin F Complex so promptly relieves the fever blisters, cold sores, brittle nails, scanty hair growth and falling hair that is characteristic of vitamin F deficiency.
>
> That is why "V-P" Vitamin G Complex so often removes the distressing symptoms in gastric ulcer, where the cause frequently is a slowing of regenerative processes because of a deficiency of specific growth factors.

In the following pages will be tabulated the known factors of each of the vitamins that have been discovered up to the present.potent, unit for unit, in the treatment of night blindness, than vitamin A from cod liver oil. The various forms and synergists are necessary for highest potency and best clinical results. Remarkable results have been reported from the use of V-P Vitamin A Complex in nephritis, hypertension, cystitis, acidosis, hemeralopia, and nyctalopia.

## NOTES ON VITAMIN B COMPLEX

Above, we have most of the known factors of the complete natural Vitamin B Complex. Although many of them have no established effect on humans, it is the experience of the clinical users of "V-P" complete natural Vitamin B Complex, No. 712, that they are necessary in natural balance to act as synergists with more specific factors. A natural combination such as this is likely, according to clinical experience, to be from ten to fifty times more potent in humans, unit for unit, than is a chemically purified or synthetic complex, or a natural complex derived from only ONE source. No ONE source contains ALL the factors of the complete vitamin B complex, and for highest potency, a number of therapeutically active sources must be tapped. Although only 22 factors and synergists are listed, ten or more in addition are indicated and are combined in such organic combinations as to make, in some cases, 50 to 100 isomers, while only one is therapeutically active. The futility of attempting to synthesize or tamper chemically with these extremely complicated food factors is thus obvious.

In clinical substantiation of the above information, are the remarkably successful results and higher potencies exhibited by "V-P" Vitamin B Complex in the treatment of cardiac fibrillation, arrhythmias, dilatations, and myocardial weakness.

CHART OF THE COMPLETE
NATURAL VITAMIN A COMPLEX

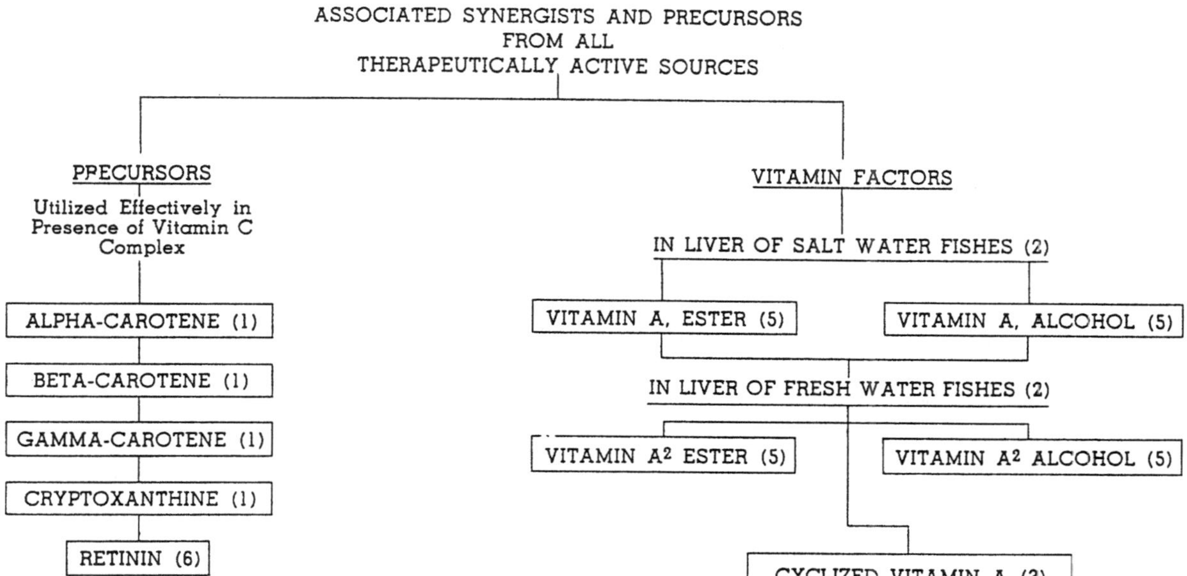


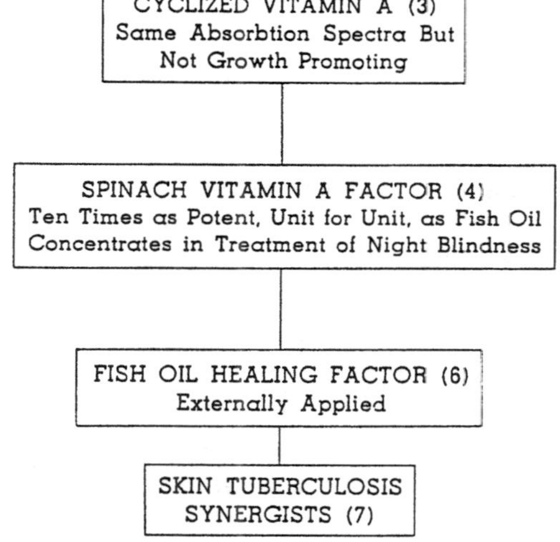


## BIBLIOGRAPHY


(1) McLester, Nutrition and Diet in Health and Disease, W. B. Saunders Co., Philadelphia, pp. 81, (1939)

(2) Nelson and Tolle, Fat-soluble Vitamins, Vitamin A, Ann. Rev. Biochem. 8;415.1939

(3) Embree, Jol. Biol. Chem. 128:187.1939

(4) Abstract, Frederichsen and Edmund, Studies of Hypo-vitaminosis A: II A New Method for Testing the Resorption of Vitamin A from Medicaments, American Journal of Diseases of Children, 53:89-109, January 1937; Clinical Experiments in the Vitamin A Balance in Children after Various Diets, ibid, 53:1178-1201, March 1937

(5) Emmett and Bird, Comparative Biological Value of Vitamin A as an Alcohol and Ester, (Abstract) Scientific Proceedings of the Society of Biological Chemists 119,1: xxxi, June 1937

(6) Stepp, Kuhnau, and Schroeder, The Vitamins and Their Clinical Application, English Translation, the Vitamin Products Company, Milwaukee, 1938

(7) The Badger Quarterly, 1,1:6. January 1939, Madison, Wisconsin

(8) Fraps and Kemmerer Texas Agricultural Experiment Station, Bulletin #560, February 1938, Relation of Spectro-Vitamin A and Carotene Content of Butter to its Vitamin A. Potency Measured by Biological Methods.


(NOTE) Clinical Experience with V-P Vitamin A Complex (the complete natural complex from various therapeutically active sources) has indicated that a combination of factors gives greater effectiveness in humans than vitamin A from any ONE source. Vitamin A is particularly hard to measure in units. The vitamin A of butter is two or three times as potent, unit for unit, as vitamin A from cod liver oil. (8) Spinach vitamin A is ten times more potent, unit for unit, in the treatment of night blindness, than vitamin A from cod liver oil. The various forms and synergists are necessary for highest potency and best clinical results. Remarkable results have been reported from the use of V-P Vitamin A Complex in nephritis, hypertension, cystitis, acidosis, hemeralopia, and nyctalopia.

COMPLETE NATURAL VITAMIN B COMPLEX AND ASSOCIATED SYNERGISTS FROM ALL THERAPEUTICALLY ACTIVE SOURCES

- THERMOSTABLE COMPONENTS
  - UNADSORBED
    - Chick Dermatitis Filtrate Factor — 1935 (1)
    - Anti-Gray-Hair Factor — 1938 (1)
    - Pantothenic Acid — 1933
    - Unknown Unadsorbable Factors (1)
  - ADSORBED
    - Nicotinic Acid — 1937 (1) (Pellagra-preventive factor)
    - Vitamin $B^6$ Anti-acrodynia, and Anti-dermatitis Factor 1938 (1) Dog Anti-anemia Factor
    - Riboflavin — 1935 (1) (Rat-cataract preventing) (Growth promoting)
    - Unknown Adsorbable Factors (1)
- THERMOLABILE FRACTION
  - STRONGLY ADSORBED
    - Thiamin (Vitamin $B^1$) 1936 (1)
    - Pigeon-Weight Factor (Vitamin $B^3$) (1)
    - Rat Anti-paralysis Factor (Vitamin $B^4$) (1)
    - Factor W (Rat Growth) (1)
    - Anti-gizzard-erosion Factor — 1928 (1)
- VITAMIN B COMPLEX FACTORS SEPARATED BY OTHER MEANS AND ASSOCIATED SYNERGISTS
  - Pigeon-weight, rat-growth Factors (Vitamin $B^5$) (2)
  - Extrinsic Factor (Anti-anemic) (3)
  - Anti-egg-white-injury Factor (Vitamin H) 1934 (3)
  - Heart-block Factor — 1930 (5)
  - Vitamin $B^7$ for normal function of intestinal mucosa and muscles — 1935 (2)
  - Grass-juice Factor — 1940
  - Choline (1)
  - Organic Zinc (4)
  - Vitamin M (6) (Anti-pellagra)

## NOTES ON THE VITAMIN B COMPLEX

Above we have most of the known factors of the complete natural vitamin B complex. Although many of them have no established effect on humans, it is the experience of the clinical users of "V-P" complete natural vitamin B Complex, No. 712, that they are necessary in natural balance to act as synergists with more specific factors. A natural combination such as this is likely, according to clinical experience, to be from ten to fifty times more potent in humans, unit for unit, than is a chemically purified or synthetic complex, or a natural complex derived from only ONE source. No ONE source contains ALL the factors of the complete vitamin B complex, and for highest potency a number of therapeutically active sources must be tapped. Although only 22 factors and synergists are listed, ten or more in addition are indicated and are combined in such organic combinations as to make, in some cases 50 to 100 isomers, while only one is therapeutically active. The futility of attempting to synthesize or tamper chemically with these extremely complicated food factors is thus obvious.

In clinical substantiation of the above information, are the remarkably successful results and higher potencies exhibited by "V-P" Vitamin B Complex in the treatment of cardiac fibrillation, arrhythmias, dilatations, and myocardial weakness.

Bibliography on other side.

## BIBLIOGRAPHY


(1) Williams, R. R. and Spies, T. D., Vitamin B[1], The Macmillan Co., N. Y., 1938.

(2) Stepp, W., Kuhnau, J. and Schröder, H., The Vitamins and Their Clinical Application, F. Enke, Stuttgart, Germany, 1936 (translation by Vitamin Products Company, 1938).

(3) Matthews, A. P., Physiological Chemistry, Sixth Edition, Williams & Wilkins Co., Baltimore, 1939.

(4) United States Department of Agriculture Yearbook (1939), U. S. Govt. Printing Office, 1939.

(5) Carter, C. W., Maintenance Nutrition in the Pigeon and Its Relation to Heart Block, Biochemical Journal, 1934.

(6) Journal of the American Medical Association, Editorial, 112,13:1258, 1939.


## BECAUSE OF ITS INTEREST IN THIS CONNECTION WE ARE REPEATING THE FOLLOWING MATERIAL FROM PAGE 130 OF VITAMIN NEWS.

The difference between complexes and the pure vitamins is very well indicated by their value in supplying nutrition to yeast. The yeast plant requires vitamins of the B and G groups to live. It takes up these vitamins from the media it lives in, and concentrates them to some extent thereby. We offer graphic charts to show the great difference in the life-giving properties of our "V-P" Complexes as compared to the chemically pure substitutes, unit for unit.

There is much the same variation in results in the use of these vitamin products in treating human vitamin deficiencies. That is why the unit offers no reasonable basis for comparing the nutritive value of different vitamin products, or their therapeutic values either.

Effect of "V-P" Vitamin B Complex on Yeast Growth

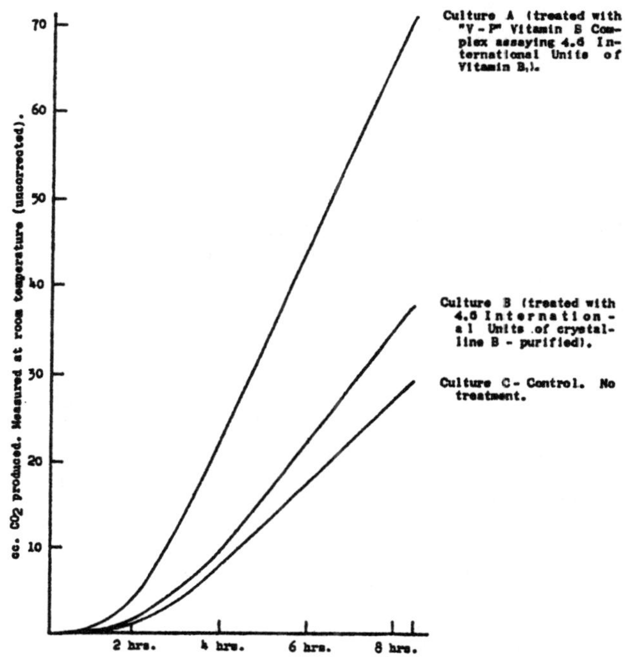

## VITAMIN C COMPLEX

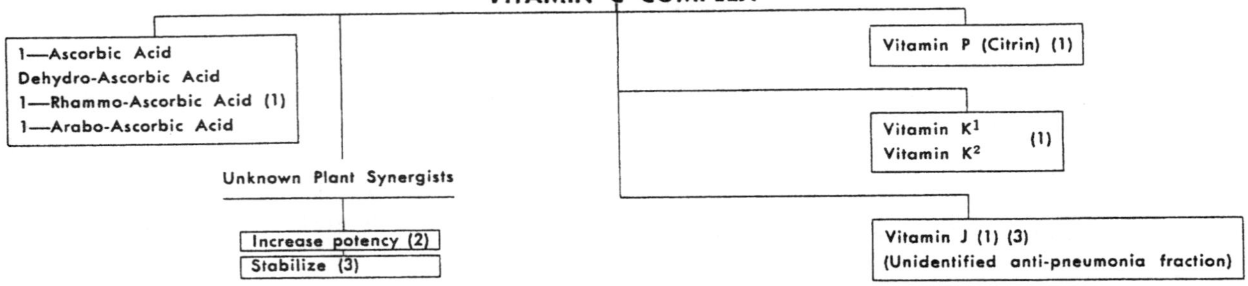


**NOTES ON NATURAL C COMPLEX:**—The most serious symptom of Vitamin C deficiency is susceptibility to infection. (4) This may precede actual scurvy. The anti-pneumonia factor (Vitamin J) has not yet been isolated or identified. Absorption and retention of the various ascorbic acid factors from food is greater than from synthetic sources. (2) This indicates that, milligram for milligram, natural ascorbic acid complexes are more potent than synthetic ascorbic acid. Synthetic vitamin C will not cure scurvy, because other factors of the complete complex are necessary. V-P natural vitamin C complex has always been more productive of clinical results than synthetic vitamin C, especially in promoting phagocytic activity.

## VITAMIN D COMPLEX

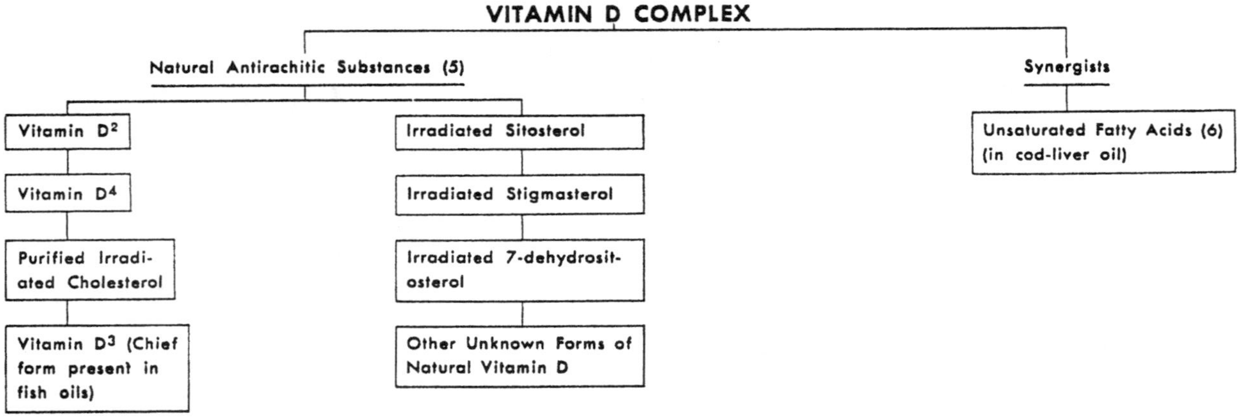


**NOTES ON NATURAL D COMPLEX:**—What we call vitamin D is not a single identity but a complete complex of known and unknown factors. (5) The toxicity of irradiated synthetic preparations, as Viosterol (7), is not present in natural forms containing the synergists. The vitamin D unit is not a reliable criterion of potency, there being species variations of as much as 100 to 1. (5) (8)

## VITAMIN E COMPLEX

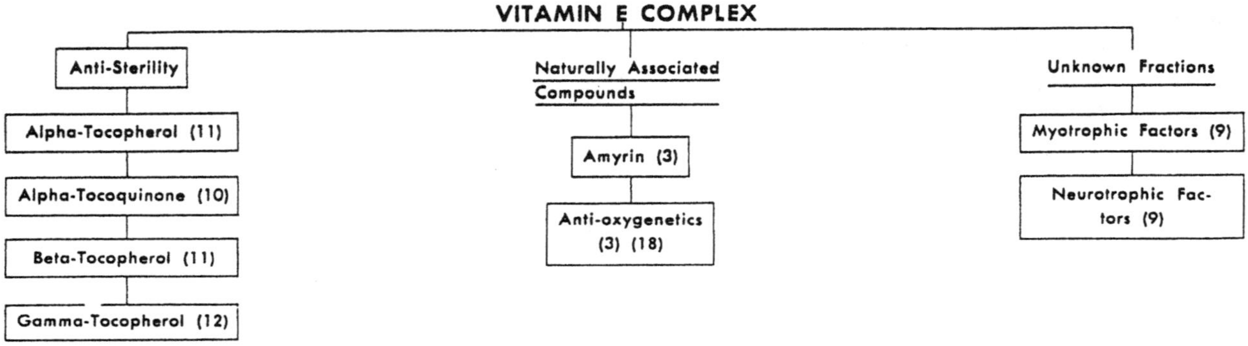


**NOTES ON NATURAL E COMPLEX:**—Drs. Gordon and Sevringhaus (13) suggest that vitamin E will be found to be a complex, requiring the combined action of all factors for proper action. They also review our inability to establish human requirements or determine potency in units.

## VITAMIN F COMPLEX

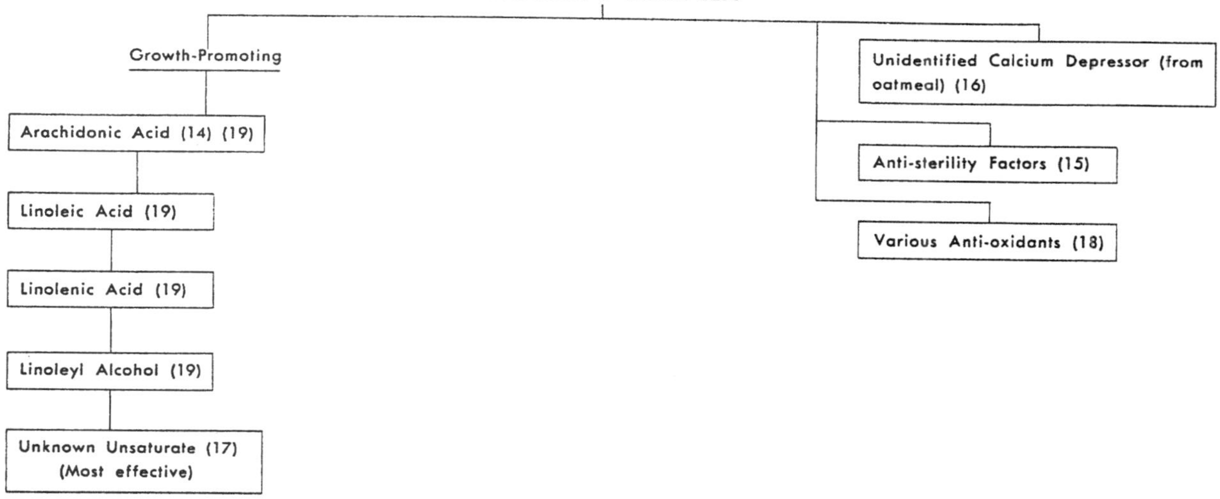


**NOTES ON NATURAL F COMPLEX:**—The chemistry of vitamin F compounds is not well developed except that we know they are unsaturated fatty acids. Their complexity can readily be imagined when we realize that arachidonic acid can have 256 isomers, of which only one might be clinically effective. Clinical reports on the effectiveness of V-P vitamin F complex in cold sores, fever blisters, scaliness of the skin, falling hair, and dandruff have been particularly encouraging. Its effect in lowering the serum calcium make it a logical protector against vitamin D toxicosis, thus explaining its presence as a synergist of vitamin D in cod-liver oil. (6) Vitamin F also is phenomenally rapid in its action of raising the blood iodine. (20)

## VITAMIN G COMPLEX

**NOTES ON NATURAL G COMPLEX:**—The factors composing the vitamin G complex are present in the vitamin B complex. Both B and G complexes are soluble in water, but the G factors are precipitated out in 85% alcohol. These factors embrace the entire thermostable components of the complete B complex, plus other unknown synergists (shown on page 135 of Vitamin News).

Clinically, V-P vitamin G complex has been most productive of results when used in relieving the distressing symptoms of peptic ulcers. The G complex is basically a combination of growth and regenerative factors, thus accounting for its efficacy in various gastrointestinal degenerative inflammations. The unknown parts of this complex from cereal seedlings and grass juice are probably the most therapeutically active in this respect.

## BIBLIOGRAPHY


1. Eddy, W. H., What Are the Vitamins? Reinhold Publishing Company, New York, 1941.
2. Hawley, Estelle E., Daggs, R. G. and Stephens, D. J., The Effect of the Administration of Acid and Alkaline Salts upon the Ascorbic Acid Content of Guinea Pig Tissues, Journal of Nutrition, 14,1:1-8, July 10, 1937.
3. Stepp, Kuhnau and Schroeder, The Vitamins and Their Clinical Application, Ferdinand Enke, Stuttgart, Germany. Translation by Vitamin Products Company, Milwaukee, Wisconsin, 1938.
4. Proceedings of the Society for Experimental Biology and Medicine, pages 1089, 1157, April, 1935.
5. Reed, C. I., Struck, H. C. and Steck, I. E., Vitamin D, The University of Chicago Press, 1939.
6. Burr, G. O. and Burr, M. M., On the Nature and Role of the Fatty Acids Essential in Nutrition, Journal of Biological Chemistry, 86:587-621, 1930.
7. Brehm, Potential Dangers of Viosterol during Pregnancy with Observations of Calcification of Placentae, Ohio Surgical and Medical Journal, 33:990, 1937.
8. Bunker, J. W. M. and Harris, R. S., The Clinical Status of Vitamin D Milks, New England Journal of Medicine, 211, 25:1140-1147, December 20, 1934.
9. Goettsch, Marianne and Ritzmann, Johana, The Preventive Effect of Wheat-Germ Oils and of Alpha-Tocopherol in Nutritional Muscular Dystrophy of Young Rats, Journal of Nutrition, 17,4:371-381, April, 1939.
10. Emerson, Oliver H., Emerson, Gladys A. and Evans, Herbert M., The Vitamin E Activity of Alpha-Tocoquinone, Journal of Biological Chemistry, 131,2:409-412, December, 1939.
11. Evans, Herbert M., Emerson, Oliver H. and Emerson, Gladys A., The Isolation from Wheat Germ Oil of an Alcohol Alpha-Tocopherol, Having the Properties of Vitamin E, Journal of Biological Chemistry, 113:319, 1936.
12. Emerson, et al, Science, 84:421, 1936.
13. Gordon and Sevringhaus, Vitamin Therapy in General Practice, pages 133, 139, Year Book Publishers, Chicago, 1940.
14. 1939 Yearbook of Agriculture, Food and Life, page 158, U. S. Government Printing Office, Washington, D. C.
15. Harris, Leslie J., Vitamins, 4:331-382, Annual Review of Biochemistry, 4:371, 1935.
16. Biochemical Journal, 24:233-238, 1938.
17. Journal of Biological Chemistry, 97:183, 1932.
18. Lea, C. H., Rancidity in Edible Fats, pages 164, 169, Chemical Publishing Co., New York, 1939.
19. Turpeinen, Osmo, Further Studies on the Unsaturated Fatty Acids Essential in Nutrition, 15,4:351-366, April, 1938.
20. Hart, James P., unpublished correspondence, Los Angeles, California to Vitamin Products Company, Milwaukee, Wisconsin.


Form 1408-CG
Printed in U. S. A. 4-41

Vitamin Products Company,
Milwaukee, Wisconsin.

# NOTES

VITAMIN NEWS

VITAMIN PRODUCTS CO. • MILWAUKEE, WISCONSIN

VOL. 9

# THE LEAST APPRECIATED FUNCTION OF VITAMIN C

Vitamin deficiencies are now becoming recognized as specialized forms of starvation. Even overweight persons getting their full quota of calories, carbohydrates, fats, and proteins, are very often starving to the danger point of disease from vitamin deficiencies.

As civilized intelligent people we as utterly fail to appreciate the widespread occurrence of vitamin starvation that is obvious to the student of nutrition who appraises the American dietary situation.

Let us investigate this situation question from the point of vitamin C deficiency alone. We discover that according to the latest opinions on this subject, the preliminary outstanding effect of mild deficiency of vitamin C is loss of resistance to infection.

> "In fact even when there is not a single outward symptom of trouble, a person may be in a state of vitamin C deficiency more dangerous than scurvy itself. When such a condition is not detected, and continues uncorrected, the teeth and bones may be damaged, and what may be more serious, the blood system is weakened to the point where it can no longer resist or fight infections not so easily cured as scurvy."
>
> *Food and Life,* p. 236, 1939 Yearbook
> U.S. Dept. Agriculture U.S. Printing Office,
> Washington, D.C.

Next to degenerative diseases of old age, (also no doubt accelerated prematurely by deficiencies), infectious diseases kill the most people, all the way from whooping cough and diphtheria to pneumonia and influenza, to say nothing of the common cold that wears us down to the point that we contract the more deadly forms of the communicable scourges.

In all probability we can chalk most of the deaths up to the lowered resistance to infection resulting from vitamin starvation.

Let us see what clinicians have to say on this subject.

Here are two of great interest,

"We are thoroughly convinced that vitamin C particularly is of inestimable value in both acute and chronic infections ... The more fulminating the acute infection and the longer a chronic infection has continued, the more is the need for vitamin C. In the presence of infection, vitamin C is rapidly destroyed and its deficiency also predisposes to infection so that a vicious circle is set up."

Albee, Fred H., *Jol. Inter. Coll. Surgeons III*, 5:425-430, Oct. 1940

"If we can, by the use of vitamins, favorably influence the course of a disease such as pneumonia, nephritis, myasthenia, even eventually to cure them, what would have happened if, before becoming ill the patient would have absorbed the right quantity of vitamin? The probable answer to that question is that the patient would never have been diseased if he had provided himself with the right vitamin!"

Szent-Gyorgi, *LaPresse Medicale*
p. 995, June 25, 1938

On the subject of specific diseases due to vitamin C deficiency the U.S. Department of Agriculture says:

"In the most recent review available on this subject, rheumatic fever, pulmonary tuberculosis, diphtheria, and pneumonia are listed as infectious diseases in the prevention and cure of which vitamin C 'undoubtedly plays a significant part' although 'there is no unequivocal evidence that this nutrient has a specific role in the prevention or cure of any of them.'

" ... Evidence is increasing, however, that vitamin C does play an important part in the immunity defenses of the body and that increased allowances are necessary when these defenses are called into action to combat infections."

*Food & Life,* p. 253

The clinical use of vitamin C in pneumonia has a very sound foundation. There is an increased need for this vitamin in this condition. (Wright, *Ann. Int. Medicine,* 12, 4:516-528, Oct. 1936.) In experimental tests, monkeys kept on a vitamin C free diet all died of pneumonia while those with adequate diets remained healthy. (Sabin. *Jai. Expel. Mod.*, 69:507-515, 1939.) clinical recovery from pneumonia is favorably affected by administrations of vitamin C. (Weymuller, *Medical Times*, 67, 11, November, 1939.)

Not the least important of the uses of vitamin C is in febrile diseases of children. In a clinical test the administration of vitamin C gave relief in whooping cough in 24 out of 26 patients as reported by Vermillion and Stafford, in the *Kansas Medical Society Journal,* Topeka, 39:469, Nov. 1938. It is known that vitamin C deficiency occurs in all febrile diseases in children. (Bumbalo, *Am. Jol. Dis. Childr.*, 55:1212-1220, 1938.) The lowering of fever temperature from the administration of vitamin C has been proven in both laboratory controlled animal tests and by clinical experience on human patients with febrile diseases. (Tislowitz, *Compt. Rend. Soc. de Biol.* 121:916-917, 1936, and Hasselbach, *Schweizerische Med. Woch.*, 67:877, Sept. 11, 1937.)

Vitamin C will inhibit the growth and lower the virulence of diphtheria bacteria in a test tube. (Gagyi. *Klin. Wchnschr,* 15:190-195, Feb. 8, 1936.) The susceptibility to diphtheria is markedly increased in vitamin C deficiency. (Booth and Hanson, *Jol. Lancet. LVII*, 12:151, Dec. 1937.) Clinical observations in a large series of necrotic diphtheritics showed substantial reduction of mortality under vitamin C therapy. (Kumagai, Yamagami, Nikai and Imai, *Kiln. Woch.*, 16:987, July 10, 1937.)

Stepp, Kuhnau and Schroeder (*Die Vitamine*, Ferdinand Enke, Stuttgart, Germany, 1935) state that lowered immunity and lowered resistance to infection occur months before scurvy symptoms are manifest. No cause is known for susceptibility to infection other than malnutrition in general and vitamin C deficiency in particular. Therefore every case of infectious disease should be given vitamin C as a primary remedy whether or not other remedies are used. Clinical tests on the administration of vitamin C show that it tends to increase resistance, hasten recovery and lower fever in infectious disease, especially pneumonia, whooping cough, diphtheria, and child febrile disease.

In the face of such overwhelming evidence why has not the use of vitamin C been hailed as the physiological competitor of sulfanilamide and the sulfa-drugs? Certainly the use of a natural physiological remedy with no toxic effects should be employed in every infectious case and hopeless cases. The use of natural foodstuffs in place of sulfa-drugs in children is especially to be desired in order to eliminate toxic effects tending to anemia and kidney disturbance.

Why treat starvation with a drug? Why not hail the discovery of vitamin C as the food to remedy this starvation? Because pure ascorbic acid has failed to do the job.

Szent-Gyorgyi himself throws some light on the matter in his book, *Oxidation* (Williams and Wilkins, Baltimore, 1939) on pp. 73-74, as follows:

> "I am talking in such detail about this substance because of a small accident that happened to us at that time. I had a letter from an Austrian colleague who was suffering from a severe hemorrhagic diathesis (vascular type.) He wanted to try ascorbic acid in his condition. Possessing at that time no sufficient quantities of crystalline ascorbic acid, I sent him a preparation of paprika that contained much ascorbic acid and the man was cured by it. Later with my friend, St. Rusznyak, we tried to produce the same therapeutical effect in similar conditions with pure ascorbic acid but we obtained no response. It was evident that the action of paprika was due to some other substance present in this plant."

Here is the most striking example of the necessity of obtaining vitamin knowledge from clinical experience. It is tragic how many times the reputation of a valuable therapeutic agent has been destroyed when the so called "active" principle has been isolated by the chemist and tested for clinical usefulness. Even such definitely specific principles as thyroxin and the digitalis glucoside are being relegated to discard in favor of the whole gland and whole leaf powder containing the unknown complex which is productive of clinical results where the so-called active principles failed.

Now, in dealing with a food product, such as vitamin C, what possible necessity is there for throwing away the associated factors of the natural vitamin complex? Let us not lose the important anti-infective therapy of vitamin C simply because we employ the chemically purified ascorbic acid rather than the natural complex.

Most of our vitamin C deficiency is a result of the oxidation in the storage and transportation of our fruits and vegetables, plus the reduction in those vegetables occurring because of depletion of such minerals as manganese from the soil. (It has been shown that the use of manganese may double the amount of vitamin C in tomatoes grown on this soil. (*Science News Letter*, May 3, 1941.)

In supplying vitamin C complex to a patient with a fever secondary to bacterial or virus invasion the resistance of that patient is apparently being built up and the vitamin is absorbed. The prompt reduction in fever is the indication of its physiological effect. The only failures reported are in such patients as have a severe calcium deficiency often to be seen in growing children, and the parallel use of calcium lactate is then indicated. Definite symptomatic relief in as short a time as an hour is often observed.

**Edited by Royal Lee, DDS**

# NOTES

# VITAMIN NEWS

VITAMIN PRODUCTS CO. • MILWAUKEE, WISCONSIN

VOL. 10


## THE PHYSIOLOGICAL BASIS OF VITAMIN C

Primarily, vitamin C is known as a protector of endothelial and connective tissue. (Dalldorf, Gilbert, The Pathology of Vitamin C Deficiency, The Vitamins, A Symposium, American Medical Association, Chicago, 1939.) Observers of scurvy usually call attention to the marked deterioration of the mucous membrane and gum tissues of the mouth which become lacerated with the slightest stress. We now know that this is brought about through the loss of activation of the constructive phase of the protein-building enzymes, which activation is normally furnished by vitamin C. (Editorial, *Journal of the American Medical Association*, 117, 11:937-938, September 13, 1941.)

In *Time Magazine*, Nov. 17, 1941, page 60, the experience of Dr. Bartlett of Harvard shows that wound healing with plenty of vitamin C present is several times faster than in deficient tissue and the tensile strength of the new skin is much greater. Drs. Hartzell and Stone of Detroit, are also quoted as stating that vitamin C aids in weaving cells more tightly together.

This protein protecting and building effect is quite likely the reason why vitamin C is so effective in combating the destructive action of bacterial infections. These bacterial toxins produce their damage through their proteolytic effect. The leukocyte carries more vitamin C than any other cell in the body. It is thereby enabled to protect its own protein structure. It also attempts to digest the foreign bacterium which is at the same time fighting for its life by secreting proteolytic enzymes designed to act upon its enemies and not upon itself.

It has been demonstrated that bacterial toxins produce deamination, decarboxylation, and oxidation of the amino acids and proteins in the blood stream. (Peters, John P., and Van Slyke, Donald B. *Quantitative Clinical Chemistry*, page 298, Williams and Wilkins Company, Baltimore, 1935.) This action can be achieved either through the action of the toxins themselves as destructive proteolytic enzymes, or more probably through the activation of the destructive phase of the reversible enzymes present in the blood stream.

It must not be forgotten that most, if not all, enzymes may be either constructive or destructive depending upon the relative concentration of actuators, end products, and nutrients in the substrate (Waksman, Selman A., and Davison, Wilburt C., *Enzymes*, page 31, Williams and Wilkins Company, Baltimore, J926.)

The vitamin C present in the white cell is really its armor to maintain its own protein controlling enzymes in the constructive phase in the face of the attack of the bacterial toxins which tend to augment the destructive phase. This, in effect, gives us a better insight into the biochemical battle between the leukocytes, the defenders of the body, and the invading microorganisms.

The following statement to the effectiveness of Catalyn in combating the toxicity of arsphenamines was made by a physician in Ohio (1938):

> "You can get a very severe condition of dermatitis in those patients susceptible to neosalvarsan ... I

> had a patient that showed this susceptibility ... and I was afraid that we were going to have to stop the administration and therefore leave her with syphilis ... I gave her Catalyn and she is able now to take the full dosage of neosalvarsan and the last report we got was that it was effective ... the point is that we would have had to stop that treatment unless we had found some way of rendering her less susceptible to the neosalvarsan ... She takes just two tablets the day before her injection ... and then she maintains it ... for two or three days. That alleviates all her sickness ... "

In this connection it is interesting to note the article in a recent journal of the American Medical Association describing experiments showing that vitamin C tends to prevent the toxic effects of neoarsphenamine and marpharsen, the anti-syphilitic drugs. (*Journal of the American Medical Association*, 117, 20:1692, Nov. 15, 1941.) Other publications have shown similar results.

French investigators have also shown that vitamin C prevents the reactions to arsphenamines. It is interesting to note that this effect may be due to two factors of the vitamin C complex. (Dainow, I., *Intolerance of Arsphenamines and Vitamin C*, Presse Med. 45:1670, 1672, Nov. 24, 1937.)

Physicians reporting from clinical experience have noticed that although the use of the sulfa-drugs is spectacular in combating the primary infection, often times the patient develops a secondary infection, sometimes difficult to locate.

Apparently such drugs deplete the vitamin C reserves of the tissues and leukocytes with resultant infections and other symptoms of vitamin C deficiency. It should be emphasized that rational therapy demands the addition of vitamin C concentrate schedule whenever the sulfa-drugs or arsphenamines are used.

It should be borne in mind that our comments are confined to natural vitamin C complex consisting of more than one factor. In most cases synthetic vitamin C (ascorbic acid) does not have the same effect as the natural complex. We may point out the experience of Szent-Gyorgyi, where he discovered that synthetic vitamin C will not cure scurvy. (Szent-Gyorgyi, *Oxidation,* pp. 73-74, Williams and Wilkins, Baltimore, 1939) and also the above described comment of Dainow that two factors of the C complex have the detoxifying effect on arsphenamine.

The useful action of vitamin C in combating the effects of hyperthyroidism has been reported to us by many physicians. It may be remembered that thyrotoxicosis is merely another name for the deamination of proteins by thyroxine (Muyer, Hans H., and Gottlieb, F., *Experimental Pharmacology*, p. 387, J. B. Lippincott, Philadelphia, 1926.) Thus the protein-maintaining effect of vitamin C also explains the often reported clinical value of vitamin C in thyrotoxicosis.

Today it is a demonstrated principle that the production of histamine and other end products from deaminized cell proteins released by injury to cells, such as trauma or burns, are a cause of shock. The well-demonstrated clinical value of vitamin C in combating shock is explained when we realize that the deaminizing enzymes from the damaged cells are inhibited by vitamin C. (Editorial, J*ournal of the American Medical Association*, 117, 11:937-938, September 13, 1941.)

It has been shown that mechanical damage to a cell results in pH changes which reverse the destructive phase of the cell enzymes from constructive to destructive activity. These pH changes spread to other cells. (Chambers, B., and Pollock, H., *Journal of General Physiology*, 10:739, 1927.) This destructive activity releases histamine and other shock producing end products. The presence of vitamin C inhibits this enzyme transition into the destructive phase.

("Vitamins for Pain and Shock" was briefly discussed on page 5 of *Vitamin News* in this file, published September 4, 1933, and "Vitamins and Resistance to Infections" was discussed on page 7, published September 18, 1933.)

Another protein protecting effect of vitamin C is seen in its demonstrated effect of preventing the decomposition of adenyl-pyro-phosphoric acid of heart muscle as a result of undue thyroid stimulus. (Berg, H., *Arch. Exptl. Pharmakol.*, 185:359-367, 1937, abst. Chem. Abstracts, 32, 16:6297, August 20, 1938.) Vitamin C in this action evidently combats thyroid tachycardia.

The utilization of oxygen is impaired in vitamin C deficiency. The capacity of the blood to carry oxygen is apparently lowered. (Peterson, I. M., *Science News Letter*, 40, 9:137, August 30, 1941.) This explains the exceptionally good clinical results vitamin C complex and Catalyn have produced during the past eleven years which have been particularly obvious in coronary cases. The first issue of *Vitamin News* (August 7, 1933, page 1 of this folder) makes the statement that shortness of breath and rapid heart action are the specific consequences of vitamin C deficiency in the heart patient: the tachycardia, being due to aggravation of thyrotoxicosis, is caused by a lack of vitamin C. Here is a good example of how clinical facts antedate explanations.

Clinical facts are often put to work and justly deserve to be, whether or not the explanation is known. In checking through the older literature, we are struck with the canny powers of observation the old-timers possessed. For example, the early mariners preferred the water of the central lake in the Great Dismal Swamp of Virginia for their stock of drinking water when starting on a long voyage. They found that their crews remained free of disease for longer periods than if well water were used. This water, brown with vegetable extractives, no doubt, contained appreciable quantities of vitamin C. (The Great Dismal Swamp, Webster, Prof. N. B., *The American Naturalist*, May, 1875, page 262.)

If you care to follow this idea further we refer you back to page 127 of *Vitamin News* entitled, "Food Facts or Theories — Which to Follow? ... The wrong path leads to an untimely death."

**Edited by Royal Lee**

# NOTES

# VITAMIN NEWS

VITAMIN PRODUCTS CO. • MILWAUKEE, WISCONSIN

**VOL. 11**


## A FEW FACTS IN REVIEW

A new term has been coined to describe and identify vitamin factors that produce a single effect, where this effect may be obtainable in various degrees of activity by a number of chemically different factors, or where different factors are necessary to produce the same effect in different species of life. The term that has been adopted is "vitamer," derived from the chemical term "isomer," which is a substance differing from another in molecular construction, but the same in proportions of its content of the elements. (*Science*, January 15, 1943 reporting the action of the Gibson Island Conference, July, 1942–p.57.)

"Whereas isomers are compounds with a given molecular formula, vitamers are compounds with a given vitamin activity and usually possess different molecular formulas."

Vitamins for ten different vitamin categories are listed: $B_1$ vitamers, D vitamers, K vitamers, niacin vitamers, pantothenic vitamers, pyridoxine vitamers, para-aminobenzoic acid vitamers, and various biotin (H) vitamers are now known.

The word "vitamer" was necessitated by the growing recognition of the fact that a specific vitamin effect in different species of animals (or plants) was often produced by quite different compounds, chemically considered. Therefore, the word "vitamer" means only that unless the species of animal that is to be fed a vitamer in discussion is also specified, the vitamin is not yet identified. We reiterate the principle: animal tests are indispensable to determine what the symptoms of vitamin deficiency are, but are worthless to determine what will cure those symptoms when observed in the human species." (*Vitamin News*, Vol. 8, p.133, November 6, 1940.)

It is apparent that to describe a vitamin and offer a standardized "unit" for use in the determination of a schedule of treatment for a deficiency disease, it is necessary for the manufacturer to have some kind of idea from clinical experience as to the effects of his product in treating human cases.

The products of this company always have had their vitamin activity determined by tests upon human subjects, and have been only from sources that were found, by ages of experience, most suitable for human food.

That is why so many later discoveries of vitamin uses were anticipated by physicians prescribing our products. Back in 1934 we stated in *Vitamin News* (p.31) that our vitamin E complex was effective in the relief of certain muscular pains, apparently of neuritic or arthritic origin, that seemed to originate from "small centers of activity," and were not variable in location.

This seems to be a fairly exact description of the pains of fibrositis, now known to be usually relieved with vitamin E concentrates. Dr. Steinberg, in an article in the *New York State Journal of Medicine* (April 15, 1942) described the treatment of fifty cases of fibrositis; he says that forty-eight cases were completely relieved of all symptoms on treatment with a vitamin E complex or wheat germ oil. Fibrositis is defined as a "rheumatoid disorder characterized by a non-suppurative inflammatory reaction in the white fibrous connective tissue, any where in the body, with a swelling and proliferation of the fibrous tissue in response to chilling, toxic influence, trauma, or fatigue. Acutely tender fibrous bands and nodules frequently form in the nerve sheaths, and press on arterioles and nerve filaments, causing muscle spasm and secondary pressure effects."

Where the fibrositis was secondary to arthritis, the value of the vitamin E was less definite. Dr. Steinberg classifies various forms of the disease that "masquerades under various titles" as lumbago, torticollis, muscular rheumatism, tendinitis, myositis, myositis ossificans, myasthenia gravis, and various other forms.

We recall that back in 1933 an Ohio physician reported to us the cure of a distressing case of myositis ossificans with "Catalyn." In 1933 there was no recognized unit assay method for vitamin E. But the same clinical test can be made without animal test units, and the drug store shelves are full of products carefully engineered to produce specific results in test animals, but sold without tests to determine what they will do to the human species. One thing is definite. The use of our products has always been limited to recommendations that involve the use of no more than the daily requirement (except in acute cases) of any vitamin complex we have. We have not found it necessary to go over this amount where the natural synergists of the vitamin are present. (That is the "complex.")

"This ... brings out the fact which is true for most of the vitamins, namely, that several related compounds may have similar biological action but the degree of their activity varies." (Elvehjem, *The Scientific Monthly,* Recent Advances in our Knowledge of the Vitamins, p.99, February, 1943.) Personally, we believe further that these members of a complex varying activity are of selective value to various tissues and organs of the body, for various separate purposes, so that to substitute a single synthetic factor for the group is a most unwise and futile attempt to simplify a problem on which our future well-being hinges. It is undoubtedly the lack of such synergists that causes the use of synthetic vitamin B (thiamin chloride) to have such startling effects as to create sterility in the succeeding third generation. Barnett Sure, (Influence of Massive Doses of Vitamin $B_1$ on Fertility and Lactation, *J. of Nutrition,* 18, 2:187-194, August 10, 1939) says that two or three times the daily requirement of $B_1$ will in effect "castrate the grand children" of his test animals, long before they are born. But the makers and purveyors of thiamin have no more heeded this discovery in 1939 of Sure's than the sellers of Viosterol heeded Steenbock's discovery that it was not vitamin D in 1933. We know now that natural forms of vitamin D such as cod liver oil contain enough vitamin F to synergize and normalize the toxic effects of vitamin D to the point that no toxic symptoms appear. No doubt, natural vitamin B complex is also harmless in overdosage if not denatured by the elimination of natural synergists. Stepp says the anti-paralysis factor cannot be removed from natural vitamin B, even by repeated crystallizations. (Stepp, Kuhnau, and Schroeder, *The Vitamins and Their Clinical Applications,* p.24.)

There is an epidemic today of commercial promotion of "anti-gray hair" vitamins, including para-aminobenzoic acid. It is here too that the dangers of a single synthetic factor are great. This factor has a characteristic shared by other constituents of cells that shows up when a pure concentrate or synthetic form is clinically tested. Para-aminobenzoic acid, gluthathione, and betaine to some extent, all tend to stimulate the growth of microorganisms as well as to stimulate the patient. Any focal infections such as appendix, tonsils, tooth abscesses, gingival pockets, etc., may flare up explosively after a few relatively small doses of any of these factors are taken. (Two to ten grains can do it.) Or if you are fighting off a cold, it will really get the upper hand on taking one dose of these products. All these factors have the highly desirable effect of increasing endurance and vigor and are powerful anti-fatigue food elements. But they do the same thing to the germs, unless you at the same time get more of the specific things that keep the germs under control, and of which the C complex is the main representative. Lately it has been shown that the vitamin K factor of the C complex is a valuable preventive of tooth decay, in that its presence in the saliva stops the growth and activity of the acid forming bacteria that are responsible. It is interesting to recall that the sugar cane juice is naturally loaded with both vitamins C and K and the minerals that build teeth, but they are all eliminated in refining.

This finding is of particular interest to your editor, as he commented in 1923 as follows: "Sajous has demonstrated that vitamin C is always present in normal saliva where it sustains the defensive oxidation which renders bacteriolytic and anti-toxic enzymes effective." (The Systemic Causes of Dental Caries, December, 1923.) It appears that the facts are not so hard to find, if we are really looking for them. If this information as first established by Sajous (*Dental Cosmos,* 1923) had been put into practice at that time by requiring that all sugar made and sold in the U.S. had to be so processed as to retain its minerals and vitamins, can you imagine what disease and degeneration could have been headed off? Not that it is even yet possible to make such sugar, but if we were as energetic in prosecuting the war against disease as we are in prosecuting the war against those who object to our tariff system, the solution would soon be found. The saving in the elimination alone of the vast array of dental carpentry necessitated by the tooth damage would pay off the bill of research cost a thousand times over, no doubt.

"Thus the present generation suffers for the sins of the past and we die because our ancestors dissipated their wealth in armies and navies, in the foolish pomp and circumstance of society, and neglected to provide us with a knowledge of natural laws. In this sense they were the murderers and robbers of future generations of unborn millions and have made the world a charnel house and place of mourning where peace and happiness might have been. Only their ignorance of what they were doing can be their excuse, but this excuse puts them in the class of boors and savages who act according to selfish desire and not to reason and to the calls of duty. Let the present generation take warning that this reproach be not cast on it, for it cannot plead ignorance in this respect ...

"Where then, are the great laboratories of research in this city, in this country, nay in the world? We see a few miserable structures here and there occupied by a few starving professors who are nobly striving to do the best with the feeble means at their disposal. But where in the world is the institute of pure research in any department of science with an income of $100,000,000 per year? Where can the discoverer in pure science earn more than the wages of a day laborer or cook? But $100,000,000 per year is but the price of an army or a navy designed to kill other people, just think of it, that one per cent of this sum seems to most people too great to save our children and descendants from misery and even death! ... " (Rowland, Henry A., President's Address to the American Physical Society, October, 1899, *Science, X,* 825-833, 1899.)

**Edited by Royal Lee**

# NOTES

VITAMIN NEWS

VITAMIN PRODUCTS CO. • MILWAUKEE, WISCONSIN

VOL. 12

## HEART DISEASE —
## OUR NATIONAL DISGRACE

Because of our national malnutrition, heart disease is our leading cause of death.

How is this brought about? What special deficiencies do this?

First is the deficiency of vitamin C. The C complex is one of the factors necessary in the blood stream to maintain its capacity to carry oxygen to the tissues from the lungs. With a depleted reserve of this vitamin, the heart is called upon to pump blood at a faster rate to keep up the necessary flow of oxygen to the tissues. This is, of course, automatic. If we develop this condition, we feel an increased force of heart beat and in time complain of "shortness of breath." The heart itself is simply overloaded. In time, it breaks down from the overload. It may become dilated, valves begin to leak, the patient complains of "heart pounding."

To recommend citrus fruits to supply the vitamin C is not good as the acid in them is not at once oxidized, and depletes temporarily the alkali buffers in the blood. This in itself lowers the oxygen-carrying capacity of the blood stream. The various proprietary alkalizers on the market are helpful in cooperating with the vitamin C to take the load off the heart. Persons who go to high altitudes from relatively low altitudes often find that they are unduly fatigued, their heart may "pound," and they yawn often and feel short of breath. All this means oxygen deficiency in the blood. A few days are required for acclimation and the body adjusts itself to the light air.

Visitors to Mexico City usually feel this influence quite definitely because of the 7,500 foot altitude. One railroad company in South America made a practice of having a physician check the heart conditions of each passenger before accepting them for passage on their line over the Andes. Going quickly into high altitudes in an airplane is not so detrimental. The blood stream seems to maintain its oxygen content long enough to avoid trouble from sudden changes of altitude. Several hours apparently are required for the development of distress signs.

The adrenal glands control our balance of potassium-sodium in the blood and blood pressure. The latter by adrenal medulla secretion of adrenalin, the former by the effect of the hormones of the adrenal cortex, and we must recall here that to accomplish this, the adrenal gland must be supplied with vitamin C in particular and some vitamins A and B, too.

Adrenalin contracts the blood vessels of the general body circulation, but relaxes the bronchioles in *the lungs*.

A deficiency of adrenal activity causes a general loss of vascular tone (low blood pressure) obvious fatigability, but a high blood pressure in the lungs with congestion and possible tendency to asthmatic conditions.

This hypertension in the lungs is obvious in an endocardiogram of the sound taken from the pulmonary position of the microphone. The aortic and mitral positions may show an almost imperceptible second sound indicating low blood pressure. The second sound is made by the closing of the valves after the heart impulse ceases. This closing is abrupt and forceful if the pressure is normal or high, otherwise it is not. But the sound of the closing of the valve leading to the pulmonary artery is often greater in magnitude than the first sound where this pulmonary hypertension exists. There is apparently no other convenient way to detect the pulmonary pressure. (See endocardiograms below.)

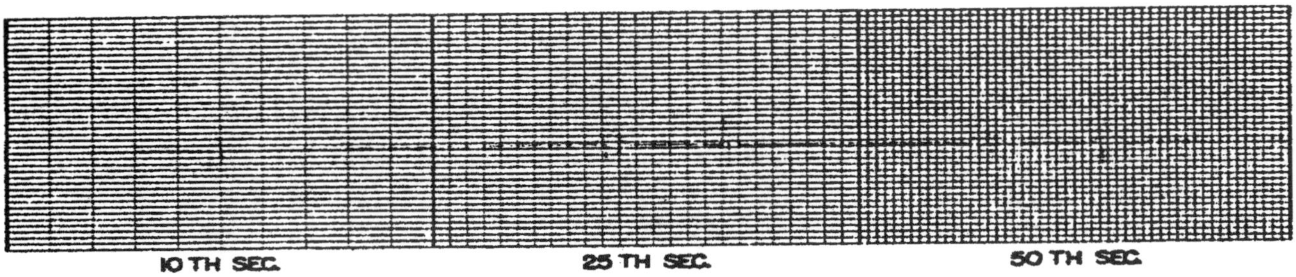


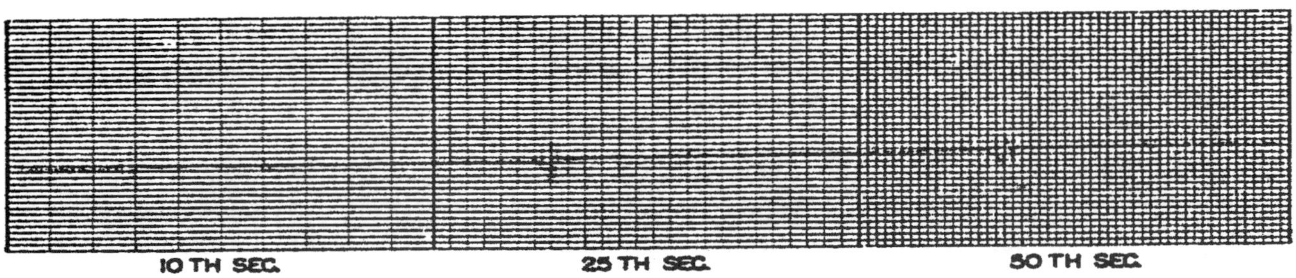


It has been found that all the effects of adrenalin are also effects of potassium. Adrenalin, therefore, apparently does its work by mobilizing potassium which normally is stored, or at least is present only to any extent, inside the body cells. Adrenalin brings it out into the blood stream where it produces the reactions commonly known as adrenalin effects. No doubt a deficiency of potassium in the diet aggravates any tendency to hypoadrenalism. A potassium deficiency is also brought about by the excessive use of white flour and white sugar. There is plenty of potassium in whole wheat, sugar cane juice, molasses and raw sugar.

The deficiency of vitamin B complex is specifically productive of loss of tone of the vascular system and tends to demoralize nerve functions that coordinate body activities. An atonic bowel sets the stage for constipation and protein decomposition is enhanced. Here we find an alarming new set of circumstances. Some strains of colon bacillus have been found to produce histamine from some proteins, animal foods particularly, and histamine is an organic toxin if out of place, but also normally acts as a hormone that regulates the secretion of gastric juice as a normal "messenger substance" between the pyloric and fundus areas of the stomach. (Also known as gastrin.)

Now, when histamine is free in the circulation, it destroys the normal balance of this stomach control mechanism. The fundus glands are stimulated to secretion of hydrochloric acid by the histamine which is in the entire blood stream. The messages now did not originate from the pyloric end of the stomach. They do not cease when the need for digestive fluids is passed. The hyperchlorhydria thus created is considered a cause for stomach ulcers (*Jol. A.M.A.*). But the primary cause is deficiencies of the various vitamins and minerals as above listed. (Clinically, the prompt relief for hyperchlorhydria is usually obtained by the use of vitamin G complex, one or two tablets with each meal.)

The histamine group of toxins, others are thought to accompany it from the same protein hydrolysis, is suspected to cause various systemic disorders. Arthritis is at the top of the list. Various obscure symptoms, even multiple sclerosis, may be end results of such absorption of intestinal toxins. We recall a case diagnosed as multiple sclerosis, in which all the various medications and treatments failed to halt the progress of the paralysis until an x-ray disclosed a colonic condition permitting a stagnation of bowel contents. The removal of this colonic disorder resulted in a prompt reversal of the progress of the paralysis, with apparent complete recovery.

Histamine in the blood in undue amounts quite probably causes a tendency for contraction of the bronchioles in asthma and probably acts in many allergic reactions as a primary sensitizer.

To understand this, we must recall that histamine relaxes capillaries, contracts bronchioles, just the opposite of adrenalin. It causes a lowered blood pressure of the general circulation and a higher blood pressure in the lung circulation. "Adrenalin and histamine are marked antagonists in their effects on the circulation." (Grollman, p. 268.) If we accept this tentative hypothesis, we may consider the patient who is absorbing protein toxins from a stagnate bowel should therefore show some of the following indications:

1. Gastritis, tendency to stomach ulcers.
2. May be allergic, asthmatic, arthritic tend to have neuritis, hives, or even possibly paralysis (multiple sclerosis).
3. Hypotension and pulmonary hypertension, as indicated by a relatively reduced second sound over the aorta and an accentuated second sound over the pulmonary artery.
4. Fatigability and a generally lowered physical condition.

NEWS ITEM ... "*The London Lancet*," for August, carried an article by Dr. Alan Moncrieff, to the effect that he had found that nicotinic acid was a valuable remedy for angina pectoris and also for cerebral thrombosis.

V. P. vitamins have been used for these purposes successfully for twelve years; "Catalyn" for the cerebral thrombosis case, vitamin E complex in addition for the angina pectoris case. We believe an unisolated sex hormone will be ultimately found to be a specific remedy for the angina syndrome. The known sex hormones aggravate the condition, but the vitamin E complex usually produces gradual improvement, and it is probable the results are due to a more normal balance in the output of hormones by the gonadal cells. It is significant that the male sex incurs angina pectoris about six times as frequently as the female, and it has been concluded that all the sex hormones, except progesterone, are common to both sexes. So we think there is some hormone in the female gonad that is secreted in higher amounts than in the male that prevents angina pectoris, and that the vitamin E complex aids in promoting the secretion of this hormone.

# NOTES

# VITAMIN NEWS

VITAMIN PRODUCTS CO. • MILWAUKEE, WISCONSIN

VOL. 12

## CORONARY DISEASE, ONE CHARACTERISTIC END RESULT

## OF THE USE OF DEVITALIZED FOODS

Many more people are dropping dead from heart disease today than ever before.

When Dr. Morgan,[1] of the University of California, put two groups of dogs on a diet of white flour "enriched" with synthetic vitamins and compared their behavior with another group fed on the same white flour, not "enriched," the surprising result was that the dogs on the "enriched" flour died first, and tended to die, after their actions became that of "sedate senility," by sudden heart failure. The human patient becomes definitely "sedate" when he begins to feel angina pains upon exertion. Can it be that — as in those dogs — the consumption of "enriched" flour by humans has an equally direct bearing on the fact that heart diseases and cancer are nowadays listed as the predominating causes of "sedate senility" — and death — while there is a general decline in other causes?

Dr. Morgan concluded that the addition of the synthetic vitamins to flour increased the demand for some of the unknown factors in the diet which, as a consequence, became acutely deficient sooner than with the diet with the non-"enriched" flour. These unknown factors could, therefore, quite appropriately be called the "heart protective group."

This would strongly indicate that the vitamin fractions so far available from synthetic sources have failed to do anything towards relieving or preventing heart diseases: in fact, Dr. Morgan's experiments tend to show that they have done the opposite.

With the above data in mind, it is interesting to reflect upon the accumulated clinical evidence, already reviewed in the *Vitamin News* (pp. 1, 99, 100, 124, 125, 126, 142, and 145), regarding the relative value of our "Catalyn" and "Cataplex B" vs. other vitamin products, especially synthetics. The favorable results obtained with "V-P" products are, no doubt, due to the presence of some of the, as yet, unidentified factors in our natural complex concentrates.

Some of the earlier literature offers some interesting clues on the subject:

> "When a cardiac crisis appears, as evidenced by precordial pain, palpitation, breathlessness, and cyanosis, prompt action is necessary, as this condition is responsible for most of the fatalities that occur in beriberi. In the past, nitroglycerin and amyl nitrite have been used ... it is needless to say, however, that this treatment is merely palliative and does not permanently relieve the cardiac distress which is liable to recur at any time and thus end the patient's life ...
>
> "Chamberlain and Vedder found that the administration of an alcoholic extract of rice polishings to infants suffering from infantile beriberi resulted in an immediate alleviation of the serious cardiac disturbance which is one of the main symptoms of that disease.
>
> "Vedder and Williams found that the same extract, when administered to an adult case of pernicious cardiac beriberi, afforded quite as prompt relief from the distressing cardiac symptoms. Since, as will be

seen later, the extract in this form is quite incapable of relieving the nervous or paralytic symptoms of beriberi, it follows that there is some substance in this extract which exerts a direct and immediate action on the heart ...

"The infants were all given twenty drops of the extract of rice polishings every two hours while awake, and the results have been truly marvelous. Improvement is immediate. Vomiting stops in 24 or 36 hours. The child who has not passed any urine for several days urinates five or six times freely. The edema disappears in the course of a few days. Usually, on the first night after treatment is begun, the infant falls into a deep sleep, although it may have been practically sleepless for several weeks. The dyspnea and palpitation cease after two or three days ...

"We may now inquire what relation does this substance bear to Funk's vitamin ($B_1$) ... there is evidence that this cardiac vitamin is not identical with Funk's vitamin. The alcoholic extract which relieves the cardiac symptoms so promptly is equally efficacious in dispelling the dropsy in cases of wet beriberi, but is quite ineffective in curing the paralytic symptoms of dry beriberi, while the administration of Funk's base promptly cures this paralysis ... "

*Beriberi*
Edward B. Vedder, M.D.
William Wood and Co.
1913
Pages 257-315

(Note that Stepp et al says that the antiparalysis factor $B_4$ is not separable from $B_1$ — page 24, *The Vitamins and Their Clinical Application* — therefore, the antiparalysis effect is probably due to the B associated with the thiamin and not to the thiamin.)

Now, just what fraction of the B complex is needed in these cases?

First note this: Acetylcholine is a substance which, as a consequence of a stimulus arriving through the nerve, is produced at the myoneural junction causing the muscle to contract. After it has accomplished its purpose, it is generally destroyed by an enzyme, cholinesterase. Prolonged acetylcholine administration, however, will consistently cause coronary disease and death in experimental animals.[2]

Now, the maintenance and control of enzyme activity is a characteristic function of vitamins, especially many of the factors of the B and G group.[3] To determine just which one of these may be useful to promote the maintenance of cholinesterase, we have for some years conducted an investigation of clinical observation and tests of vitamin B and G concentrates from various sources to find one that was most effective in accomplishing consistent relief in cases of coronary disease and angina pectoris. We finally found a combination of extracts from calf brain, yeast and sprouted barley which appeared to be quite dependable in acting as a "physiological nitroglycerine" for relieving anginal pains and coronary spasticity.

Since, in view of the known value of nicotinic acid in coronary cases, the vitamin G group was the natural subdivision of the B complex to promote this action; we have improved our "Cataplex G" by the addition of these concentrates. The biggest uses of the old "Cataplex G" were in the relief of peptic ulcers and in cataract cases. We believe this new product, by reason of the added extract, will now be more effective for these same purposes; and that in addition, it will be found of indispensable value in coronary and angina pectoris cases. Gastric disturbances are common concomitants of heart and coronary disorders, suggestive of a common cause.

The relationship of the sex hormones, as mentioned in *Vitamin News,* page 146, to the cause of angina pectoris is also apparent in the gastritis and ulcer cases. Ulcers are far more common in men, just as angina pectoris is six times as frequent in men as in women. Boyd says that: "Pyloric hypertonus by preventing the normal regurgitation (of alkaline duodenal contents), is the great cause of gastric hyperacidity."[4] Here we seemingly have the identical spastic reaction of an accumulation of acetylcholine. Hyperacidity is considered one of the chief causes of ulcers and gastritis.[5] In the writer's humble opinion, we here have a basic reason for this whole picture of coronary disease, angina pectoris, gastritis, thrombosis of coronary or cerebral vessels, and arteriosclerosis in general.

On this basis, the cases would differ, both in kind (location) and degree, as to the relative deficiency of the enzyme cholinesterase, or as to the degree of overwork of the nerve endings in the organ involved. Nerve tension and nervous shock as discussed in these pages before can, as is well-known, bring on the gastritis, etc., even coronary collapse. Where such spastic reaction reaches tetanic proportions and invades areas of sensor innervation, anginal pains can be created.

This hypothesis would explain why nervous strain and nerve shock can be so detrimental to the angina and coronary cases. These events simply cause the secretion of more acetylcholine at the nerve endings and pile up biochemical dynamite. At last the tetanic attack is possible, and the final setting-off impulse need not be particularly violent. The size of the flame that ignites a store of gunpowder is not important, but the amount of explosive is. The accumulation of the explosive here, in coronary disorders, is dependent on two factors: the intensity and frequency of stimulation of the coronary nerve-endings which generate the acetylcholine and the amount of cholinesterase available to remove that acetylcholine. When the balance favors the accumulation of acetylcholine, danger is ahead for the patient for he is now loaded up for an attack likely to end in some form of coronary breakdown.

General arteriosclerosis has also been produced clinically by the administration of acetylcholine when tried for its remedial action on arthritis.[6] Its success in this disease was found to be offset by the serious consequences of arterial degeneration. Here, then, we might have the explanation for the up-to-now baffling situation of the coronary artery often being the first one in the body to show signs of sclerosis. It is a most overworked artery; its walls, as a consequence of emotion and exercise, are constantly subjected to acetylcholine-producing nerve stimuli. Therefore, the liberation of acetylcholine would be greater there than elsewhere, and the need for cholinesterase would also be greater than elsewhere.

Sajous pointed out how the muscle wall of the arterioles regulated the blood flow to the capillaries.[7] He also explained how adrenalin could dilate arterioles by contracting the vessels supplying the arteriole wall thereby causing the arteriole wall muscle fiber to relax by reason of the choking off of this nutrtion. (Doctors Lutz and Fulton, of Boston University, have announced their verification of this regulative function of blood flow to capillaries, according to an Associated Press release of June 12, 1944.) The anatomical makeup of a vascular area thereby determines whether it would be contracted or relaxed by adrenalin; and the opposite effect of this agent on different kinds of tissue is made rational. Hypothetically, then, if acetylcholine were not destroyed by cholinesterase promptly after a contractive impulse as it normally is, and a relatively chronic state of contraction were created, the effect would of necessity be permanent damage to those arterioles which were thus deprived of sufficient nutrition. In each case, the extent of this nutritional deficiency would determine the rate and final degree of degeneration of the muscle fibers and their subsequent replacement by connective tissue, all of which appears to be the process involved in the development of arteriosclerosis.

Without cholinesterase there can be little free choline in the tissues. Without free choline there is a tendency for the development of papillomata;[9] the vagus function is impaired;[10] and lactation is impeded.[11]

Choline is also available from the splitting of ingested lecithin; this splitting is done by another enzyme, lecithinase. Often lecithin administration fails to do what is expected, fails to relieve fatty liver, fails to relieve arthritic pains, fails to correct psoriasis, all of which it may successfully accomplish in other cases. These failures are probably due to lack of lecithinase or cholinesterase, as either should render choline available.

Bee venom contains lecithinase, so do calf brain and rice bran.[8] That may explain why bee venom is a success in some arthritic cases. It theoretically would fail where lecithin is in too low a content in the blood stream. Lecithin often relieves arthritic pains, but we can see why neither bee venom nor lecithin has received much acceptance as a useful remedy, for neither can work where the other is missing. The lecithinase of bee venom would release free choline in the blood if lecithin is available. If lecithin is not present and the naturally occurring lecithinase of the tissues is present, lecithin administration should be effective in yielding choline.

To get at the real and basic cause, we must replace the nutritional deficiency that impaired the formation of cholinesterase and other enzyme systems in the body. We reaffirm a principle once before stated in these pages:

> Correction of faulty nutrition permits natural balances to recur in the endocrine and biochemical systems of the body. The baffling complexity, not to say confusion, of present-day therapeutics should serve as a caution against the hasty introduction of additional complexities, at least as long as more rational theories and simpler remedies prove applicable and effective.
>
> The average physician, no matter how learned and courageous, can hardly find any great comfort in prescribing more or less theorized substitutes for hypothetical deficiencies, be it hormones or otherwise. The honest physician feels his responsibilities keenly, and prefers to move about on more solid ground, whenever possible. Therefore, where food-stuffs are needed and their replacement will correct the existing trouble, he gladly avoids hormone therapy and its dangers of misdiagnosis and over-dosage.
>
> (Violation of this rule brought about the death of patients given acetylcholine injections for their arthritis.)

In our extractions of the sources of natural vitamin B Complex, we try to carry enzymes through intact; no heat destructive to enzymes is used at any time. Vitamins are often conjugated with heat labile proteins, often of special nutritional values, very probably as enzymes. These considerations serve to explain the entirely different action of a "vitamin accompanied by its natural synergists" as shown by the line of "V-P" products. The new "Cataplex G" again demonstrates the soundness of this principle. As an experimental* treatment, its uses are:

1. As a remedy for the coronary and angina pectoris type of heart disease.
2. As a factor to combat fatty degeneration and cirrhosis of the liver.
3. As a possible remedy for arthritic pains.
4. For the relief of psoriasis.
5. As a physiological remedy for papillomatous growths.

See, also, *Vitamin News,* page 142, on the value of "V-P Cataplex C" in reducing the load on the heart, and page 126 on the value of "Cataplex B" in heart arrhythmias.

It happens that we have available at this time the sphygmographs of two interesting cases (which are reproduced herewith), taken a few hours apart, showing the effect of two tablets of "Cataplex G."

Mrs. M. B. had a racing heart, apparently no control from the vagus (otherwise known as the parasympathetic branch of the autonomic nervous system) which normally acts as the governing instrument and which is put out of commission by potassium deficiency, as well as by deficiency of the G group of vitamins. V-P "Minaplex" is ordinarily very effective in bringing such over-running hearts under control by reason of its content of potassium, which we should obtain in sufficient quantities from the green leaf vegetable part of our diet. In this case, the restoration of function of the vagus was apparently very efficiently accomplished by the "Cataplex G."

In addition, there were evident occasional extra systoles, commonly called "skipped beats." The first graph shows four or five in the one-minute period. The second shows only one. Also, the muscular condition was evidently quite bad, fatigue being evidenced by the varying amplitude of the pulsations. In fact, it practically resembles the so-called "water-hammer" pulse of aortic regurgitation. The heart is obviously struggling under a terrific handicap, in this case nothing more than vitamin starvation. The next polygram, made 14 hours later, is hard to believe to be the same case. The single extra systole is the only indication of anything abnormal, with the exception of a perceptible fatigue waver in the amplitude. The pulse rate has dropped from 120 to 64.

The next case, Dr. B. M., has a rapid, but very weak and wavering pulse. The tracing is typical of "auricular flutter," considered as being due to the inability of the ventricle to follow the auricle. Where this is a result of an impairment of conduction of impulses from the auricular-ventricular node, it is no doubt a situation that is partly a result of deficiency of the vitamin B vomplex component known as the "anti-paralysis factor," $B_4$. V-P "Cataplex B" owes its merit in controlling heart block, fibrillation, and similar arrhythmias to its content of this factor, we believe. (See *Vitamin News,* page 126, for cardiographic evidence of this.)

The polygraphic curves made the next morning show a great improvement, some tachycardia being still present. Probably a "Minaplex" tablet or two would have been useful in getting the vagus function back to normal; a potassium deficiency is very persistent in keeping up the pulse rate. Most of us are low in our intake of this essential element, which is considered to be most vital in heart function. Meyer and Gottlieb, in their *Experimental Pharmacology,* J. B. Lippincott Co., Philadelphia, page 416, state that potassium is the sole radio-active element of the body, and that it owes its effect to this property. Potassium is known to be the activator of the cells that set up the timing frequency of the heart.

[1] Morgan, Agnes Fay, *Science,* March 14, 1941.
[2] Hall, Ettinger and Banting, F. G., *Canadian Medical Jol.,* 34:1, 9-15, Jan. 1936.
[3] Evans, E. A., Editor, "The Biological Action of the Vitamins," (A Symposium), C. A. Elvehjem, University of Chicago Press, Chicago, Illinois, 1942, pages 5, 30, 60.
[4] Boyd, William, *Pathology of Internal Diseases,* Second Edition, page 278, W. B. Saunders Co., Philadelphia, Pennsylvania.
[5] "Acid Factor in Peptic Ulcer," *J.A.M.A.*, (Sept. 9) 1933, page 857.
[6] Bodansky and Brindlev, *Proc. Soc. Exper. Biol. And Med.,* 35:547-548, Jan. 1937; Sarrony and Raynaud, *Paris Med.*, 2:111-114, August 7, 1937.
[7] Sajous, Charles E. de M., *The Internal Secretions and the Principles of Medicine,* Vol. 1, pages 248-257, F. A. Davis Co., Philadelphia, Pa., 1911.

[8] Sumner, James B. and Somers, G. Fred, *Chemistry and Method of Enzymes*, pages 52-53, Academic Press.
[9] *Biological Symposia V,* Jacques Cattell Press, page 181.
[10] Ibid., pages 180 and 223. Ibid, page 181.

**We say experimental to comply with the federal law which permits no claim for a new product until it is accepted by the consensus of medical opinion. Naturally, such a consensus of opinion cannot exist until the product has been generally accepted by the medical profession. This usually requires several years.*

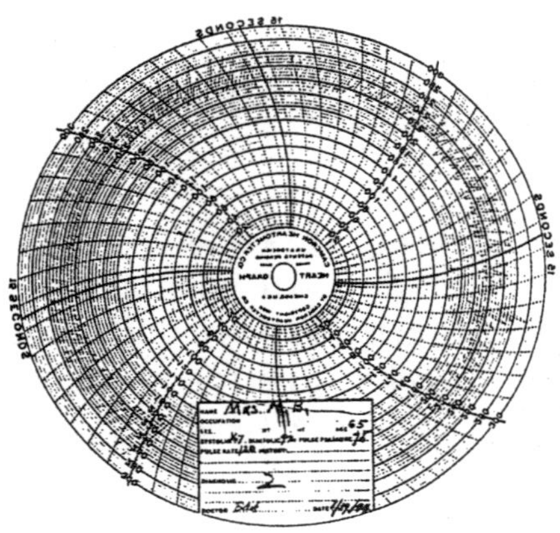


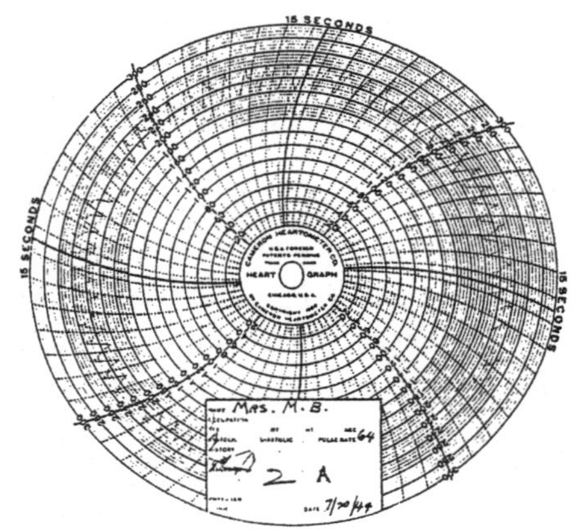


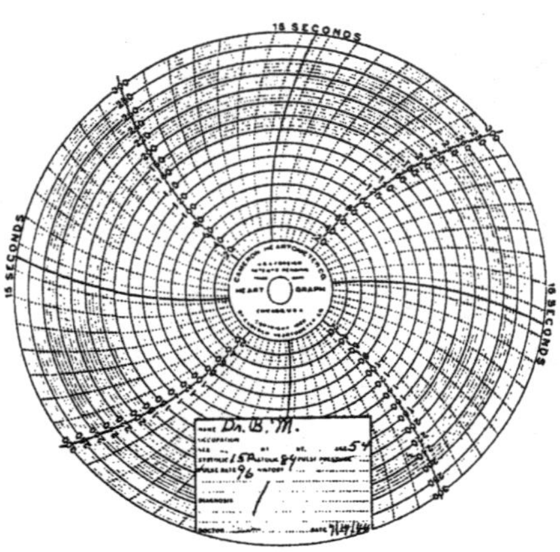


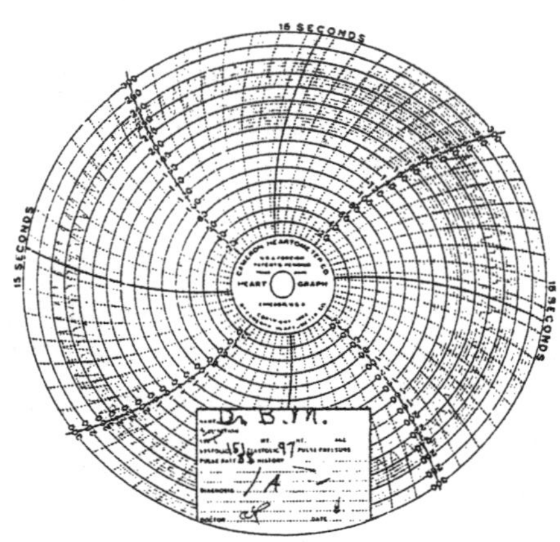

VITAMIN NEWS

VITAMIN PRODUCTS CO. • MILWAUKEE, WISCONSIN

VOL. 12

# THIS BARBAROUS AMERICAN FOOD SITUATION

1. Diseases of the heart, arteries and kidneys cause the majority of deaths in this country, 536,745 to be exact, in 1940.

2. Cancer killed half as many.

3. Seventeen cents per death, or $93,835.00 was spent that year on research to find the causes of heart, vascular and kidney disease.

4. $525.00 per death was paid the same year for research into the causes of infantile paralysis.

5. Did you know that in China, where the people cannot get our white flour, refined sugar, soft drinks and pasteurized milk (pasteurized so it need not be produced under strictly sanitary conditions, pasteurized so dirt and all can be bottled and sold), there is very little arthritis, heart disease, high blood pressure or cancer? In Hong Kong, the death rate from cancer is 8 per hundred thousand deaths. In San Francisco, it is 102.

Note well this quotation from Dr. Snapper's book, *Chinese Lessons to Western Medicine*, Interscience Publishers, 1941.

> "The rarity of coronary thrombosis in North China is the more striking because the increase ... of this disease in America and Europe is appalling ... The rarity of arteriosclerosis is proved by the scores of middle-aged patients dying of all sorts of diseases showing hardly any sclerosis at autopsy ... This explains why the genuine angina pectoris syndrome ... and ... coronary thrombosis are rarely encountered."

The difference in these diseases in this country as compared to China is a monument to the advertising skill and the political power of the American devitalized food industry.

For a complete expose up to that date, read Dr. Harvey W. Wiley's book, *The History of a Crime Against the Food Law,* (1929) at your public library. He lost his job as head of the Food and Drug Administration apparently because he tried to stop the sale of bleached flour, declared to contain poisonous substances by the U.S. Supreme Court. (Notice of Judgement 722 and Notice of Judgement 3398.)

Most of our vitamin authorities apparently take orders from these interests and lend their aid to keep the public in the dark. The value of vitamins in saving lives by correcting heart lesions was proven by users of V-P products fifteen years ago, published twelve years ago in the first issue of this publication, and proven by cardiographic records constantly, first shown in *Vitamin News* in 1936.

Why has so little attention been shown to these remarkable facts?:

The value of vitamin B complex as a "Cataplex B" in helping to correct extra systoles, heart block or fibrillation.

The value of vitamin C as "Cataplex C" in improving the oxygen assimilation by the blood, to relieve the overload on the decompensated heart.

The value of the vitamin G group as "Cataplex G" in relaxing the spastic distress of the coronary case.

Is it because synthetic vitamins fail to produce results of this kind? What do *you* think?

## ITEMS OF INTEREST FROM RECENT REPORTS

"A finding that certain sulfa drugs can increase the vitamin C content of calves' blood may cast a new light on the mechanism through which sulfa protects against disease, according to Norman Lundquist and Paul Phillips."[1] (He writes checks on the vitamin balance)

"This Station previously developed a method of preventing or curing nutritional ... (dysentery) ... in young calves by giving them extra vitamins, including vitamin C. Other experiment stations have reported good results in treating the infectious ... (dysentery) ... with sulfa drugs. Now it appears that the effects of these treatments are the same in one respect — both increase the vitamin C content of the blood."[2] (Sulfathiazole caused a 27 percent increase in blood vitamin C content in a week's time.)

The administration of the drug chlorobutanol causes a mobilization of the body reserves of vitamin C into the blood stream, according to Lundquist and Phillips, after observing tests on cows.[3]

A study of the symptoms of sulfonamide poisoning and C-Avitaminosis suggests the possibility that toxic reactions to the sulfonamides may be manifestations of an accentuated latent vitamin C deficiency. The author says, "I have found that concurrent administration of large doses of vitamin C in sulfonamide therapy not only prevents toxic reaction but apparently enhances its bacteriostatic efficacy." This investigator suggests precautionary chemical or physical tests for C-Avitaminosis preliminary to sulfonamide therapy.[4]

In animal feeding tests, butter fat was much superior to vegetable fat in causing growth where there was a relative deficiency of the vitamin B complex, in a diet mainly of milk, sugar and fat. "These findings serve as a warning against the use of 'filled' milk in which the butterfat is replaced by cheaper fats. If the principles indicated here apply to human nutrition, then infants — living entirely or largely on milk, and hence dependent on lactose for carbohydrate — would have their health seriously jeopardized by the filled type of milk."[5] (And how about oleo for children?)

Experimental animals become paralyzed from excessive dosages of vitamin A, Herbst and Elvehjem.[6] (We have always said beware of high potency vitamins in which more than the nutritional requirements are suggested — that is where nutrition stops and drugging begins.)

The idea that too much sugar promotes dental decay now is supported by experimental evidence in rat tests, in which large numbers of cavities appeared in the molars within 14 weeks when placed on a synthetic diet containing ordinary sugar as the only carbohydrate. It remains to be seen whether these findings apply to man. (Shaw, Schweigert,

McIntyre, Elvehjem and Phillips)[7]

(The same rats showed no cavities when fed on natural cereal foods.)

Coffee is a fairly rich source of the pellagra-preventive vitamin, niacin, say Teply, Krehl and Elvehjem.[8]

Calves are usually born with a vitamin A deficiency, which predisposes to dysentery.[9]

Vitamin C is helpful in preventing calves from incurring navel infection and pneumonia.[9]

Two new vitamins, $B_{10}$ and $B_{11}$ were found in yeast and liver, that are required by chicks, apparently necessary to reproduction, and hatchability of eggs.[10]

Hens will not produce eggs with good hatchability without ample quantities of $B_6$ and biotin, normally obtained in the insect part of the hen's diet.[11]

The vitamin content of oatmeal is not dependent upon the variety of the oat, but upon the fertility of the soil, according to Cooperman and Elvehjem.[12]

That honey contains a fairly good amount of B-complex vitamins, is a finding of Schuette and Elvehjem.[13]

The new vitamin, folic acid, (found in leafy vegetables and liver, a member of the B Complex) is required by the monkey; without it, it develops dysentery and leucopenia. Monkeys also require biotin; without it, they become baldheaded. (Waisman, Elvehjem, Clark, and Rasmussen)[14]

Lettuce and Swiss chard may lose half their vitamin C content a few hours after cutting, before reaching the grocery store, unless refrigerated.

Monkeys require a new, unnamed vitamin of the B complex for prevention of dental caries. Liver supplied the protective factor, according to Shaw, Phillips and Elvehjem.[14]

The same investigators found that in test animals, coarsely ground cereals caused a greater incidence of tooth decay than finely ground products.

THE STATEMENTS HEREIN MAY NOT AGREE WITH CURRENTLY ACCEPTED MEDICAL OPINION. NEVERTHELESS, THE PUBLISHER BELIEVES THEM TO BE SOUND.

## REFERENCES

[1] *61st Ann. Report of Univ. of Wis. Agricultural Experimental Station,* p. 38.

[2] Ibid., p. 39.

[3] *60th Ann. Report of Univ. of Wis. Agricultural Experimental Station,* p. 3.

[4] McCormick, W. J., "Sulfonamide Sensitivity and C-Avitaminosis," *Canadian M. A. J.*, 52:68, Jan., 1945.

[5] *61st Ann. Report of the Univ. of Wis. Agricultural Experimental Station*, p. 22.

[6] Ibid., p. 25.

[7] Ibid., p. 21

[8] Ibid., p. 15.

[9] *60th Ann. Report of Univ. of Wis. Agricultural Experimental Station,* p. 1.

[10] Ibid., p. 10.

[11] Ibid., p. 11.

[12] Ibid., p. 17.

[13] *60th Ann. Report of Univ. of Wis. Agricultural Experimental Station,* p. 18.

[14] Ibid., p. 48.

VITAMIN NEWS
VITAMIN PRODUCTS CO. • MILWAUKEE, WISCONSIN

VOL. 13

## V-P VITAMIN C AND DIABETIC GANGRENE, A TEN YEAR SCOOP ON MEDICAL SCIENCE

Drs. Wirtschafter and Widmann in the March 1 issue (1947) of the *Journal of the A.M.A.*, tell how they have discovered a new treatment for diabetic gangrene, and with its help they have saved five veterans from imminent amputation of their feet, at the Veteran's Administration Hospital, Los Angeles.

Their treatment is practically identical with that recommended 10 years ago by the Vitamin Products Co. as described in the case below. They used injections of vitamin C and histamine. We recommended "Cataplex C" and "Catalyn." (Catalyn and Cataplex C both contain vitamins in combination with their naturally associated amino acids including histidine.) (Most natural vitamins are linked with proteins.)

Here is our case report as received from the surgeon who had decided to try the vitamin treatment because the patient refused to consent to amputation.

Dr. – H.
St. Paul, Minn.

February 6, 1937
Dr. Royal Lee
Vitamin Products Company
2023 West Wisconsin Ave.,
Milwaukee, Wisconsin

My Dear Dr. Lee,

Thank you very much for the fresh supply of a dozen bottles of Catalyn tablets which came Monday to be used for clinical investigation in charity cases.

I also want to recount briefly to you a rather dramatic experience I had in the case of a diabetic woman, age 72, with a history of diabetes of 4 years' duration, insulin dosage 30 units daily for the past two years, who came to my office in September with an ulcer between the toes, treated in the hospital with vaso-dilators and intermittent negative pressure with no improvement. Blood sugar under 80 units of insulin a day was 130 mg.; without insulin 200 mg. An X-ray of the blood vessels showed no calcareous deposits.

A stay in the hospital of one month brought about no amelioration of symptoms and no reduction of pain in the foot. In fact, the ulcerating spot began to develop a gangrenous scab on it, which increased in size to 3 x 5 cm. And pain was quite constant. Then resort was had to the expedient of soaking the arms to the elbow twice daily in water 115 degrees in temperature for 20 minutes duration. This brought about some amelioration in symptoms, considerable improvement in color of the foot and some modification of the pain. The improvement, however, did not last; the spot of gangrene began to spread, pain became quite severe, so that by the first of January, our resources were exhausted, and because of pain and debility, amputation of the affected toe was advised and this was refused by the patient.

January 6th the treatment was begun with tablets of Catalyn, three times daily. January 15th one tablet each of vitamin B and C were added daily. January 25th the foot was less painful, although there were periods of lancinating pain from time to time, and for the first time in three months, the spot of gangrene showed some shrinkage in area and the contiguous tissues to the scab showed a healthy pink color. At this time, an attempt was made to continue three Catalyn tablets a day and increase the vitamins B and C to two each day, making a total of seven tablets a day. January 27th patient complained of nausea and all vitamins were discontinued for 24 hours. Then a gradual return was made to two tablets of Catalyn a day and two tablets of vitamin B and two of vitamin C.

On this regime, the patient continued to do well, and when seen February 3rd, her general condition had improved. There was an increased interest in food. She had a better control of the bladder sphincter which had been incompetent. The extra systoles in her heart were almost eliminated, and the gangrenous scab had partially separated from its base and was trimmed away, except at either end where it was still slightly adherent. When the scab was removed, healthy looking granulation tissue was evident.

I am quite convinced in my own mind that it was the action of the vitamins and nothing else that brought about this improvement.

Very truly yours,
Dr. – H. (M.D.)

Such is medical progress. The synthetic vitamin C has received little recognition for the treatment of capillary diseases because it alone failed to have any beneficial effect. As stated by Abt & Farmer in *The Vitamins* (Published by the A. M. A. in 1939), that although scurvy was characterized by capillary breakdown, ascorbic acid was useless in capillary disease other than scurvy. In the same book, the statement is made, "The claim by Szent-Gyorgi that a new factor called vitamin P is responsible for the anti-hemorrhage effect attributed to vitamin C has been shown to be erroneous. The postulated vitamin P apparently does not exist."(Page 336)

However, later search *did* prove its existence. At the Scientific Assembly of the A. M. A. — San Francisco, July 1-5, 1946 — Drs. Griffith et al showed how the new form of vitamin P, (Rutin) from buckwheat, cured capillary fragility specifically according to the Gothlin Test. Followed by an article in *Collier's* of March 11, 1947 entitled "Block That Stroke," intimating that no one need suffer a cerebral hemorrhage now that the new vitamin was available.

Well, take a look at this case report of May 27, 1937, also 10 years ahead..

**CASE NO. 11707**
**5-7-37**

Diagnosis — Purpura Hemorrhagica with Blood Findings Similar to Secondary Anemia.
Female, age 55.
Case of 15 years standing of gradually increasing intensity to cause usual routine of five blood transfusions. Patient did not respond.
TREATMENT: "V-P Catalyn and "V-P" Vitamin C Complex given at the rate of one tablet each per hour.

After the third day, patient showed signs of returning vitality.
Fourth day dosage reduced to four tablets of "Catalyn" and four tablets of Vitamin C Complex per day.
Eighth day patient was able to sit up in bed.
Same Dosage continued.
Twelfth day patient up in convalescent's chair.
Dosage continued at four "Catalyn" and four Vitamin C Complex tablets per day.
At the end of third week, patient resumed light household duties.
Dosage continued at four "Catlayn" and four Vitamin C Complex tablets per day.
Treatment was begun eighteen months ago.
Patient now is active and in very good health.

Signed _____________ Patient
Signed _____________ Physician

It seems that publicity is pretty well controlled as to vitamin deficiency consequences, timed as to release so as to coincide with commercial availability. As to Rutin, our investigations so far indicate it has severe limitations, again because it is processed and purified so as to eliminate its associated factors. Recall how even drugs like digitalis are rendered dangerous and unduly toxic by attempts to isolate the active principle, and how tincture of the green leaf was found best? Well, we believe that the best Vitamin P is the green buckwheat juice, entire, vacuum dried into a powder and tableted. It was once listed in botanical tests as very good in treating Erysipelas, a capillary disease associated with various infective agents (none being specific causes). But it was not capable of poisoning normal healthy animals, so it was thrown out of the *Materia Medica* as an old woman's dream. (As were all the other vitamins in their natural forms, like cod liver oil.) (We note that gelatin capsules of cod liver oil were mentioned by Stille's *Materia Medica* in 1868, and were listed in *Merck's* index in 1896.)

In the last issue of *Vitamin News*, the effect of the sulfa drugs in promoting depletion of the tissues of their vitamin C was pointed out. Now, the outstanding after effect of the sulfa drugs is to cause hemorrhages in the tissues. So ascorbic acid is not the answer again, maybe? And refer back to where we argued that vitamin C complex should be called "the physiological competitor of sulfanilamide and the sulfa drugs."

How does vitamin C act to destroy infection?

"Vitamin C acts like Popeye's spinach when the vitamin gets into the blood. The white blood cells take a 'bite' of the C then grab and literally squeeze the life out of disease germs by engulfing them, which is a natural process known as phagocytosis." (Associated Press item of May 14, 1947, describing the discovery of Dr. Nungester of the University of Michigan, as announced at the meeting of the Society of American Bacteriologists at Philadelphia, May 13.)

Well, we scooped that discovery a little, too. See *Vitamin News,* page 8, September 1933. In our discussion of the role of the various vitamins in combating infection, we listed as the function of C "to promote phagocytosis."

Now, maybe you would like to know what we think the next big "discovery" will be in the vitamin field.

It may be the "discovery" of the necessity for vitamin E to prevent heart disease. (I mean the natural E with its phospholipid synergists, chiefly lipositol.)

When vitamin E is removed from cattle feed, (like the degermination of our flour and other cereal foods) the cattle begin to drop dead in the pasture without previous signs of disease (just as our leading businessmen for years have been getting front page notices for the same reaction) according to tests reported in *Science,* October 4, 1946

Why? Simply because muscular dystrophy and paralysis are end results of vitamin E deficiency. And in the sedentary man what muscle does the hardest work?

The iron curtain has for some time been screening off from the public any mention of vitamin E as an essential nutrient for the human family. The Federal Trade Commission as far back as 1938 stopped Sears Roebuck & Co. from advertising that the average diet might not be adequate in its vitamin E content, and from "implying that any substantial proportion of persons are exposed in this country to a vitamin E deficiency." (*Drug Trade News*, Sept. 26, 1938.)

Apparently, the time is not yet ripe for an unveiling of the necessity for a campaign to "Block That Heart Attack." But it almost is, is my guess.

The FTC was in no position of involuntary ignorance in this matter, for I assume they have access to the Congressional Library. In *The New York Physician* for November 1935, an editorial ably sets forth some basic facts. Among them: "For some unexplainable reason, the fallacy continues to be reiterated that vitamin E is widespread and sufficiently abundant in food. Hardly is this consistent with the editorial comment appearing in the Oct. 26, 1935 issue of the *Journal of the American Medical Association*; that in the case of all the vitamins, the tendency for harm is to be sought in their under rather than in their over-supply. Obviously, the physicians of the country see through the damages that afflict processed foods. Natural foods may be rich in vitamins, E included, but processed foods are more than likely to be vitamin poor.

"Take the case of milk. Human breast milk is vitamin-E poor, presumably because the food of the mother is vitamin-E poor. Cow's milk is vitamin-E poor; clearly because the food of dairy herds is vitamin-E poor. Canned milks are vitamin-E free because they are evaporated in copper-lined and other metallic vessels and begin with a vitamin-E poor milk to start with.

"Take the case of eggs. It has been shown that vitamin-E poor feeds make for a low vitamin E content of the yolk; and this makes for infertility and non-hatchable eggs. The average hatchability of eggs over the country is about 66 per cent. Does this look like abundantly and sufficiently widespread vitamin E?

"Take the case of lettuce. It is reputed to be a very rich source of vitamin E — providing it be the fresh garden variety. Etiolated lettuce contains barely a trace of vitamin E. Thirty heads of etiolated lettuce were required to do the work of 3 minims of a pure, fresh wheat germ oil. Is this widespreadness?"

> "Examples can be multiplied, and each new example brings out still more forcibly the danger from 'too little rather than from too much' vitamin availability in foods as obtained by the public – not as grown in the agricultural college laboratory farm."

From the *New York Physician*

Vol. 5, No. 4, pages 48-9, Nov. 11, 1935

With heart disease the commonest cause of death in this country and plenty of synthetic as well as natural vitamin E available, certainly the discovery soon will be officially made that it all can be prevented by taking "ethically prescribed" food supplements, as advertised and recommended in the proper medical journals.

# NOTES

VITAMIN NEWS

VITAMIN PRODUCTS CO. • MILWAUKEE, WISCONSIN

VOL. 13

# THE VITAMIN P GROUP
# OF THE C COMPLEX

The promotion of rutin from buckwheat is another revival of an old household remedy.

Millspaugh's *American Medicinal Plants* (1887) states that the only uses on record of the buckwheat plant are that an infusion of the leaf is useful as a remedy for erysipelas, and that the flour of the seed, made into a paste with sour milk, is useful as a poultice to the mammary glands to increase the secretion of milk.

It is not too much of a coincidence, then, to find that today the juice of the plant is found to be a valuable source of the vitamin C component that is important in stopping capillary hemorrhages, and that the buckwheat meal is now known to be a source of a fraction (as is rice and barley) that is very useful in increasing tissue permeability and thereby lowering blood pressure.

When we look into the erysipelas background, we find it is not a disease with a definite cause, but "the most common excitant is Streptococcus pyogenes"[1] "It is usually accompanied by constitutional disturbances, the most marked of which is fever ... aside from the local lesions, there may be a toxemia marked by petechiae in the serous membrane, swelling of the spleen, focal necroses, and albuminous degeneration in the kidney and liver."

Sajous, in his *Analytical Encyclopedia of Practical Medicine,* says also "From its etiology, therefore, erysipelas is a nonspecific disease." That, of course, means to us that the cause is not any one type of germ. The real cause, then, may be deficiency, just as the cause of capillary breakdown in scurvy is deficiency. Here, we have the added complication of infection, the infective agent being incidental, not the basic cause, just as it is in tuberculosis. Both can only occur in a subject who has lowered resistance due to malnutrition.

Erysipelas should be called "fulminating scurvy" as distinguished from the better known slower form of the disease. Various infective agents can convert a case of sub-clinical scurvy where the symptoms may be relatively inconspicuous into this type. The commonest of course, is streptococcus progenies. Bacteriologists and followers of Pasteur believe that the microorganism is the *only* cause. Bechamp, the French professor whose research Pasteur appropriated without credit as his own,[2] had other ideas. He believed that diseased cells gave off, "microzyma," fragments as it were of chromosomes that recombined in other forms and, in effect, became disease "germs." (These fragments are now known as "chromidia.") This he said, accounted for the species specificity of most infectious disease.

Florence Nightingale said "The specific disease doctrine is the grand refuge of weak, uncultured, unstable minds, such as now rule in the medical profession. There are no specific diseases: there are specific disease conditions."[2]

Bechamp's program was to "treat the patient, not the disease." Pasteur has led us up a blind alley, it is apparent, by his overstressing of the infective agent, and understressing the condition or the state of the patient that made him susceptible.

Pyorrhea is a "germ disease," but it cannot be cured by germicides, and only malnutrition can cause it. Cats fed on pasteurized milk invariably develop pyorrhea and lose their teeth, get constipated and suffer from gastric ulcers, finally dying of arthritis or heart disease.[3] Sounds familiar, does it not?

The vitamin in milk that is destroyed by heat processing happens to be one that keeps the blood calcium levels from dropping with advancing age.[4] When pituitary and sex glands regress in middle age (before, malnutrition is present, no doubt), calcium levels in the blood drop, as these hormone sources complete the calcification of the skeleton at maturity, and are essential to keep it calcified.[5] It is obvious how pasteurized milk can promote physical decay in middle aged people, and hasten the advent of "store teeth," atrophic arthritis, etc., etc.

Since vitamin P is also a factor aiding in maintaining a high blood calcium,[6] it is no mystery how deficiency can contribute to a drop in tissue resistance to infective agents, and open the door to pyorrhea, erysipelas, and all the other infective diseases Dr. McCormick has listed as now being on the wane because we are eating more fresh vegetables and fruits, not because medical science knows more about how they may be controlled.[7]

This high level of blood calcium, or possibly specially earmarked calcium due to the vitamin P, seems to have the special function of promoting the formation of fibrin in blood clotting. This fibrin is biochemically identical with connective tissue fibers, and the same biochemical substrate is essential to the formation of both.[8]

Here is where we can go back to the old, once stressed function of vitamin C. The "participation," in a still unknown manner, is the formation of colloidal intercellular substances, which comprise those of cartilage, dentine, and the matrix of bone and, furthermore, the collagen of all fibrous tissue and non-epithelial cement substances. These phenomena are in close relationship to the disturbance of the calcium metabolism during times of vitamin C depletion, which directs growth and maintenance of bones and teeth and which sometimes appears similar to that observed during vitamin D deficiency."[9]

It becomes quite evident why synthetic ascorbic acid failed to perform as "vitamin C." Since both ascorbic acid and vitamin P are partners in the function, the observed alterations in the ascorbic acid levels afforded a rough index of deficiency of the C complex. The blood rise in ascorbic acid or increase in excretion, following the administration of sulfa drugs,[10] antipyrin,[11] chloretone,[12] amidopyrine or codeine[13] is no doubt a clue to the effect of these drugs. They simply mobilize the vitamin into the blood, where its effects are attributed to the drug, and ultimately leave the patient more debilitated than ever. Just another one of those common asininities of trying to cure the effects of starvation with a synthetic drug or poison. We hear that the U.S. Army medical authorities have abandoned the use of sulfra drugs because of the after-effects. We might class these after-effects as a new kind of scurvy.

The natural vitamin C complex has not had the fanfare and publicity of sulfra drugs, but as Dr. McCormick has shown, has accomplished far more in ridding us of infective scourges, tuberculosis alone having dropped to one-tenth its incidence of a hundred years ago. He quotes the great English physician, Dr. Leonard Williams: "The discovery of the vitamins has altered our conception of the causes and origins of disease. Until lately disease was regarded as a sin of commission by some unseen and subtle agency. The vitamins are teaching us to regard it, in some degree at any rate, as a sin of omission on the part of civilized or hypercivilized man. By our habit of riveting our attention on microbes and their toxins, we have sadly neglected the side of the question which concerns itself with our own bodily defenses."

McCormick remarks "After all, we should recognize that natural resistance to disease is developed by fundamental improvement in nutrition and hygiene. Such resistance gives protection to all diseases. Artificial immunization, on the other hand, is dependent upon the conversion of a portion of this latent general resistance to a specific resistance, such as toxoiding for diphtheria. The injection of an attenuated virus or bacteria toxin elicits a reaction of the organism to that specific morbific agent only, and drawn upon the reserves of natural immunity to meet this conversion demand. If repeated demands exceed the supply we are left physically bankrupt." And that is just why the Army found the sulfra drugs impractical, no doubt. Borrowing immunity from the future? What next may we expect in wonders of science?

Sulfathiazole too, promotes vitamin K deficiency.[13]

Vitamin K is an integral part of the C complex, found associated with it in most green plant sources, but has the solubility of chlorophyll, so is removed in concentration as a member of the chlorophyll complex. Its function is to promote the synthesis in the liver of the prothrombin that is essential to the formation of the fibers of fibrin or connective tissue laid down by the other reactions depending on the intact vitamin C complex. So the overdosage of a patient who may have many deficiencies including that of vitamin K, with too much vitamin C complex, especially that of the buckwheat vitamin P, may theoretically aggravate the latent K deficiency. Venous congestion and enlarged veins are the symptoms. It is very interesting to see the "Road Map" faces and many the erythematous and xanthomatous skin lesions of the chronic type gradually clear up under treatment with these concentrates. Diabetics are particularly prone to these complications, especially in the eyes, where vascular breakdown is really serious. A general improvement in the sugar metabolism is common to, the need for insulin often becoming progressively less.

Potassium bicarbonate is another factor needed by the diabetic, he tends to drift to acidosis and his alkali bases become depleted. Potassium is required to combine with sugar in the phosphagen molecule (di-potassium-creatine-hexose-phosphate) which is the form in which sugar is fixed in liver and muscle cells. Potassium deficiency can impair sugar absorption thereby, is known to cause paralysis in both human subjects and in dogs. The general use of sodium bicarbonate as an alkalizer is physiologically unsound. Sodium ions normally cannot enter the cell.[16] The physiological dosage of potassium bicarbonate is not over one gram (15 grains) per day.

## REFERENCES

[1] Delafield & Prudden: *Textbook & Pathology,* 15th ed., Wm. Wood & Co., New York.

[2] Hume, E. D.: *Bechamp or Pasteur,* 3rd edition, C. W. Daniel Co., London, 1947.

[3] Pottenger, F. M., ":The Effect of Heat-Processed Foods and Metabolized Vitamin D Milk on the Dentofacial Structures of Experimental Animals." *Oral Surg.* 32(g): 467-485, August 1946.

[4] Van Wagtendonk, W. J. and Freed: *J. Biol. Chem.* 167: 219-224; 225-228, 1947.

[5] Baker & Leek: *Am. J. Physiol.* 147: 522-526, 1946.

[6] Raunert, M.: *J. Urol.* 32: 630, 1938.

[7] McCormick, W. J.: "The Changing Incidence and Mortality of Disease in Relation to Changed Trends in Nutrition." *Med. Rec.*, p. 533, September 1947.

[8] Lee, R. and Hanson, W. A.: *Protomorphology,* P. 167. Lee Foundation for Nutritional Research, Milwaukee 3, Wis., 1947.

[9] Rosenberg, H. R.: *Chemistry and Physiology of the Vitamins*. P. 330, Interscience Publishers, Inc., New York, 1942.

[10] *61st Annual Report of University of Wisconsin Agricultural Experimental Station*, page 38.

[11]. Frommel, Favre & Aron: *Helv. Physiol. Acta* 5:15, 1947.

[12]. Roy & Guha. *Nature,* 1946, 158, 239.

[13] Ztschr. *Vitamin forsch*. 1946, 17, 84-88.

[14] *Nutrition Abst. & Rev.* No. 3187, p. 636, January 1949.

[15] *Nutrition Abst. & Rev.* No. 3214, 3215, p. 641, January 1947.

[16] Fenn & Cobb: *J. Gen. Physiol.* 17: 629.

THE STATEMENTS HEREIN MAY NOT AGREE WITH CURRENTLY ACCEPTED MEDICAL OPINION. NEVERTHELESS, THE PUBLISHER BELIEVES THEM SOUND.

VITAMIN NEWS

VITAMIN PRODUCTS CO. • MILWAUKEE, WISCONSIN

VOL. 14

# "CATALYN" — A REAL
# HIGH POTENCY VITAMIN PRODUCT

"High Potency" is a much abused term. Vitamin and other food supplements are often loaded with low cost ingredients in quantities far greater than any physiological requirement; the high cost, more rare, components which may be much more important are ignored and the product promoted as a "high potency" — supposedly "highly effective — agent.

Agnes Fay Morgan, the celebrated nutritional authority, once made a test of the high potency vitamins used to "enrich" foods like white flour. The test animlas on the high potency enriched diet did not live as long as those on the same low vitamin diet without the "enrichment."

This is proof that a high potency in milligrams cannot be compared to a high potency in clinical test. Why not? Simply because the nutritional requirements for humans or test animals includes too many factors to be easily thrown together from a few sources of single vitamin, mineral, or amino acids, selected because of commercial availability.

A real high potency product will contain the vitamins with their natural synergists as found in unrefined foods..

For example, "natural forms of vitamin E (as alpha tocopherol) lose up to ninety-nine percent of their potency when separated from their natural synergists, (tannins, fatty acids and phospholipids)."[1] We interpret this to mean that tocopherol without synergists ceases to be vitamin E, if it means anything. It means exactly what Dr. Morgan discovered, that fractions of vitamin complexes were not vitamins in effect, that such fractions cannot act as the whole any more than the case and face of your watch can keep time.

How, then, can the potency of a food concentrate be determined?

Simply by the clinical performance. Here is what a celebrated, internationally known physician says about CATALYN — "It will interest you to know that I rechecked a patient yesterday who had undergone a complete physical and mental breakdown as a result of a rapidly fulminating senescent process. He has been treated for the last eighteen months and he is now normal in mind and, for his age (63 years), in his body. Examinations of his retina show a complete disappearance of the arteriosclerotic process, with a return of the silver streak in the arteries. He was treated through dietary measures, colonic irrigations, and eight Catalyn tablets per day. This sort of improvement is dramatic and is proof that pathological senescence is fundamentally a matter of improper nutrition — not alone a matter of food deficiencies, but also a matter of excesses of processed foods."

This patient had the good fortune to meet a physician who knew how to use physiological remedies. A physician who knew that improving the elimination and correcting the nutritional deficiencies were the first principles of restoring health.

"High potency" vitamins may actually reverse in their effects and perform the opposite of what the physician prescribing them may want to accomplish. Bicknell & Prescott in their new book *The Vitamins in Medicine* (Grune & Stratton, New York) page 735, tell how bone decalcification, a reaction to vitamin E deficiency, can also be caused by large doses alpha tocopherol. They recommend no greater concentration of alpha tocopherol than is found in wheat germ oil for any therapeutic use. High potencies defeat their purpose here, just as in Dr. Morgan's tests.

We believe that the first and commonest symptom of deficiency requiring "Catalyn" is fatigue. Truly, we consider "Catalyn" as "fine food for fatigue" Often, one or two tablets will afford a great relief in fifteen or twenty minutes. Two or three tablets a day often mean the difference between enjoying one's work, or finding it unbearable drudgery.

Why? Simply because it contains such a variety of scarce nutrients, not a high content of a few. It contains practically every trace mineral needed in nutrition, according to spectographic tests. They are not added by us. They are normally present as an integral part of the food concentrates, in organic combination, and inseparable from the vitamins and enzyme factors of which they are activators.

How can we tell you what the potency of such a product may be? It is something you or your patient must experience. The factors that you may need may be as yet unknown to science or medical arts. We kept ourselves alive with wheat germ and rice polish before they were discovered as essential. (the hard way, by observation of victims dying of starvation for years before anyone had wit enough to decide that maybe the meddling with rice and wheat had something to do with the situation.) One authority in tracing the history of polio discovered that the first cases reported were in Vienna in 1840. He stated that it was no probable coincidence that the first roller for making white flour was set up in Vienna in 1839.[2] Polio has many of the earmarks of beriberi, even down to the virus accompanying it, which was also found in beriberi by Dr. McCarrison, as related by him in his book, *Studies in Deficiency Disease.*

We believe that in terms of clinically demonstrable potency, it is the lowest cost nutritional supplement on the market. It was engineered to produce results, not to exhibit a "high potency" label.

When you have to lose sleep, try it as a fatigue dispeller. Its effect is physiological, the benefits are not borrowed from the future.

Trace mineral deficiency is today becoming recognized as the cause of undulant fever; trace mineral feeding is the first successful treatment for the disease whether it appears in cattle or human victims.[3] This is another example of how unknown factors work for us, being unsuspected until we blunder into their field of action. Undulant fever becomes now a deficiency disease. (Raw milk is cleared of suspicion, as it should have been long ago when statistical studies showed that there was more undulant fever where pasteurization was required by law than where it was not. Raw milk users get more vitamin C, and thereby have a higher resistance to all infections.) We see now that the real cause of these infectious diseases is low resistance due to malnutrition.

**REFERENCES**

[1] *Annual Rev. Biochemistry,* 1943, P. 381.

[2] W. J. McCormick, M.D., "Observations on the 1941 Outbreak of Poliomyelitis and Encephalitis in the Midwest," *Medical Record*, Feb. 4, 1942.

[3] "What About Trace Minerals?," Ed Rupp, *Missouri Ruralist*, April 9, 1949.

**Excerpts from Reference No. 3**

What about those trace minerals? Are we getting anywhere in learning more about them?

A little more than a year ago, *Missouri Realist* reported certain experiments taking place in the vicinity of Springfield, Mo., on the relationship between trace elements and health — human health, animal health and health of plant life.

Dr. Ira Allison, Springfield, had treated several undulant fever patients with trace element therapy as the background for his experiments. Results were almost incredible. Public attention was given to the experiments thru a clinic arranged by Dr. Allison in December of 1947.

There was another similar clinic last month in Springfield. A group of about 76 persons representing a varied field in everyday life was present to see for itself, ask questions of the patients as well as the doctors and others seated around the questioning table.

Beginning with patients whose blood tests were definitely positive, the trace element therapy seems to work an almost immediate improvement. After four or five months on trace element therapy and improvement of diet, blood tests became negative to undulant fever. Not only that, but patients questioned at the clinic said they felt better. In some cases, they were able to get up out of bed and go to work.

Testimonials of the undulant fever patients were so similar that one transcribed record would nearly suffice for each case. First the symptoms: alternating fever and chills, loss of weight and strength, despondency, fear of imminent danger, pains and aches in muscles and joints and others. After treatment by Doctor Allison, each testified to general improvement and relief.

Between 45 and 50 of Doctor Allison's patients had volunteered to tell their individual stories. Ages of patients ranged from about 12 to nearly 80 years. Patients came to the conference room one at a time. But time ran out. Only 15 or 20 of the patients could be heard in one day.

In about two years' time, approximately 1,800 patients have been treated, Doctor Allison says.

In the meantime, the Nicholson dairy herds are being fed trace mineral in their normal ration. Results, although incomplete, so far are quite astounding. In the first place, there was breeding trouble. Calf crop a year ago was despairingly low. This year, the calf crop was in the upper percentage bracket.

Possibly the most interesting moments during the clinic came during the discussion periods when no patients were in the conference room. It was during these times that indictments were heard of our dietary habits as a civilization. Habits which have led food processors into extracting nutritive qualities by the barrelful from normally good foods and putting back a pinch of synthetic nutrition. All to satisfy the taste of the public rather than their nutritional needs.

One bone of contention was our favorite, white bread. Actually these men and women claimed white bread is so low in actual good quality that rats and mice won't even tear open the wrapper. If a grocer would stock whole wheat bread made from whole wheat flour, rats and mice would invade the shelf from miles around. Still, they would leave the white bread alone, nutritionalists claim.

Then there was another indictment against pasteurization of milk. Heating milk thru pasteurization to the point where harmful bacteria is killed will also destroy beneficial bacteria they claimed. In other words, clean low bacteria count raw milk carried more nutritive qualities than the milk pasteurized.

Then, too, habits of cooking and food preparation as well as balanced meal planning came in for body blows, as a high level of carbohydrates or of sweets could be detected running thru the diets of the patients.

THE STATEMENTS HEREIN MAY NOT AGREE WITH CURRENTLY ACCEPTED MEDICAL OPINION. NEVERTHELESS, THE PUBLISHER BELIEVES THEM SOUND.

**Edited by Royal Lee** **June 1949**

# VITAMIN NEWS

VITAMIN PRODUCTS CO. • MILWAUKEE, WISCONSIN

VOL. 14

## VITAMINS

## F AND $F_2$

Vitamin F is now officially recognized as a member of the vitamin family. (See page 422 of the 1949 volume of the *Annual Review of Chemistry*.

Vitamin F was so named and described by your undersigned editor in these pages, issue of June 15, 1934, as follows:

"Vitamin E from different cereal sources has been found to ... have quite different characteristics. This we consider to be due to the (presence of) varying proportions of two distinct vitamins. We have taken the liberty of designating the new one vitamin F ... We consider this "F" to be identical with (blood) calcium depressor found in oatmeal. It is also present in considerable amounts in rye, but there appears to be little in wheat."

It was suggested that the physiological effect of vitamin F was opposite to vitamin D on the serum calcium, and that it might be found a preventive of sunstroke, or an antidote for the toxic effects of overdosages of vitamin D, and a physiological synergist of D, present in natural vitamin D complexes.

On August 15, 1935, the comment was made that the main use so far developed for vitamin F was in the treatment of prostate enlargement. Later, Hart and Cooper reported more exact data on this use.[1] This has put prostate enlargement definitely into the category of a deficiency disease.

Studies in French Indo-China showed the natives to be completely free of prostate disease, whereas the white population showed the usual incidence, indicating the possible effect of other factors than age in the cause.[2] Vitamin A deficiency also has been suspected to be a factor in causing prostate trouble.[3]

Prostate hypertrophy with great frequency becomes carcinomatous,[4] so it is with great interest we note that the current issue of the *Annual Review of Biochemistry* (1949) states that vitamin F destroys carcinogens, and that this may be one of its functions in living tissue (page 422).

The vitamin F complex (the fatty acid group known to carry vitamin F activity) was found to prevent increased susceptibility to malarial infection, and blood fractions rich in this F Complex inhibited malaria multiplication.[4,5,6].

These effects of stimulating resistance to infective agents by vitamin F are in all probability the effect of the diffusible form of calcium that the F promotes.

The vitamin F effect is associated with certain fatty acids, arachidonic acid commonly being highest in activity, especially if from mammalian sources. Even then, it varies from organ to organ, the liver, kidney and adrenal fat being highest.

Recently, we have found that fatty acids in phospholipid combination (available from liver) have greater potency and a different activity than the free unsaturated acids. We have provisionally termed this new form of this vitamin complex as $F_2$.

$F_2$ acts as a protector of certain vital tissue components, possible as a part of the phospholipid complex in nerve structures, but more definitely as a protective monomolecular layer for the determinant factors that are essential to the repair and regeneration of all tissue. (We refer the reader to *Protomorphology*, by Lee and Hanson, for detailed information of the theories of cell physiology that are responsible for the discovery of $F_2$.) vitamin $F_2$ promotes tissue repair to judge from the clinical results. Skin, which is one tissue that must constantly be replaced, responds at once, where a deficiency has caused an induration and degenerative effect.

The most spectacular results, however, are seen in some cases of atrophy of muscular tissue, commonly suspected to be of multiple sclerosis type, but apparently due to a deficiency of $F_2$. (We cannot state as yet whether all muscular dystrophies are specific results of $F_2$ deficiency. We assume not.)

It will be noted that here we are encroaching on territory of vitamin E. Let us recall, however, that vitamins F and $F_2$ are really members of the E complex. The tocopherols are simply anti-oxidizing agents and may be limited to this function. They may act mainly to prevent oxidation and destruction of the fatty acids and their linkages.

The F effect may be mainly in preserving the tissue determinants without which new cells or cell repair cannot take place. These determinants seem to be the catalysts that promote the formation of the specific proteins of the cell, and include trace mineral patterns that are part of the enzyme systems essential to cell metabolism.

It begins to appear that osteoarthritis is a disease partly, at least, a result of determinant loss, because the bone changes seem particularly of the type attributable to a determinant paucity. F, in clinical tests, seems to greatly enhance the action of other antiarthritic vitamins such as the Wulzen factor, found in unpasteurized milk and sugar cane juice. The new adrenal gland hormone, cortisone (compound e), is already known to be a determinant conserver — it may be its only function — and has been stated to be the longsought specific remedy for arthritis. (This theory of arthritis was elucidated in *Protomorphology* two years ago, pages 219, 298.)

The regeneration of red cells in the bone marrow seems to be dependent upon the presence of determinants, too, and pernicious anemia seems to be specifically a state of erythrocyte determinant paucity. The same adrenal factor helps in the treatment of pernicious anemia (*Protomorphology*, page 295), and a liver extract (apparently $F_2$) was effective also (page 295).

We have received some clinical reports suggesting that Vitamin $F_2$ is the missing link in liver therapy for pernicious anemia.

The effect of vitamin A concentrates from both vegetable and animal oil sources has been found to be useful in the treatment of some types of hypertension. This effect was traced to the unsaturated fatty acids in the less refined concentrates, apparently the vitamin F fraction. (Grollman, *Recent Progress in Hormone Research*, Academic Press, Vol. 1, 1947, page 383.) The purified vitamin A had lost the effects . (As is usual with any food product — the more refined, the less useful.)

Zaicsek and Weiser of Budapest discovered in 1934 that feeding rye to test animals caused muscular lines of development in distinction to the fatty type of growth in wheat fed animals, and attributed the difference to a then unknown vitamin present in rye. That vitamin was no doubt our old friend vitamin F. For vitamin F (as the physiological combined form of $F_2$) acts as a protector of the determinants which are the catalytic activators of cell mitosis, and which, if permitted to be enzymatically removed too freely, will result theoretically in a failure of development or of maintenance of any organ. (See *Protomorphology* for details.) Guanidine is a fatigue poison, an end product of muscle activity, and vitamin F is known to activate the conversion of guanidine back into the muscle component known as phosphagen, with the help of thyroid hormone. (Morse, 2nd Edition, Saunders, 1927, page 585. Morse attributes the cooperative effect to the unsaturated fatty acid component of cod liver oil — vitamin F Complex to us.)

Here we have the explanation of why some symptoms of F deficiency are also listed as those of thyroid inactivity — dry skin, loss of hair, constipation, muscular pains and eczematous tendencies. Maybe vitamin F is the missing link in getting the conversion of fat to muscle that we so long have expected thyroid to accomplish. No wonder we got toxic reactions instead of what we wanted.

Many users of vitamin F tell us that it eliminates the after-effect of stiff muscles often following unusual muscular activity. It should, if it aids in the reconversion of muscular waste products that are as toxic as guanidine.

Remember, the Finns habitually eat rye bread, and they walk away with first place regularly in the Olympic games. In 1924, Finns took the ten first places in the distance races. "Men of Iron," said Alfred McCann in his book *The Science of Keeping Young*. (Published in 1926, now suppressed by the copyright owner, we believe by reason of McCann's clear indictment of white flour.)

The new vitamin found in sugar cane and raw milk, known as the anti-arthritic factor or the Wilson-Van Jendonk factor, seems to have a parallel effect to the $F_2$. It promotes the availability of easily hydrolysable inorganic phosphorus to form phosphagen and adenosine triphosphate. (*Journal Biol. Chem.,* 165:449, 1946; and United States Patent #2439914.) It should probably be considered as a special form of vitamin F as found in the milk complex with vaccenic acid, and in sugar bearing plant juices.

The clinical experiences with the anti-arthritic factor in treating arthritis are parallel with results of tests with our F complex — some are benefited and some report an aggravation of symptoms. At the moment, we are inclined to believe those that find aggravation of the arthritic symptoms are low in phosphorus, and need to get their phosphorus-calcium balance adjusted before relief is possible. Low phosphorus states in test animals are uncommon because they are not fed refined sugar products or white flour. That may be the reason the animal tests do not apply here to the human subject.

The clinical uses of vitamin F complex as CATAPLEX F, and the new vitamin $F_2$ may be tabulated as follows:

## Uses of CATAPLEX F

(1) As synergist of vitamin D, to insure delivery of calcium to bones, teeth, muscle, nerve or phagocytes in a form that is diffusible — probably as calcium bicarbonate.

Chalky teeth in children usually become hard and translucent if the F is supplied with calcium lactate (one tablet of F and three of five-grain Calcium Lactate, taken on arising in morning, 15 minutes before food). Vitamin C aids this effect. A 60-day treatment will demonstrate this reaction.

(2) As a palliative (and often affording complete relief) in cases of prostate enlargement. Apparently, this disorder is a deficiency state, for it very consistently clears up under treatment with vitamin F — three tablets per day.

Vitamin C again is synergistic, probably by its promotion of capillary circulation.

(3) All states requiring more diffusible calcium in the tissues.

### Uses of VITAMIN $F_2$

(For experimental use — a new product)

(1) Diseases where there is a definite failure of tissue regeneration. Muscular dystrophies, creeping paralyses, anemic states, weakness and atrophy. To be used in connection with all known physiological remedies, such as vitamin E, amino acids, special diets, with definite restrictions on refined foods, processed cereals, soft drinks, all white sugar products, favoring raw foods, rare meats, vegetable juices.

## BIBLIOGRAPHY

[1] *Report #1*, Lee Foundation for Nutritional Research, Milwaukee, 1942.
[2] Le Roy des Barres, A., *Bulletin Academy de Medicine Paris*, 117:367, 1937.
[3] Moore and Mark, *Journal Experimental Medicine,* 64:1, 1936.
[4] Trager, W., *Proc. Soc. Exper. Biol. & Med.*, 64:129-34, 1947.
[5] Axelrod et al, L. *Biol.*, 175:265-74, 1948.
[6] Trager, W., L. *Exper. Med.*, 85:663-83, 1947.



Edited by Royal Lee October 1949

VITAMIN NEWS

VITAMIN PRODUCTS CO. • MILWAUKEE, WISCONSIN

VOL. 15

# TRUTH vs. PROPAGANDA IN NUTRITION

This is the eighteenth year of publication of *Vitamin News*. Your editor has made every effort to offer reliable information on the relation of malnutrition to disease, and in many cases offered information greatly in advance of other sources.

Possibly the most outstanding is the reporting of the value of natural vitamin C complex as a prompt builder of resistance to infection, and its probable action through the promotion of phagocytosis (an opsonic effect), in the issue of September 18, 1933. The confirmation of this statement was reported in *Vitamin News* of December 1947. Meanwhile, many physicians had reported results definitely confirming our definition of the natural C complex as the "physiological sulfanilamide." The sulfa drugs in fact were later shown to actually do part if not all their work by mobilizing vitamin C from the tissues into the blood stream; and if C is not present, the sulfa drug fails in clinical experience to act as a germ killer.[1]

Advance knowledge of this kind is of the highest value to the physician. The doctor who used the vitamin C complex to treat infections had no regrets of poisoning his patient, as many learned to their dismay after seeing the effects of sulfa dosing.

Again, in September 1934, attention was called to the fact that the cause of arteriosclerosis is vitamin deficiency and lack of the mineral elements lost in flour milling. Multiple vitamins plus the phytates in orthophosphoric acid solution was recommended as a treatment. Today we find that the only known successful treatment of arteriosclerosis is in the use of inositol (from that same phytate), and in the lipotropic vitamins of the B complex as found in wheat germ. We have had the pleasure, meanwhile, of having hundreds of people tell us how their lives have been extended by this treatment.

In *Hygeia* for August 1949 appeared an article on this very subject of cardiovascular disease and arteriosclerosis. Our position has been years ahead of the best authorities in reporting progress, for the author, Paul H. Fluck, M. D., heads his article "Natural Causes, the Great Killer." He sees no reason to assume that cardiovascular disease has any possible relation to malnutrition, but is simply the accidental form of the manifestation of the ravages of wear and tear, namely old age.

Now, it is somewhat strange that Dr. Fluck is less well informed than the science writer for the *American Weekly,* G. B. Lal, for Mr. Lal, in the July 1949 issue of that layman's journal, carried a very good article on the use of choline, inositol and methionine for cardiovascular disease. It seems that Dr. Lester M. Morrison and his colleagues at the County Hospital in Los Angeles had reported their success in treating indigent victims of John Barleycorn who had liver cirrhosis and other blood vessel diseases that had been (up to that time) 90% fatal: they were cured if given these food factors that are lacking in our usual foods by reason of refining and processing. This disparity in Dr. Fluck's position and that of your editor is apparently due to the ineptness of the former in keeping abreast of and informed of the latest far-reaching discoveries in medicine and nutrition.

Another writer in the same issue of *Hygeia* is also frightfully behind the times. He is Dr. Wesley X. Spink, writing about "Today's Knowledge of Undulant Fever," who actually has not heard that undulant fever is a disease caused by trace mineral deficiency, and has been cured by trace minerals. This has long been known, since Dr. Oscar Erf of the Ohio State University tested the discovery by two spectroscopists (Drs. Irene Levis and F. H. Emery of Cleveland) in 1939 that only cows with deficiencies of manganese, copper, iodine, and cobalt in their tissues were susceptible to the infective agent in brucellosis. Dr. Erf was unable to get cows to become infected if they had proper nutritional supplies of these elements. Since then, Dr. Allison and Dr. Albrecht at Springfield, Missouri, have conclusively proved that the addition of these minerals to the food of animals or human patients ends their disease just as quickly as brown rice can cure beri-beri .[3]

Since *Hygeia* had reported in September 1947 that undulant fever was a serious matter, being exceeded in importance only by tuberculosis and venereal diseases, certainly a far reaching discovery like this should deserve announcement with headlines and all the trimmings of a major medical scoop. Dr. Spink in other statements exhibits a very antiquated viewpoint, too. He says, for instance, that raw milk is capable of carrying the infection to human victims, in addition to its common avenue of inoculation, through skin abrasions or wounds, from the handling of infected meat or diseased animals. He evidently never heard of the account in *Nelson's Encyclopedia of Medicine* (Chapter 44, Volume 2, section by Strong), where the raw milk from 2000 cows that had been accidentally inoculated with a live culture of brucella organisms (instead of the killed culture intended as an immunizing agent), had been sold and used for six months without a single milk consumer being infected. Most authorities accept the fact that disease germs are in general destroyed in the stomach, with few exceptions (such as typhoid).

Dr. Strong, in his report in this medical encyclopedia, says "Undulant fever is not contagious to man."

Dr. Spink says "People living in ... areas where only pasteurized milk is sold are not victims of brucellosis except when they travel and drink unpasteurized milk or milk products." This statement has never been supportable by scientific evidence, but is frequently made in such articles. Mrs. Darlington, in her complete exposure of the pasteurization racket that permits the safe sale of unsanitary and filthy milk without restriction, offers ample proof of the way the undulant fever scare has been used to cover up this unsavory business.[4] Probably the most valuable food principle in milk is vitamin C complex, which activates phagocytes and builds resistance. One authority reminds us that pasteurization destroys more of this vitamin than all the citrus trees in the country can replace with their fruit.[5] So pasteurization, in fact, can make us even more susceptible to brucellosis, and cooperate with mineral deficiency in undermining our health.

The quicker we get the truth, the sooner we can apply the remedy. Here we need to realize that all our feed for animals susceptible to brucellosis must be fortified with 100 parts per million of manganese, 0.1 of copper, 0.1 of cobalt, 0.1 of iodine, 6.0 of magnesium, and 1.5 of zinc.** That brings up the point that man cannot assimilate cobalt as a salt, but the ruminats can. Man must get his as vitamin $B_{12}$, now claimed as the main constituent of the anti-anemic complex in the liver. $B_{12}$ might be better known as the organic form of cobalt required by the human economy.

Here is one of those cases where a mineral element must be in an organic form to be useful. And it is of interest that only a fe v short years ago our best authorities were telling us that no mineral element for nutrition needed to be in an organic form. (Statement of Drs. C. A. Elvehjem, F. E. Bear and E. L. McCollum at the McCollum-Pratt Seminar, Johns-Hopkins University, April 12-13, 1948; reported in *The Land*, Summer, 1948, page 301.) These men admitted that 99% of the people differed from their opinions, had no evidence to support their own dissenting viewpoints, and still used their professional prestige to promote the pronouncement that no mineral needed to be in an organic form to be nutritionally effective. Within months, the discovery that cobalt had to be in the proper organic form to be useful in the human dietary (as vitamin $B_{12}$), and that man cannot live without it, proved the ridiculous nature of their untenable position.

Again, your editor can modestly claim priority in this idea. Here is a reprinted review of a few ideas on trace mineral activities, originally published in 1947: [6]

> We are just beginning to recognize some of the important functions of trace minerals. The activation of enzyme activity of manganese, cobalt and other trace elements is one important feature of trace mineral physiology, but many other minerals, fluorine in particular, may inhibit enzymes. Some stimulate enzyme action at one concentration or hydrogen ion level, and reverse their action at other ranges of concentration or hydrogen ion level. This field is not well explored, but in time may throw light on many obscure reactions both normal and abnormal.
>
> But the biggest new fact about trace minerals is their distribution in such cell organs as show that they probably are responsible for hereditary characteristics. It seems that the trace mineral in the chromosome is in a way, the "ink on the blueprints." No derangements that follow deficiencies of some trace minerals — boron, zinc, manganese or copper — show changes that seem to be definitely due to impairment of the hereditary mechanism, changes indicating that somewhere some record is lost, some structure is incomplete. These minerals are undoubtedly attached to protein molecules, and as such very probably assimilated by the higher forms of life only after metabolism by lower forms. Here may lie the secret of "organic gardening." Yeasts, molds, and bacteria act as sub-contractors for plant life, live only where organic compost is available, but obtain part of their mineral nutrition from inorganic soil sources. It is the same partnership in microscopic life we see in all the balances of nature in the higher animal kingdoms, a mutual partnership that the human family has funded to destroy by overcropping the soil and removing too great a proportion of not only trace minerals but also failing to maintain the compost bed that supports these forms of cell life that perform the first step of conversion of inorganic mineral substances to the organic state.

Before we get too enthusiastic about getting our heavy doses of nutritional minerals like manganese, let us check into the clinical experience. We find that inorganic salts of manganese "in small, repeated dosage" to the human patient causes liver cirrhosis.[7] We know that choline and inositol prevent and cure liver cirrhosis. In natural foods, we get manganese, choline and inositol in the same complex, such as cereal germ. Feeding manganese to cows which get plenty of bran and middlings from flour mill by-products is a lot different from feeding manganese to human patients eating white flour. That is the same mistake as fortifying foods with a few syntehtic vitamins expecting to get the same results as leaving in the flour all the natural vitamins. It should be no surpise to find the same result: the result of aggravating the maluntrition instead of relieving it.

Here we see how impairment of tissue integrity by poor nutrition can and does set the stage for the invasion of the infective agent, which is the secondary cause of disease in most cases, the primary cause being the deficiency-starvation of tissue in the face of an excess of proteins, fats and carbohydrates, especially the latter.

As we write this, Dr. Irene Diller announces at the A.A.A.S. meeting in New York her discovery of various forms of fungus in cancer tissue.

The same old story. The susceptibility of malnutrition. Did not Dr. Davidson years ago prove that mice could be made susceptible to cancer by imposed malnutrition, and afterward rendered immune by improving their diet? [8]

## REFERENCES

1 Bicknell, F., and Prescott, F., *The Vitamins in Medicine.* Second edition, New York: Grune and Stratton, 1948. P. 585.

2 Under, F. E., and Grove, R. D., *Vital Statistics Rates in the U. S., 1900-1940.* U.S. Public Health Service, National Office of Vital Statistics. Washington, D. C.: Government Printing Office, 1947. Table 14, P. 253.

3 Wischhusen, 1. F., "Bang's Disease and Undulant Fever are Nutritional Deficiencies," *The Polled Hereford Magazine,* July, 1948.

4 Darlington, Mrs. Jean B., "Why Milk Pasteurization?" *The Rural New-Yorker* March 15, May 3, and July 5, 1947.

5 Rorty, J., and Norman, N.P. M.D., *Tomorrow's Food.* New York: Prentice Hall, Inc. P. 158.

6 *Journal of the Academy of Applied Nutrition*, Winter, 1947. P. 112.

7 Cushny, *Pharmacology and Therapeutics,* Tenth edition, Philadelphia: Lea and Febiger, 1934. P. 712.

8 Davidson, J. R., "Cancer, a Nutritional Deficiency." *Question Mark* magazine, February, 1943. Published by the Science Department of the University of Manitoba.

---

*Some columnists on medical subjects tell us that the terrific incidence of cardiovascular disease is not to be worried about; it is simply because more people are getting older now, thanks to the reduced deaths from preventable disease; and because doctors are now classifying more deaths as heart disease formerly classified as nephritis and cerebral hemorrhage. But this is a form of guess work unverified by any conclusive evidence, and amounts to an attempt to "argue away" a very probable increase in cardiovascular deaths. Reliable federal statistics show a 14% increase in the death rate from heart diseases between 1900 and 1940 for the ages 35 through 44: a 62% increase for the ages 45-54; and a 72% increase for ages 55-64, during the same period in the U.S. death registratoin area.[2] (These increases are based on age-spcific rates : deaths per 100,000 population in the age group, thus eliminating the argument of "more deaths because of more old people" by placing each age group on a common denominator of 100,000 persons.)

THE STATEMENTS HEREIN MAY NOT AGREE WITH CURRENTLY ACCEPTED MEDICAL OPINION. NEVERTHELESS, THE PUBLISHER BELIEVES THEM SOUND.

**Edited by Royal Lee** **June 1950**

VITAMIN NEWS

VITAMIN PRODUCTS CO. • MILWAUKEE, WISCONSIN

VOL. 15

# CHLOROPHYLL:
# A FOOD ESSENTIAL

Chlorophyll is a fat soluble pigment, the green coloring material in plant leaves. It is naturally associated with the fat soluble vitamins of the leaf, the vitamin E complex, the K complex, the A complex, and the F complex the most important factor of which is also known as the X factor of Dr. Weston A. Price (only found in young seedlings during the period of rapid growth).

If the chlorophyll is to be made water soluble, it must be separated from these synergistic factors, reduced to a chemically pure (refined) form, and the magnesium molecule it carries be partly substituted by copper. The chlorophyll then becomes of a bluish hue instead of green, but will dissolve in water. The natural form is insoluble in water..

Paul de Kruif in August (1950) "*Reader's Digest* writes about chlorophyll as "nature's deodorant." He tells us that 100 milligram pills of the water-soluble form counteract B.0. and halitosis if used regularly, and are "harmless." This amount of the synthetic copper-chlorophyll could well be toxic, and we feel that 10 milligrams a day would be the limit of use for such a product, if to be taken day in and day out as it were. The natural fat soluble complex, we believe, would fall under Paul de Kruif's idea of a harmless product. Copper is a dangerous trace mineral to gamble with in dosages of more than a few milligrams a day. Foods or water contaminated with copper are known to be specifically destructive to the optic nerve, blindness having been caused by the use of hot tap water (used to make coffee) carrying traces of copper from the coils of the water heater. (The makers of these heaters tell us not to use the hot water for cooking, as some kinds of water take up copper more readily than others.)

Chlorophyll has two definite effects when taken into the human economy. It destroys guanidine on contact, and promotes the elimination of cholesterol.[2]

Guanidine is a poison that is produced by the breakdown of phosphagen. It precipitates calcium[2] and the function of the parathyroid is to eliminate guanidine and restore the presence of the otherwise precipitated calcium in the body fluids. The guanidine is disposed of by its anabolic regeneration into phosphagen. Phosphagen is dipotassium-creatine-hexote-phosphate, and is the energy source for all mammalian dynamics. The male sperm, for instance, is loaded with phosphagen as a power source, just as a loaded torpedo has a compressed air tank or charged storage battery to take it to its destination. That is why the male economy never wastes creatine in the urine, while that same creatine is a normal component of the urine of the female. (Here is the first explanation offered for this heretofore mysterious phenomena.) (More information on this in *Protomorphology*, Lee & Hanson, Lee Foundation, Milwaukee.)

Phosphagen is so easily broken down that simple mild trauma or heat releases its components, which are highly irritating to nerve endings. The prick of a pin or a drop of hot water causes pain by this reaction, we believe. (Discussed in *Vitamin News*, pp. 5 and 6, 1933.) Free guanidine is probably the main toxic agent in severe burns. Chlorophyll acts much like Vitamin F in treating burns. It nullifies the pain; the quicker it is applied after the burn the less the severity, for the toxic agents are destroyed before they can do much damage. Chlorophyll applied to extracted tooth sockets stops the same type of pain; the agonizing, irritating pain that keeps the patient awake, that is so hard to alleviate with narcotics. Vitamin F restores the diffusible calcium that is precipitated by guanidine, so its parallel action is rational. Vitamins D and F operating as a complex, as in cod liver oil, are obviously paralleling the action of parathyroid, both protecting the blood calcium levels (heretofore known to be parallel but without a clue as to the biochemistry). Another puzzle is cleared up — castrated animals are known to be immune to tetanic seizures if their parathyroids are removed. Since the male hormones promote the retention of creatine and guanidine for building phosphagen for the sperm cells, the parathyroid is essential as a creatine catalyst — and as this catalysis of guanidine into creatine and the prevention of excretion of creatine take place in the kidney, we here have the reason for the mysterious fact that parathyroid function is confined to kidney reactions. Prostate phosphatase is probably a partner in this phosphagen synthesis. It is significant that prostate disease seems to be a Vitamin F deficiency state in most cases. (See *Lee Foundation Report No. 1*, "Vitamin F in the Treatment of Prostatic Hypertrophy," 1941.) (We wish to report that vitamin F is now a recognized member of the vitamin family — see the *Annual Review of Biochemistry,* 1949, page 422. First introduced by the Vitamin Products Company in 1934 as a calcium metabolizer and synergist of vitamins D and E.)

The other known effect of chlorophyll — the elimination of excess cholesterol — is of great interest. Cholesterol is the material used in cell activity as a regulator (with lecithin) of cell wall permeability. If an excess becomes deposited by reason of a failure of the proper balance of the body fluid fat controls (the lipotropic factors), there is an increase in blood pressure, and an increase in sedimentation rate. (Betacol is a concentrate of the lipotropic factors from beet and cane molasses. Its major use is for control of high sedimentation rate.)

The sedimentation rate is high in most toxic states — pregnancy, chronic constipation, arthritis, infectious disease. Chlorophyll seems to be a synergist of the lipotropic factors. These include the cereal phytates (the rice diet for hypertension is a success we feel only because it supplies phytates that afford inositol and orthophosphoric acid after digestion), inositol, betaine, choline and lecithin. We feel that the natural complexes of these lipotropic factors are far more potent, quantitatively, than the pure forms. It is hard to get a patient to take enough choline to accomplish the desired purpose. But the natural complex is not needed in more than one tenth the volume to get the same result, according to our findings.

## SPECIAL NEWS ITEM — POLIOMYELITIS NOW PROVEN TO BE A DISEASE OF MALNUTRITION JUST AS DEFINITELY AS BERIBERI OR PELLAGRA.

Dr. Benjamin P. Sandler of Asheville, N. C. has been working since 1931 on the theory that an excessive amount of glucose in the diet promotes susceptibility to virus or bacterial disease.

Tuberculosis patients rapidly improved when put on a non-sugar and glucose diet.[3]

Monkeys and rabbits were made immune by similar means.

But here is the final proof. After Asheville and other North Carolina papers gave his views considerable publicity, the incidence of polio in North Carolina dropped from 2402 cases in 1948 to 214 in 1949. One ice cream distributor in North Carolina sold one million gallons less of ice cream in the season following Dr. Sandler's news release. Ice cream and soft drinks, or rather the synthetic glucose and sugar in these counterfeit foods, are the causes of polio and do not believe propaganda to the contrary. Dr. Sandler has previously shown how glucose is the most potent offender of all the sugars in undermining resistance, and that the natural glucose in the blood stream formed by conversion in the body from starches or proteins is not the same as the synthetic glucose sold us in adulterated foods.[3,4] This is headline news, but you will not see much about it in papers carrying soft drink advertising or cnady and sugar ads. It is very unhealthy to condemn sugar as a cause of disease. One dentist who has been studying this problem thoroughly, and has been getting phenomenal results in improving calcium assimilation in his patients by inducing them to eat no glucose or refined sugar, suddenly found himself arrested for practicing medicine without a license, in a state where the medical practice law specifically stated that its restrictions did not apply to dentists. His trial is still pending after dragging along over a year, his defense having cost him many thousands of dollars. Some malignant influence is obviously behind this. It savors of the kind of justice we heard about in the dictator-ridden countries. Who is dictating here? We would like to know. Dr. Wiley warned us long ago that the makers of counterfeit foods had taken possession of the law enforcement agencies. They seem to have been entrenched well ever since they ousted him in 1912. Let us all beware; get the facts for yourself.

[1] *Chemurgic Digest*, June 30, 1946, p. 215.
[2] *Acidosis & Nutrition,* Royal Lee, 1947.
[3] B. P. Sandier and R. Berke, *American Review of Tuberculosis,* 46:238-261, 1942.
[4] *Prevention,* June 1950, Rodale Press, page 44.

## MORE SIDELIGHTS ON GLUCOSE

Dr. Harvey W. Wiley, the first head of the Federal Food & Drug Administration, suspected glucose to be a dangerous adulterant of food, because it was a synthetic imitation of the natural sugars, made by the conversion of corn starch by acid treatment in which all mineral and vitamin factors were destroyed during the synthesis of the "corn" sugar. Dr. Wiley thought the use of the word "corn" as a descriptive adjective was fraudulent for the new sugar or syrup, as it inferred that they were natural products of corn. Corn syrup is no more a corn product than oleo made by hydrogenating a vegetable oil is butter. Both are hideous insults to the intelligence of the food buyer, synthetic counterfeits deliberately designed to undersell the genuine products they simulate.)

Glucose is a first class adulterant for soft drinks, canned fruits, and dried fruits because it is so cheap, puffs up the weight, and saves real sugar.

Refined cane sugar cannot cause diabetes in test animals. Glucose does (according to tests made by Drs. Lukens and Dohan at the Univ. of Pa.).

One form of cancer fails to respond to treatment until diabetic symptoms are under control, according to Dr. Quigley of Omaha. Synthetic glucose therefore may very definitely contribute to cancer. (*Am. Jour. Roentgenology & Radium Therapy,* Vol. 34, No. 1, p. 83.)

Glucose causes low blood sugar as well as diabetes (Ref. 4 above), and this state results in a predisposition to heart disease, lassitude, brain fatigue, high blood pressure, overweight, irritability, mental depression, to list the findings of a current report. (*Newsweek* of July 17, 1950, p. 45.)

Glucose present with proteins when they are cooked results in a destruction of the most important of the Amino Acids — Tryptophane, Lysine, Threonine, and Methionine. (See *Journal of Nutrition,* Vol. 40, No. 2, Article by Friedman & Mine.) "Relatively small losses in amino acids were associated with drastic changes in availability to animals ... "

Calcium assimilation, too, is blocked by the presence of glucose, while some other sugars like lactose (milk sugar) encourage calcium assimilation. (See *The Vitamins in Medicine,* page 641. This is a new English reference book for the physician; no doctor who wants to keep abreast of this subject can afford to be without it.

Calcium has so many functions it is hard to say how vital its importance is. There are good reasons to believe that no virus infection can occur unless the calcium levels of the body fluids have dropped below a certain limit. No doubt here is where the insidious relation of soft drinks and ice cream to polio is to be found. Since vitamin P increases the calcium content of the body fluids (Rosenberg, *The Vitamins,* p. 517), it is easy to see how orange juice is better than ascorbic acid to protect against polio, as found in tests. (See *Prevention* magazine, June 1950, p. 15.)

Here, then is the case against glucose (alias corn syrup, grape sugar, dextrose, corn sugar). It contributes, according to positive tests in animal feeding and clinical findings in human observation: to the cause of diabetes, cancer, hypertension, lassitude, brain fatigue, overweight, irritability, mental depression, impairs the assimilation of calcium, and destroys vital amino acids if they are cooked in its presence.

The calcium deficiency can cause reduced resistance to infection, can cause the loss of teeth by decay or pyorrhea, and can predispose to a long list of chronic disease including forms of arthritis.

Was Dr. Riley right when he opposed its free use without even label declaration of its pernicious presence?

Was Dr. Riley right when he said that the enforcement personnel of the food & drug law were protecting the law violators instead of the people who pay their salaries

The monkey in the jungle knows better than to eat poisonous fruits and insects. He has learned the hard way. Why cannot we learn the hard way too?

THE STATEMENTS HEREIN MAY NOT AGREE WITH CURRENTLY ACCEPTED MEDICAL OPINION. NEVERTHELESS, THE PUBLISHER BELIEVES THEM SOUND.

Edited by Royal Lee September 1950

# VITAMIN NEWS

VITAMIN PRODUCTS CO. • MILWAUKEE, WISCONSIN

VOL. 16


## CHOLESTEROL, CANCER, CARDIOVASCULAR DISEASE, AND ALUMINUM

Various items are appearing in the scientific journals and the newspapers about cholesterol, its bad effects if permitted to collect in the human body. It is blamed for hardening of the arteries and hypertension as well as old age in general. Blakeslee, the Associated Press science writer, called inositol the *"Youth Pill"* in a release of September 5, because it is known to aid in cholesterol elimination. Many persons, reading this type of literature, become alarmed, and try to reduce their cholesterol intake by restricting the amount of eggs, butter, milk, cheese and fat meats. They are not aware that these sources of cholesterol also carry the best antidote for it, the phospholipids and lecithins which are always naturally associated with cholesterol, that the loss of these phospholipids is more certain to cause serious trouble than any excess of cholesterol.

The phospholipids, (which include lecithins), in food are a part of the vitamin E complex. The E complex loses as much as 99 percent of its potency, (measured as antioxidant stability), if the associated phospholipids are removed along with the other synergists from the tocopherol.[1] The E complex is also known to facilitate cholesterol transport and metabolism.[2]

So we can see that a deficiency of vitamin E complex can increase trouble from cholesterol in the tissues. Lecithin as a biochemical balancer for cholesterol is shown by the fact that a high cholesterol content of the tissues predisposes to cancer,[3] and a high content of lecithin protects from cancer.[4]

Just how this takes place is explained in more detail in other references.[5] The vitamin E and associated factors seem to act by protecting the chromosome units in the cell. These units are the "blueprints" for the designs of life; the guiding determinants that insure that healing or regenerating tissue is like that which is being replaced. If the blueprints are destroyed, say by oxidation or enzymatic digestion, because the protective phospholipid wrappers are injured by reason of nutritional deficiencies of the vitamin E complex and phospholipids, it is easy to understand why cancer can occur, or the walls of the blood vessels become patched and degenerated. Sudden death, that well-established penalty for vitamin E complex deficiency, is easily understood. (A group of 28 cattle put on rations having the E complex removed during the first year of a three-year test, lost 13 of their number by heart failure during this time.)[6]

Whole wheat carries a liberal content of the vitamin E complex and phospholipids. Commercial flour, both white and whole wheat, is treated with oxidizing chemicals in proportion to the vitamins present, four times as much for the whole wheat flour as the white. As a result, test animals die much quicker on commercial "whole wheat" bread than on white bread.[7] So we can readily see why such foods predispose to cancer, sterility, cardiovascular disease, creeping paralysis and a host of other chronic degenerative changes. (Vitamin E complex is also essential to the maintenance of the integrity of the insulating films in nerve fibers, the same function as the protection of the chromosome wrappers.)

Flour bleaches destroy phosphatase in flour, which otherwise would release inositol from the phytates during the yeast-raising period of bread-making. Therefore, they contribute to all the diseases that are suspected to follow inositol deficiency (arteriosclerosis, fatty degeneration of the liver, susceptibility to cancer, inhibition of lactation in mothers, loss of hair or impairment of its growth, muscular degeneration).

There is another specific destroyer of phosphatase and phospholipids that should be taken into account. That is the element aluminum. Any form of soluble aluminum is destructive to any phosphorus linkage found in food. When it is desired to observe phosphorus deficiency in test animals, the easiest way to block the assimilation of phosphorus is to give them some aluminum salt in their food. The blood phosphorus drops quickly to a minimum level. Aluminum has a greater affinity for phosphorus than for any other element, except one. That is silicon. So sodium silicate becomes an antidote for aluminum. Sodium silicate becomes an antidote for aluminum. Sodium silicate is one of the remedies sometimes used to relieve arteriosclerosis. Probably its only functions as such in those cases where the arteriosclerosis is being produced by aluminum poisoning.[8] It is of interest that silica poisoning (silicosis) of the lungs from inhaling silica is successfully being treated by the inhalation of aluminum dust.[9]

In the only test on record that purported to show that animals were unharmed by feeding aluminum salts, sodium silicate was administered in their "mineral ration," and served as an antidote.[10] Rat poison is harmless too, under similar circumstances. Soluble aluminum salts are poisonous to plants too, but most soils have enough silica to control their effects.[11]

The inept personnel of our enforcement agencies (FDA and FTC) see nothing bad about aluminum. In fact, the FTC suppresses anything it finds and issues orders to cease any discussion of the toxicity of aluminum against health lecturers who bring up the subject.[12] The penalty for violation is ten thousand dollars; and with no opportunity to fight the despotic order in court, if you do not happen to know. This is one of the examples of the decay of democracy, and its degeneration into totalitarianism. *It is happening here.* The public ear must not hear both sides of these matters.

The notorious incidence of ill health in the "baking powder belt" where hot biscuits and corn bread are made with alum baking powder is another national disgrace. The victims of such poisoning surely act as if the insulation on their nerve trunks were faulty. They have not the energy to lift a hand, very often. Typical "mountain boys" who let "Grandma" do all the work. We call it "pellagra;" but we never have found the remedy to control it properly. Certainly, various better food components do a lot of good. But the real answer is not in sight. It is a conspicuous fact that foods high in phospholipids are essential in the treatment of pellagra — eggs, wheat germ, milk. No vitamin pattern alone is able to cure the disease. Alum is used in baking powder simply because it reduces the cost to about one-fifth of that of a tartrate powder. (Tartrates are wine by-products.)

The substitution of synthetic fats for natural ones, and oleo for butter, has brought into use another large group of cheating foods. They lack the phospholipid content of natural fats. So they must contribute to premature aging, cardiovascular disease, sterility, sudden death and cancer. They are also suspected of causing the partial castration of both sexes, and to make boys develop into sissies, and girls into narrow-hipped, broad shouldered freaks that can only bear babies by the cesarean route,[13] and about as capable of nursing the new arrival as the father.

These remarks may sound very cynical and harsh to the uninitiated. Please believe me when I say that they are not intended to be more than a plain report of the facts. When we are faced by an unscrupulous situation, we had better recognize the facts. To gloss over their harshness is to really become one of the "poor, deluded souls." The makers of flour bleached with poisonous bug-killing chemicals are advertising a product unfit for food. No flour miller I have met eats the stuff himself. Drop in any mill and ask the superintendent about it. Read the answers to the questionnaire sent out in 1906 by Ladd and Stallings to the millers. Even in those days they admitted it was a dishonest fraud, long before the facts were known about its poisonous effect on dogs and other animals.

These bleached flour makers know their business would be difficult to carry on in competition with small local mills if they did not use bug-killing bleach. Why is its use continued in spite of the law? Why is the law not rigidly enforced? Their attitude is well expressed by the writer of the history of the Washburn-Crosby Co., in the book *The Medal of Gold* (William D. Edgar, The Bellman Co., Minneapolis, 1925 p. 40):

> "Those who mourn for old process flour, as for the unattainable, and lament the lack in modern flour of the old, 'nutty flavor,' may find consolation in the knowledge that this delectable flavor was not imparted by the method of grinding, but by the crease dirt adhering to the wheat from the field in which it was grown and not removed by the old process. They can easily secure the long-lost flavor which they crave by simply mixing a small quantity of ordinary earth, well powdered, with the beautiful wholesome white flour they find on the market. Street dust would answer the purpose admirably, and probably add somewhat to the nuttiness they yearn for, or think they do."

Commercial "whole wheat flour" is far worse than the white. It is so much more saturated with bleach poison to block bug infestation that test animals die far quicker on whole wheat bread than on white.[7] That is why most of us shudder at the idea of eating commercial "sawdust" flavored bread. Certainly our sense of taste warns us of the unfitness of this "food."

Few people are aware that there is much evidence pointing to the conclusion that predisposition to cancer may follow the use of improper and devitalized foods. Dr. Davidson of Winnipeg proved that with animal tests years ago. His work was ridiculed and suppressed. Canadian government officials refused to permit any public money to be used to check further into his claims, or to continue his investigations. Dr. Daniel Quigley of Omaha, a veteran cancer surgeon and author of *The Conquest of Cancer by Radium & Other Methods,* D. A. Davis Co., 1929, stated in a lecture at Los Angeles two years ago that he had never observed a recurrence of cancer in patients who avoided devitalized foods, after elimination by surgery or radiation, in his thirty-odd years of practice.

We know that people who have no access to the devitalized foods of civilized man have little cancer. Dr. Weston A. Price, in his book *Nutrition and Physical Degeneration.* tells us of many cases where cancer soon appeared after the introduction of white flour and while sugar into territories where these food products had been unknown.

Dr. Duncan Bulkley, the author of another book on cancer, (*End Results of the Medical Treatment of Cancer,* 1928), and founder of the New York Skin & Cancer Hospital, considered wrong diet the cause of cancer and improved diet a most important part of the treatment. As a result of these views, it appears, he was boycotted into bankruptcy.

Other cancer specialists can be cited who have been boycotted because of their frankness in blaming bad food for their patients' plight. Remember, a cancer specialist gets his patients only by reference from other general practitioners. If the A.M.A. were to order a boycott, who would know? We do know that Fishbein's man Friday made a deal with the flour millers in 1925 to help protect their business, to propagandize both the doctors and the public in favor of white bread .[14] Some terribly malign influence is obviously blocking progress towards any intelligent investigation of the nutritional deficiencies that may predispose cancer. Dr. Davidson of Winnipeg was ridiculed as another deluded soul when he asked for government money to further investigate the nutritional cause of cancer, after he proved that mice could be made susceptible to cancer by a poor diet, and again made immune by improving the diet.[15] Millions of dollars are available to discover a fancy synthetic drug to cure disease, but not a cent to really locate the cause if it happens to be poisoned bread, poisoned meat, synthetic sugar or counterfeit butter, or other devitalized foods.

Organized medical "science" is a political and not a truly scientific activity. Behind the front, that is set up to conceal the real political apparatus for the operation of the curious commercial promotions that represent the moving power of medicine, are many different but cooperating interests.

Dr. W. R. Hadwen in the preface to his book, *The Difficulties of Dr. Deguerre*, well expresses the situation thusly:

> "No medical man during his student days is taught to think. He is expected to assimilate the thoughts of others and to bow to authority. Throughout the whole of his medical career he must accept the current medical fashions of the day or suffer the loss of prestige and place. No public appointments, no coveted preferments are open to the medical man who declines to parrot the popular shibboleths of his profession. His qualifications may be beyond reproach; he may in himself possess qualities that command respect, but unless prepared to think and act within the narrow circle of accepted dogmas, he must be prepared for a more or less isolated path.
>
> "The public press of today is largely governed by the orthodox rulers in the medical profession. The ubiquitous 'Medical Correspondent,' who draws his inspiration from the pages of current fashionable medical literature, is expected to supply only such copy as will gratify the tastes of the mysterious power that stands supreme behind the editorial chair. The views of the unorthodox are with rare exceptions refused. So rigid is the control which medical orthodoxy seeks to exercise over the public mind, that not a word upon health matters, however important and interesting, is even allowed to be broadcast by wireless unless it is approved and sanctioned by the bureaucrats of the Health Ministry.
>
> "Every now and then some new medical 'discovery' is proclaimed with clamorous voice. The public eye is arrested by commanding headlines in the leading organs of the public press. The simultaneousness of their appearance and the similarity of the announcements leave no doubt as to how the whole scheme has been engineered. It may be a new cancer germ discovery; a new serum, vaccine or chemical inoculation; a new theory concerning some old-fashioned disease or an old-fashioned disease dressed up in a new garb; a new outcry against flies, fleas, lice, cockroaches, dogs, cats, parrots, rats, or goats; but, upon reflection, it will always be found that these notorious 'discoveries' are entirely devoid of originality.
>
> "It is safe to say that, among all these flaming pronouncements, no real discovery has been made during the last half century, at least; no original medical idea has been promulgated; no permanent contribution to medical science has been furnished; no advancement in medicine achieved. The public press has been utilized for the propagation of little else than medical sensationalism, proved to be such in time; by clinical and statistical experience. While it is not to be denied that these sensational reports make interesting journalism, the time cannot be far distant when all who have not very short memories will read them with skepticism."

This was written in 1918. There is little change up to today. The sulfa drugs, so highly publicized, have been found toxic, and are now known to be effective simply by their effect of mobilization of vitamin C into the blood from the tissue reserves. Few victims of sulfa poisoning escape serious kidney damage. The use of the real agent, vitamin C complex, is still too simple and natural a proposition to accept. Even penicillin is now suspected because it sensitizes the patient and a new shot may be causative of anaphylactic shock. Too, the germs soon become immune to it.

Streptomycin no sooner was announced with great fanfare as a new answer to the problem than it was found to destroy the innervation to the semilunar balancing mechanism of the inner ear, rendering the victim as badly symptomatic of syphilis in the tertiary stage as any victim of this disease was ever able to demonstrate. Cortisone, the newest wonder drug, intended to supply synthetically an adrenal hormone to substitute for the loss of function of the patient's own glands that have been starved out of commission by devitalized foods, has already reported to have caused kidney stones, mental derangements and diabetes if used for any length of time.

Medical "Science," censored as it is, keeps these facts pretty well hidden from the public eye. A continual array of new and phony remedies are paraded before the public, each announced with all the new releases so characteristic. After the public has bought and poisoned itself with millions of dollars worth, it is found wanting, and soon is relegated to the limbo of forgotten things. Viosterol, one great phony promotion, poisoned uncounted numbers of children, (See *Jol. of the A.M.A.* "Vitamin D Intoxication with Metastic Calcification," Bauer & Freyburg, 130:1208, April 27, 1946) before it blew up in a cloud of litigation dust.

Are we probably here witnessing the crumbling of our civilization by reason of the compromise with principle that is being made by the guilty parties in government and business who have so thoroughly sold the public health down the river? "Just a *little* poison in the flour — Nitrates in meat never hurt anybody — Aluminum toxic? Are you crazy?"

This is one simple concrete example of how it works. We could cite innumerable others.


1 *Annual Rev. Biochem.,* 1943, p. 381.
2 *Arch. Path,* Adamatone, F. B., 31:711-16, (194 1).
3 *Protomorphology,* p. 279.
4 *J. Urol.*, Herbst & Bagley, 59:595 (April, 1948).
5 *Protomorphology,* "The Principles of Cell Auto-Regulation," Lee & Lianson.
6 *Annals, New York Academy of Sciences,* Vol. 52, Art. 3, p. 258. (Guilieson, 'Reproduction in Dairy Cattle')
7 *Newsletter of American Academy of Applied Nutrition*, pg. 30-31 Jan, Feb, Mar., 1949.
8 *Sodium Silicate in Arteriosclerosis,* Kuhn, Mench. Med. Woch., Dec. 16,1921.
9 *Chemical Abstracts,* 32,22:9330, Nov. 20, 1839, M. Bauer.
10 *Aluminum Compounds in Foods*, E. E. Smith, Paul Hoeber 1928,pg.294.
11 *The Nature & Properties of Soils,* Lyon & Beckman, 4th Ed. Macmillan, pg. 301.
12 *FTC News Release,* April 21, 1939, announcing that Martin W. Pretorius had agreed (under threat of prosecution) to cease representation that aluminum compounds were poisonous in food.
13 *A.A.A.N. Newsletter*, pg. 3-4, September, 1948.
14 *Baking Technology,* January, 1925
15 Davidson's *Cancer A Nutritional Deficiency.*
16. *Jol. of A.M.A.*, "Vitamin D Intoxication with Metastatic Calcification," Bauer-Freyburg, 130:1208, April 27, 1946.

# NOTES

VITAMIN NEWS

VITAMIN PRODUCTS CO. • MILWAUKEE, WISCONSIN

VOL. 16

# POISONED FOODS, PINK TOOTHBRUSH, FEEDING THE BABY

Are nitrate fertilizers dangerous? Yes, the State of Minnesota Health Department reports 139 cases of infant poisoning in 2 1/2 years from nitrate salts in well water, used in making up the baby formula. The nitrates got into the well from fertilizers used on land from which the well water drained. There were 14 deaths attributed to the poison. (*Jol. A.M.A.* June 3, 1950, p. 476.)

Babies are most susceptible to nitrate poisoning during the first two months of life. The nitrates are harmful because they are reduced to nitrites by the body metabolism. Both nitrates and nitrites are commonly used to keep unrefrigerated meat products from discoloring, (ham, sausage, etc.)

Nitrites and nitrates are old stuff in flour bleaches, too. After we have been told that flour bleaches only hurt dogs, that were unfortunate enough to develop "fits" that were often fatal if fed a little white bread, we now discover the reason the toxic reactions were not well defined in the human family. Few two month old babies are fed bread or crackers, so we haven't had the "corpus delicti" so important as legal evidence.

All this adds up to the soundness of the policy "permit no addition of poison, no matter how small, in foods." The present fad of adding fluorine to drinking water to protect us against tooth decay is a similar fallacy. A quack remedy to offset the damage of too much demineralized sugar, flour and soft drinks, candy, etc. A Texas research group has now discovered that cancer seems to be induced by fluorine salts, so the campaign to put fluorine in the water is grinding to a sudden stop.

Do you have pink toothbrush?" If so, you will be interested to find that a vitamin product is now available that stops this type of subclinical scurvy in a hurry. Two tablets of our Rutaplex A, taken at night, will show improvement the next morning in most cases, with a complete disappearance of the tendency in a few days. (Our regular Rutaplex is not the proper thing for this unless you also wish to take the anti-cholesterol fractions from the buckwheat meal — the same factors that make the rice diet a remedy for hypertension.* (Only with Rutaplex you need not take a peck of rice to get ten grains of the active principle.) The Rutaplex A is the dehydrated green leaf juice alone. There is no known contraindication we know of this form of vitamin C complex. Its rutin content is negligible, we feel rutin is a poor form of vitamin P, far less effective than its synergists in the green juice.

The hemorrhagic conditions in ulcerative colitis call for this Rutaplex A, the deficiency of vitamins P and K are now considered a major factor in the etiology of this disease.[1]

It is just a matter of time when every dentist in the country will routinely prescribe Rutaplex A for "pink toothbrush." It is the first time that such a product has been available; every dentist needs to hear about this right now.

Bleeding gums have long been called subclinical scurvy, but the use of ascorbic acid as a remedy failed dismally and completely,[2] in an official test in England on 2,962 cases of men in the R.A.F. Just why it is possible to rate ascorbic acid as a form of vitamin C when it is only a single factor of a biochemical complex is one of the century's mysteries.

The failure of ascorbic acid to relieve gingival hemorrhage has led many dentists to think that it is not a deficiency reaction. It is quite probable that the pus pockets that precede pyorrhea and the loss of sound teeth is only possible by reason of the gingival degeneration beginning as hemorrhage. The ultimate loss of teeth and their preliminary loosening are hastened by calcium deficiency, and there the major factor now seems to be the failure of cooked foods to supply the enzyme phosphatase. Even milk is pasteurized, the effectiveness of pasteurization being commonly measured by the completeness of destruction of milk phosphatase.

Common sources of phosphatase other than milk are raw bran, raw potato, raw bone marrow, all foods not commonly met within civilized circles. That is why tooth decay and pyorrhea follow civilized foods, the refined, pasteurized, and counterfeited stuff we eat instead of honest but perishable staples we once subsisted upon.

The book, *Vitamins in Medicine*, cites three cases of Pacific Islands where the establishment of steamship schedules made civilized foods available with the immediate deterioration of the near perfect teeth of the natives within a very few years.[4] Still our makers of soft drinks, white flour products and candy containing glucose jump on any dentist who warns his patient to avoid such foods, and threaten him with statements that "there is no scientific proof that refined foods cause dental disease." Just as the flour millers seem to be successful in keeping the average physician from learning that his patients drop dead from the vitamin E deficiency created by white flour. (Of 28 cattle put on an E-deficient diet, 13 dropped dead from the effects of 12 months of the deficiency ration.) (Reported in the *Annals of the New York Academy of Sciences,* 1949, p. 256 — note that this is *not* a medical journal.)

Do not forget that of the sugars, lactose aids calcium assimilation; cane sugar neither aids nor blocks calcium assimilation; while glucose, the one synthetic sugar actually blocks calcium assimilation.[5] Do not permit your baby to have its pasteurized milk sugared with glucose. Use only lactose made from milk.

To supply the tooth and bone-building elements in their most assimilable form, we make Biost, a dehydrated raw veal bone with cereal germ flour to absorb the marrow fat. (Each 12-ounce jar contains 6 ounces of raw bone.) It carries an ample amount of phosphatase, as well as the amino acids (tryptophane and lysine) commonly destroyed in cooking. Clinically, it is just as important to the edentulous patient as to the one who still has his teeth, for it toughens tremendously the supporting membranes in a few weeks if used at relatively small doses. All cooked bone products of the past have been colossal failures to actually build bone or teeth. Biost may be used in baby feeding at any age, suspended in milk, ½ teaspoonful per day. It is ball-milled to the finest powder and has a very attractive flavor. The X-ray shows regeneration of bone in the patient with bone resorption within two to three weeks, so you need not take our word for its effect, or that of he patient either. Loose teeth often tighten up, abscessed areas recalcify.

## REFERENCES

[1] "Postulating A New Concept of the Etiology, Pathology & Treatment of Chronic Idiopathic Ulcerative Colitis — Is It a Hemorrhagic Disease Caused by Multiple Nutritional Imbalances?" N. Phillip Norman, 1951.

[2] *Journal of A.M.A.*, 126:437, 1944.

[3] *The Importance of Food Enzymes in Promoting Mineral Assimilation*, Royal Lee, 1950

[4] *Vitamins in Medicine,* Drs. Bicknell and Prescott, p. 688.

[5] *Vitamins in Medicine,* Drs. Bicknell and Prescott, p. 641.

*These factors include inositol, phosphatase and the products released by phosphatase–phosphates of magnesium and calcium — protective colloids, and water soluble fractions of the vitamin B complex.

THE STATEMENTS HEREIN MAY NOT AGREE WITH CURRENTLY ACCEPTED MEDICAL OPINION. NEVERTHELESS, THE PUBLISHER BELIEVES THEM SOUND.

**Edited by Royal Lee** **July 1951**

# NOTES

VITAMIN NEWS

VITAMIN PRODUCTS CO. • MILWAUKEE, WISCONSIN

# DENTAL DISEASE,

# PROPAGANDA AND FOOD

VOL. 16

Sometimes we wonder if there is a deliberate plan to keep the medical and dental professions ignorant of the latest knowledge in etiology and treatment, where some business interests are likely to be disturbed by the facts. The immediate cause of my comment is the perusal of the latest *Merck Manual*, a 1500-page reference work for the physician. This eighth edition, just out, contains this remarkable misstatement: "Systemic conditions play an insignificant role in caries formation ... The saying 'for every child a tooth' no longer is tenable, apparently once the permanent teeth are fully formed they are little influenced by the nutritional state or the calcium demands of the body."

What monumental and colossal misinformation. Dr. Harold Hawkins in his book *Applied Nutrition*, shows conclusively how caries cannot occur in a patient who has the proper blood ratio of calcium and phosphorus, which is an exact reflection of his food chemistry.

Of all comments that have no foundation in fact, the one denying that formed teeth are immune to later influences is a prize example. Every physician has seen with his own eyes the rapid destruction of the sound and filled teeth of the pregnant and malnourished mother. How does it take place? Simply by acid destruction, the hydrochloric acid of the regurgitated stomach contents in the nausea of pregnancy very soon destroys teeth, loosens fillings and renders sound teeth sensitive by reason of the porosity produced by the acid. The drinking of hydrochloric acid often prescribed for achlorhydric patients is just as destructive, unless carefully taken through a straw, as every doctor knows.

Getting more diffusible calcium into the saliva by the use of calcium lactate and vitamin F is just as practical in restoring damage to teeth that has not progressed too far, as well as in recalcifing chalky teeth in children. In a few weeks the chalky appearance is changed into the normal translucent hard form of enamel, if the proper biochemical conditions are created.

The hyperemesis of pregnancy is purely a reaction to starvation, the specific form of starvation that follows the use of foods that are "made worse so that they can be sold for less." It promptly ceases in the vast majority of cases where a natural concentrate of multiple vitamins is used to supplement the white flour and refined sugar products that represent 60% of the average starvation diet in this strange country of sick and prosperous people who can buy automobiles enough to all go pleasure riding at the same time, but cannot afford to eat food that will protect their bodies from dissolution.

The state of mind being the result of cheapening the basic foods to where the makers of good products cannot make most people believe that is it necessary to pay twice as much for a food that is infinitely better — infinite being the term to use where one product inevitably brings death and disease, the other life and health.

The propagandists are even politically powerful enough to promote laws stopping the use of the term "health food," as it creates the true impression that the "health food" is better in building health and life.

Bleached flour, refined sugar, synthetic glucose or counterfeit fats could not possibly be legitimately marketed as foods without corruption, dishonesty and compromise at the sources of law making and law enforcement.

To get the calcium-phosphorus balance restored to the normal ratio, the hog feeder uses alfalfa meal with its alkaline ash and high potassium content in his feed to offset the acid ash and the high phosphorus of the grain or cereal part of the ration. (Potassium lowers the blood phosphorus; it leaves the body only as phosphate.) (Hawkins, p. 112) To fail to add the alfalfa may cut in half the rate of bone and tooth development and stunt the animal with corresponding loss of profit to the hog feeder. So he is far more accurately informed as to the facts than the august authorities who concoct the information in the Merck Manual.

If anyone needed proof that better food will immunize us to dental caries, we can refer him to the practical experience of such men as Dr. Fred Miller of Altoona, Pa., who has put his dental patients on such diets as to create perfect tooth structures at will. He simply eliminated all processed and refined foods from the schedules.

The *Merck Manual* goes further to say that the use of fluorine added to the drinking water (1 part per million) "in the early years of tooth formation appears to be an effective weapon in preventing the future development of caries." Here is another odd statement. Our best authorities say that such a procedure is still in the experimental stage. Further, what is fluorine but an attempt to treat a deficiency disease, a form of starvation with a poisonous drug? Such ignorant practices are common to our propaganda-guided healing professions. I again recall the definition of a medical education by a top dentist who was once president of the American Dental Association: "The warping of unsuspecting immature minds into a meticulous system of commercial superstition."

We are here dealing with a cult that makes its converts fanatics who cannot see or appraise any other idea than the one they have been inoculated with. Of all healing cults that have fastened their vicious tentacles upon the minds of men, the poison is the most horrible. It is positively malignant in its nature. Remedies for disease are defined "as of necessity poisons." To try to prevent a result of malnutrition by introducing poisons into drinking water is an exhibition of insanity, to our way of thinking.

To say that fluorine compounds are found in foods is no argument. Arsenic is a trace mineral food element too, so is cobalt, so is barium, chromium, zinc and copper. But they must be present in nutritional forms, in organic combinations, forms that have already gone through cell life otherwise they are deadly poisons. We as well as all animals must depend upon plant synthesis of foodstuffs for our existence. We tear apart the organic foods that they put together, return them to the earth in degraded forms for resynthesis into food, resytnhesis into plant cells, often assisted by microbic subcontractors in the soil

The followers of this poison cult get incurably fixed in the obsession that the physical integrity of the human body has no relationship to the materials supplied it as food. They declare that cancer has no relation to nutrition; in fact, some insist that malnutrition has no relation to disease at all. (Sworn statement of Dr. Elmer Nelson of the Federal Food & Drug Administration.)

With such warped minds supplying the entire medical and dental professions with "authoritative" textbooks, what hope is there for survival of the race? I have here a new textbook on "Human Biochemistry" by Israel S. Kleiner, PH.D (Mosby) 1951. On page 443 is a reiteration of the comment that there is no truth in "a tooth for every child," and that tooth structure cannot be recalcified once it becomes porous. And, on page 618, "saliva has no bactericidal power." Certainly, normal saliva controls bacterial activity, as do the secretions of all tissues. We have here the age-old obsession that bacterial causes are responsible for disease, not malnutrition that weakens the body and lets in the bacteria. Lowered resistance from malnutrition MUST in time be accepted as the basic cause of disease instead of the accidental encountering of swarms of bacteria — although that cause is not to be underrated once it is well established, like a forest fire that is a result of dry weather once started will burn pretty damp trees. Lowered resistance of the entire population sets the stage for successful invasion by microbes, viruses, etc.

We have before us a very recent review of periodontal disease, published by a large drug house. They fail to list any nutritional cause, or even to discuss the possibility except to say "soft foods ... favor calculus formation."

Now gingivitis we can say is vitamin P deficiency. Bleeding tendencies can usually be controlled in a day or two by the use of two tablets a day of the simple dehydrated juice of green buckwheat in tablet form. It seems to be just as specific as any good form of vitamin C in scurvy. Ascorbic acid, or course, has dismally failed to have curative effects on the hemorrhagic aspects of either scurvy or gingivitis.

Most dentists agree that with no gingivitis, no pyorrhea will develop. But an added factor aggravates the bone disease once it's established, that is the lack of the amino acids, enzymes and minerals found in raw bone. (Cooked bone is as useless to supply calcium as cooked or pasteurized milk. Remember that test animals lose their teeth very quickly on pasteurized milk by pyorrhea that ensues.)

Raw bone in flour form is now available.[3] It is just a stone age food that affords the same protection to the integrity of bone and the tooth-supporting structure as a stone age diet of bone reduced to a pulp under a stone hammer.

As a very good insight into the mental processes of the makers of unfit foods, the fellows we think are responsible for the biased "scientific opinions" here exposed, we cite the words of one of their legal counsel in *Food, Drug & Cosmetic Law Journal,* Oct. 1951, page 781: "We must not confuse the preachments of (nutritional quacks and industry baiters) with expressions of honest differences of opinion among honest men with a common objective" ... a word of caution is in order. The propaganda, which needs to be combated, cannot be successfully met by a campaign of outclaiming the fakers ... prudence dictates that a skunk be dispatched rather than engaged in contest." This from the flour millers' legal front man. Remember those millers themselves said in answer to a bunch of questionnaires that flour bleaching was a "fraud, a cheat, an abomination, a deceit, a method to sell low grade flour as a product of the finest wheat," that 99 in 100 millers were sorry that the process was ever invented?

That is the "honest men" that would cooperate with the "quacks," to advance the interests of the milling industry if they were not "skunks" to be dispatched. In order to prosecute competitors of these makers of "death foods" — the makers of "health foods" — the government has stretched the constitutional limitations far beyond the breaking point. We further quote from the same journal: "Such legislation dispenses with the conventional requirement for criminal conduct — awareness of some wrongdoing. In the interests of the larger good, it puts the burden of acting at hazard upon a person otherwise innocent but standing in responsible relation to a public danger." (Page 756) This really means that to insure the best interests of the public, the constitutional principle that an act can only be criminal when the offender is aware of the harm he is causing must be suspended.

At the same time, the makers of bleached flour are going scott-free while knowing that they are criminals and admitting to it. What a frightful perversion of law. Their competitors can be framed very easily with this constitutional protection removed. I can recall several cases, one where a conviction was obtained by the connivance of a federal judge who actually refused to permit the accused to know what his crime was until he got into court. Then after getting a conviction from a bamboozled jury, to block a successful appeal to a higher court the Federal prosecutor brazenly got away with claiming that the defendant's chief witness said the opposite of what he really did in his argument to the appeal court, the transcript apparently having been tampered with to permit this stunt. The whole thing was so cleverly covered up that it was ten years before it was noticed. The Food & Drug Administration have publicly stated that they intend to put all "health food" sellers out of business. That would leave only "death foods" like bleached flour for us to eat.

These fellows have so manipulated the law (or somebody else with parallel objectives) that it is impossible for an honest man to get a fair shake in any food and drug litigation today. It is a serious offense, punishable by a ten thousand dollar fine, to claim that a synthetic food is inferior to a natural product, according to Federal Trade Commission orders. And, no court has jurisdiction to review the justice of this edict. It is as despotic as any of Hitler's pronouncements.

A fine specimen of propaganda by commercial fertilizer interests appeared in September *Country Gentlemen.* Dr. R. I. Throckmorton of Kansas State College hysterically attacked organic principles of farming. One statement he made was that "the belief that commercial fertilizers are poison is ridiculous." Had he not read in the *Journal of the A.M.A.* (June 3, 1950, page 476) about the 14 infants who died in Minnesota by getting in their milk formula a few parts per million of nitrate chemicals that leached into wells from field soils? With 130 more who were poisoned and ill enough to instigate an investigation and a correct diagnosis?

Ammonium nitrate, after leaching into a well can be fatal to a baby in dilutions of one part in a million. Such a poison should be well enough publicized as to be known to a Dean of a College of Agriculture like Dr. Throckmorton unless he is not a dean at all — just a figurehead and front man for the Poison Cult and their partners the chemical fertilizer interests. The *Country Gentlemen* needs also to look to its own gullibility in taking in such a piece of propaganda and offering it as honest information for its readers. Let us have the scientific facts — and let us expose the deliberate racketeers who have no conscience. If we treat them like gentlemen, they will continue to rob us behind our backs of our health and life. They will continue to poison not only our wells and foods but also our sources of information like *The Country Gentlemen.*

Why has no university yet set up experiments to ascertain what merit, if any, the organic agriculture idea might have? I will tell you. It is too hard to suppress the possible adverse findings on commonly used fertilizers that would embarrass the chemical industry. Just as we have shown that no honest effort is being made to find what, if any, relation there may be between malnutrition and cancer, malnutrition and polio, etc. Millions of dollars are being spent upon frivolous and irrelevant, fundamentally unsound projects such as trying to find a poison cure for those diseases that are really forms of starvation.

Somebody is sifting these projects and blue-penciling the only ones that would find a remedy unless I am an imbecile. Of 63 projects listed in *Public Health Report* of June 1951 of the Federal Security Agency for cancer research, each calling for up to a million dollars, none were looking into possible causes that relate to malnutrition.

That state of affairs cannot be a coincidence. Neither can Dr. Throckmorton's tirade in *The Country Gentlemen.* If so, I would say "about as much of a coincidence as for a bunch of monkeys jumping on typewriters to write the *Encyclopedia Brittanica.*"

The comments in this issue are of special interest at the present time in view of the propaganda articles appearing this month (December, 1951) in the *American Magazine* and the *Woman's Home Companion.* These articles tell us that the American people are the best fed in history and that we need not worry about deficiency, disease, even while 750,000 persons a year are dying from heart disease, which is due to refined devitalized and adulterated food products (mainly bleached flour that has been deliberately deprived of its oxidizable vitamins by the chemicals added to deceive the buyer into thinking that it is of higher quality than it really is. Most wheat makes a gray flour).

More of the campaign against *health* food as distinguished from *death* food.

THE STATEMENTS HEREIN MAY NOT AGREE WITH CURRENTLY ACCEPTED MEDICAL OPINION. NEVERTHELESS, THE PUBLISHER BELIEVES THEM SOUND.

**Edited by Royal Lee** **December 1951**

# NOTES

VITAMIN NEWS
VITAMIN PRODUCTS CO. • MILWAUKEE, WISCONSIN

VOL. 17

## THIS FLOURINE FREE-FOR-ALL ...

## LOOSE TALK BY PROFESSED AUTHORITIES

The editor of the *Journal of the American Dental Association* in the April (1952) issue gets somewhat hysterical in his support of fluoridation of water, and tells us that since the program has been endorsed by all the political organizations that commonly substitute the "consensus of opinion" for the real facts whenever necessary to promote the sale of counterfeit and foodless "death foods," we should unquestioningly accept the matter as settled.

The facts up to date on fluorine are available in the *Congressional Record,* remarks of Hon. A. L. Miller. Note that in Grand Rapids, Michigan, the statistics show that after water fluoridation the deaths from heart disease doubled, the deaths from nephritis increased 50 percent and deaths from "intracranial lesions" (cerebral hemorrhage) increased 50 percent. That is the reaction of the synthetic forms of flourine used to adulterate the water, I would conclude. Natural fluorine does not do these things, as is well known.

The editor of this journal uses the typical communist tactic of personal smear in trying to discredit the motives of the opposition, apparently because he cannot meet the issue on its merits. As to the real facts in the government prosecution of myself and the Vitamin Products Co., the date of citation was 1940, not 1950, an intentional "error" (?) and the diseases that were at that time considered by the "consensus of opinion" as not due to nutritional deficiency by the august authorities marshaled by the government and for which the fine was assessed, are now in almost every list of deficiency diseases in the literature of every firm that sells vitamins. My offense was being the first to announce them. The government owes me a sincere apology and about $100,000 damages, neither of which I ever expect to get. In fact, the *1939 Department of Agriculture Yearbook* completely vindicated my statements, but it was not printed at the time of the trial, (Jan. 1939).

The dentists might do a little investigating to learn just how and why their organization is being used for such criminal purposes as promoting water adulteration, and the support of the "death food" industries, the smearing of opposition, and the propagandizing of themselves to the effect that "there is no scientific evidence to prove that dental disease is a result of malnutrition." This last is the prize lie to be promoted. It of course protects the candy industry, the soft drink industry, the white flour industry and the synthetic glucose industry. Dr. Weston A. Price and Dr. Harold Hawkins in their books, *Nutrition and Physical Degeneration* and *Applied Nutrition,* demonstrated beyond all reasonable doubt that all dental disease was due to bad food, and exactly how and why. But it is worth millions of dollars per year to the food racketeers to smear them and hide the fact. No dental college in this country has the power, the privilege or the guts to tell the truth on this subject. As I see it, the faculties of these institutions have to parrot lies to hold their jobs. And, any individual dentist who tries to tell the truth is smeared and squeezed by the politicians in charge of the profession, according to my observations.

## HOW COME THIS OVERWEIGHT STUFF?

Too many of us are having a constant battle with ourselves to avoid overweight. We know that overweight is a bad thing, a life-shortening matter, that life insurance rates should be higher for fat people. We know that overweight undermines our health, undermines our efficiency, undermines our happiness. Doctors tell us that it is just a matter of calories, that if we eat less we will stop gaining and reduce. They tell us that glandular imbalances have little to do with overweight, that the use of thyroid substance is dangerous, that only one in a thousand can reduce under thyroid treatment.

All that is half true. There is a remarkable misunderstanding about thyroid; those who are deficient may be dwarfed; children who fail to grow may be often stimulated to develop normally if fed a little thyroid. It has little to do with our state of obesity. But there are other glands that have a terrific lot to do with fat metabolism. Did you ever hear about the custom of castration to promote fat development in meat animals? Either sex develops uncontrollable tendencies to get fat if their sex glands were removed or damaged. A spayed dog becomes fat and lazy if overfed. Feed a healthy bull all you want, and you cannot fatten him for beef, he remains muscular and full of fight.

What has this to do with us? Well, it has a great deal to do. Recent discoveries tend to establish the thesis that our sex glands depend upon unrefined cereals for vitamins and precursors of sex hormones.

Precursors of both female and male sex hormones are now known to definitely exist in wheat germ oil.[1] Probably all sources of the vitamin E complex carry some of this activity. (None will be found in refined wheat germ oil, nor in the synthetic imitations of vitamin E commonly sold as the real vitamin.) Certainly, the use of foods that have been refined to the point that none of the vitamin E complex remains, can possibly support the normal function of the sex glands. The victim of such foods will gradually become castrated as efficiently as if the result were accomplished surgically. It will be just a matter of time. The first thing he or she will notice, in all probability, will be a tendency to accumulate fat. Remember, any farmer will tell you that you cannot fatten a bull by feeding him lots of calories. (In spite of the fact that man has carefully selected his breeding animals for their ability to reflect as fat in the most efficient manner all feed that he gives them.) (Wild animals are difficult to fatten by dietary means, as they have not been so selected for the development of this characteristic.)

Therefore, to defeat this tendency to convert calories to fat, we need to make a careful inventory of foods to identify those that may act as "nutritional castrating agents." That means we must avoid with great aversion all refined foods, all cereals that have been degerminated, all white flour (bleach chemicals destroy remaining traces of all vitamin E complex in white flour, and much, if not all, commercial "whole wheat flour" has been doctored with the same bleach to keep out bugs), so it is essential that you get fresh ground floured bread from such flour where possible. (It is highly significant that Dr. Daniel Quigley of Omaha, the celebrated cancer specialist, tells us that similar precautions are part of his recommendations to patients having cancer operations to prevent recurrence.)

Other than fresh ground cereals, our major source of vitamin E complex is natural fats, butter being at the top of the list, the best butter carrying ten percent as much of this vitamin as wheat germ oil.[2] As butter does not cost over one-tenth as much as wheat germ oil, it is evident that the rest of the butter is free. So you see oleo-margarine cannot possibly ever compete with butter. Oleo never carries any of the vitamin E complexes that we need to protect our sex glands, as far as I can determine. In fact, since it is made by hydrogenating oils to make them solid fats, all traces of vitamins originally in them are lost in the process. The test use of these counterfeit foods (hydrogenated fats and oleo) was found to accomplish exactly the effect I have been discussing; that of wholesale castration.

I refer to the celebrated test reported in the *Journal of the American Medical Association*[3] where test groups of boys and girls were subjected to oleo feeding in comparison to butter, over a period of years. The girls grew more than twice the annual average when fed on oleo; the boys too were taller than normal on oleo. (Castration in humans is always known to increase height.) But the payoff was in the weight figures. The annual average gain for girls on oleo was greater than the gain for boys on oleo, and far more than the normal gains on butter, which had the effect of controlling the weight of both the girls and the boys. (Girls and boys on oleo both increased 2.2 inches in height per year, girls on butter 8 tenths of an inch per year.)[4] (The "experts" who made the above test, however, missed the point. They said oleo produced as much growth as butter.)

Some years ago, a celebrated physician called attention to the effect of refined foods in causing boys and girls to become neutral in sex characteristics, and put up a group of photographs of the body silhouettes of an equal number of boys and girls of adolescent age, at a medical convention, with a ten dollar reward for the doctor who could accurately separate the sexes. He pointed out that the normal wide hips of the girls and broad shoulders of the boys were totally lacking. Is it any wonder that these castrated characters will have a lot of trouble trying to keep down their weight when they reach the age of 30 to 50?

Counterfeit foods make counterfeit bodies. Ask any army man how he likes counterfeit men. Ask any fat woman how she likes to be a counterfeit female. She doesn't, but she has no choice. You who read this do. You will be pleasantly surprised how well Mother Nature can repair the damage if you give her a chance, by giving that body of yours genuine nutrition in place of the counterfeit.

Do not assume that you will be able to get injections of hormones that will repair the damage. Such shots are all right as medical treatments where drug effects are to be accomplished, but to use them in place of nutrition may cause as much of a hullabaloo as the stilbestrol now used to castrate chickens and fatten them quick.

Minks fed such contaminated meat (minced chicken heads) were castrated too, so that their owners collected fat damages from the Federal Department of Agriculture who recommended this cheap source of mink feed. Many a doctor who tried hormone shots on his patients has been dismayed by an effect the reverse of what he intended.

Heavy doses of various vitamins as well as hormones have often been observed to have the opposite effect of smaller doses. That is why we need to be especially cautious in using synthetically prepared vitamins or hormones. Even such supposedly innocent food factors as synthetic thiamin when fed to test animals caused the castration of their offspring, and a cessation of reproduction in the families so fed this dangerous counterfeit vitamin.[4] Double the daily requirement was enough to do the harm.

Dr. Henry C. Sherman of Columbia University found years ago that increased calories from refined foods shortened the life span of test animals. But that increased calories from natural unrefined foods with their increased quantities of vitamins and minerals caused an increased life span.[5] Elvehjem has just reported that the best way to increase susceptibility to cancer in test animals is to reduce their available vitamins and minerals.[6]

These are just circumlocutory ways to say that refined foods are killing us at an early age. These are death food in contradistinction to health foods.

## REFERENCES

1 *Endocrinology* Vol. 49 Sept., 1951 No. 3 P. 289-300
2 *Dairy Council Digest* 21:6 July 1950
3 *Science News Letter* Feb. 14, 1948, Page 108
4 Barnett Sure, *Vol. Of Nutrition* 18, 2:192-193, 1939

5 Henry C. Sherman, *Food & Health,* Macmillan, 1936, Page 200
6 *Cancer Research*, April 1952

THE STATEMENTS HEREIN MAY NOT AGREE WITH CURRENTLY ACCEPTED MEDICAL OPINION.
NEVERTHELESS, THE PUBLISHER BELIEVES THEM SOUND.

VITAMIN NEWS

VITAMIN PRODUCTS CO. • MILWAUKEE, WISCONSIN

VOL. 17

# CLINICAL ACIDOSIS AND ALKALOSIS

The blood pH is supposed to remain "practically constant" according to our best textbooks. The physician who starts to check his patients, however, cannot concur. Instead of the normal figure of pH 7.3 to 7.5 he finds it varying from 7.2 to 7.8.[1]

The measurement of pH is attended with difficulty because blood loses $CO_2$, and thereby rises in pH rapidly after it has been withdrawn. In two minutes, a rise of .2 may occur.[1] Clinical pH meters are available where the electrodes are built into a syringe so the pH may be read directly before the blood is exposed to air. (National Technical Laboratories, Pasadena, California).

The importance of clinical pH tests was illustrated by the following report of a pharmacist. He had been supplying for a number of months a capsule formula of aspirin, caffeine, phenacetin and ammonium chloride to an arthritic patient where the remedy had been successful in controlling arthritic pains. The capsule dispensed was a standard formula of a pharmaceutical house, with a specific catalog number. The patient returned two days after receiving a renewed supply of capsules, complaining that they were ineffective, and different from the previously used kind. On checking the records, it was found that the original formula had been revised, and the supposedly unnecessary ammonium chloride had been omitted. On supplying capsules of ammonium chloride alone, the patient reported the usual successful results.

What was the biochemistry behind this? Simply that a high pH tends to throw calcium out of solution in the body fluids, and bursitis, arthritis, neuritis, lumbago, sciatica, and a host of other painful syndromes develop as a consequence. Cheilosis may occur and herpes simplex, and other virus type diseases become active. The low calcium bicarbonate in the body fluids seems responsible. Vitamins F and D as well as the C complex are also factors, their deficiency aggravates the situation. Allergies become acute; the calcium deficiency aspect of allergic sensitivity is well known. Normal rates of wound-healing are greatly reduced; ulcers tend to become static.

The alkalosis-correcting effect of ammonium chloride is of course due to its decomposition into ammonia and hydrochloric acid in the blood after absorption, where the ammonia becomes urea and the acid is available to reduce the pH. Calcium chloride seems to be a synergist needed; if ammonium chloride is used alone for too long a time calcium demand increases, no doubt by the conversion of other calcium forms in the blood to chloride. If the ammonium chloride is used in tablets or capsules, an equal amount of calcium chloride should accompany it. Five to twenty grains a day of the combined chlorides is the usual range of effective dosage.

Ammonium chloride is a natural constituent of gastric juice, calcium chloride is the form of calcium found in arrowroot starch, so both these materials are physiological therapeutic agents, factors common to body biochemistry and not new and foreign substances to the physiological economy (As are synthetics and antibiotics).

*Merck's Index*, Fourth Edition, says that ammonium chloride is useful in the treatment of bronchial affections, hepatic congestion, pelvic cellulitis, muscular rheumatism, gout, sciatica, chronic glandular enlargement, hemicrania, senile gangrene, dysmenorrhea and leucorrhea.

Calcium chloride is listed as useful in the treatment of hemorrhage, hemorrhagic endometritis, epistaxis, menorrhagia, erythema nodosum, tetanus, spasmophilia, blackwater fever, hay fever, asthma, hemophilia, albuminuria, nephritis, typhoid, coryza, tuberculosis, osteo malicia, scrofula, rachitis, arthritis, spasm of glottis, infant convulsions, urticaria, eczema, pruritis, among others.

All these effects are no doubt in the main simply accomplished by correcting the unbalanced state of the buffers and mineral salts in the tissue fluids. It will be noted that vitamin C complex is a desirable synergist in most of the conditions listed. Gout is mentioned as one situation where ammonium chloride may help. Recently it has been discovered that the juice of cherries contains some active agent effective in gout, 4 to 6 ounces of the juice (preferably unsweetened, but may be the canned or cooked form), promoting relief within a few days with consistent improvement. This is the first time that the possibility of gout being a deficiency disease has been suspected. We can say that the ingestion of sodium compounds — particularly sodium phosphate — is definitely aggravative. Gout patients should see that their diet contains a preponderance of potassium. Sodium promotes the precipitation of the gouty concretions of sodium urate in the tissues.

A very important aspect of alkalosis is the fact that the habitual use of milk of magnesia promotes the condition. It also tends to cause epistaxis, very specifically.

You will be surprised how many of the patients who ask for a remedy for nosebleed are using milk of magnesia as a laxative.

Citrus fruits being of a highly alkaline ash, with a high content of organic acid (citric), need special attention. The first and immediate effect of ingestion of a few ounces of grapefruit or lemon juice is to lower (acidify) the blood pH. The patient with alkalosis feels temporarily better. Later in the day, after the citric acid has been destroyed by oxidation as a fuel (it is classed as a carbohydrate) the aggravation of the alkaline state becomes apparent. The temporary effect of the citric acid is to cause calcium to be picked up, no doubt from some bone reserves — and after the pH change this calcium is deposited elsewhere — in physiologically undesirable spots. The treatment of bursitis obviously becomes simple. No longer can we recommend X-ray treatment with equanimity. Let the physiological treatment be the preferred method.

Guanidine, a fatigue and tissue poison, and end product of the breakdown of creatine (combated by vitamin B Complex which stops the loss of creatine from the tissues), is the most potent organic alkaline substance known. It specifically precipitates calcium (recall our comment that its diffusion from tired heart muscle into coronary vessels is the cause of precipitation therein of calcium), is normally reconverted into creatine by the influence of the parathyroid hormone, and with the assistance of the thyroid.[2] Blood gunaidine levels rise eight fold after parathyroidectomy.[3]

We can see where the guanidine effect as a fatigue poison is contributory to the arthritis, sciatica etc. the patient often telling us how fatigue aggravates his state of misfortune. Local inflammation also can release guanidine, its presence insuring a spastic state of blood vessels, contributing to gangrene, of necessity.

There seems no doubt that the effect of the oxygen metabolizing vitamins — the C and E complexes — is vital in combating these morbid reactions by preventing the degradation of tissue elements into guanidine. Where vitamin E deficiency has caused the tissue demand for oxygen to rise up to 250% of normal,[4] the augmented release of end products certainly includes guanidine, and we see here how the finding of Dr. Shute of London, Ontario, that vitamin E reduces capillary hemorrhage may be rationalized.

A vicious cycle is set up, the more oxygen demand the less supplied, by reason of the constructive effect of guanidine on blood vessels. Degeneration, rupture of capillaries is inevitable. As vitamin C promotes more oxygen supply, that is why it also is good in gangrene (especially the diabetic type) and in "capillary fragility." (The true antifragility vitamin is vitamin P, which provides a special calcium to promote collagen formation.)

Vitamin F opposes the toxic effect of guanidine by providing more of the diffusible calcium (from the colloidal blood reserves) that is precipitated out of the body fluids by guanidine, thereby ameliorating the spastic, nervous and irritative (allergic) reactions.

The thyroid hormone physiologically promotes the resorption and dissolution of protein structures that have reached the end of their physiological cycle (a la the theory of the dynamic state of living tissue, replaced and rebuilt at specific time intervals). That is why in children, thyroid deficiency is the cause of delayed development. In the adult, a hyperactive thyroid may again cause toxicosis by promoting more tissue poisons that the eliminative system can tolerate. In old people, this may be a critical situation, thyroid sometimes becoming a violent poison, only because the normal synergists are not available to maintain the desirable complete cycle of activity. We can see that vitamin F is vital to the prevention of this toxicosis. It tells why the thyroid puts its secretion into the blood after ingestion of vitamin F to the extent of a doubling of the iodine content of the blood.[5] The normal activity of the gland had been blocked by reason of F deficiency. In this blocking, we have apparently the explanation for prostate hypertrophy. Once the thyroid is permitted to secrete, its hormone makes quick work of the fibrous tissue collected in the prostate.

This also explains why we consider the vitamin F complex, and $F_2$ the most friendly vitamins for the older person. The $F_2$ is a more highly developed compound of the basic F (a sensitized fatty acid) in which this fatty acid is combined into a phospholipid molecule that appears to have a specific function of catalyzing protective (insulating) layers in nerve tissue and cell nuclear structures. Thereby protecting the basic controls of metabolic activity. Loss of appetite and wasting disease suggests the possible need for this vitamin. Appetite restoration is immediate where the deficiency exists. (In adults and children alike.)

There seems to be as much clinical acidosis as alkalosis.[1] The effect of acidosis may be aggravated by a diabetic state where organic acids cannot be oxidized normally, instead must be combined with reserve alkaline salts and excreted.[5]

Where sodium bicarbonate is administered to relieve diabetic acidosis, the urine should be watched and dosage stopped when a neutral urine pH is reached, according to this authority. Normally, blood glutamine provides ammonia for this purpose. Beet root and leaf are best vegetable sources of glutamine, which is very high if grown on high ammonia content soils. (Plant cells form glutamine to dispose of excess ammonia).

When an abnormal blood pH is found, it must be considered only as a sign that something is wrong. The symptoms may be entirely different with the same abnormal pH figure in different patients, in view of the fact that there is an infinite number of combinations of chemical situations that could alter pH — as many as there are different acids and alkalies. Just as a plump patient may be bloated with gas, water logged, fat, or hypermuscular, It is a preliminary classification, not a final.

The pH of the blood is a resultant of the forces acting upon it. The regulation of the blood $CO_2$ by the respiration control center of the brain is a major factor. The parathyroid by eliminating the alkaline guanidine, and the kidney, eliminating mineral salts (both acid & alkaline as may be required) no doubt exercises a supplementary control.

The clinical value of vinegar is more or less well known as an alternative of merit. Creatine is a methylguanidine acetic acid, and the regeneration of guanidine into creatine requires acetic acid. In the toxemias of pregnancy, guanidine is a critical factor, vinegar is often craved by the patient, very logically it would seem.

Cider vinegar being the preferred form, no doubt the malic acid of the apple is a factor, calcium malate being a catalyzer of polyphenol detoxification.[6]

**References:**

[1] "The Importance of the Acid Alkali Balance of the Blood" Trans. 1941-42 *AM. Therapeutic Soc.* Pp. 59-66.
[2] *Protomorphology*. Lee & Hanson, P. 213. Lee Foundation 1947.
[3] Robertson. *Principles of Biochemistry*, Lea & Febiger, p. 436. (1924).
[4] Hottchin & Matill, *Jol. Biol. Chem.*, 146:301, 1942.
[5] *Principles of Acidosis,* Sellards. Harvard Univ. Press, 1917.
[6] Robertson, *Principles of Biochemistry,* p. 466.

## VITAMIN G COMPLEX

The first intimation that the vitamin G complex existed occurred when it was found that there was doubt about the identity of the "beriberi curing complex and the growth promoting factor" in foods.[1] (1921). Note that at this early day the word "complex" was used. The growth factors were classed later as the G group of vitamins, and since they were separable by precipitation with alcohol from the beriberi-preventing complex, it was obvious that they were protein in nature. Later the proteins were found to be enzymes, and riboflavin and a dozen or so other flavins split off and identified as essential components, plus the pellagra-preventive groups and the anemia-preventive group.

Where did the idea become extant that a vitamin was a single chemical substance? Only after fractions were synthetically made, and sold with the idea that such fractions were of vitamin value. No natural vitamin has ever been made to my knowledge that was a single synthesizable fraction. It is impossible, even by repeated crystallization, to eliminate accompanying factors that also take part in physiological processes, like the case of natural thiamin which cannot be separated from the $B_4$ fraction which is essential to prevent the nerve paralysis that develops in beriberi along with the polyneuritis.[2]

The original G complex then contained that entire group of B vitamins that were linked with enzyme systems. Today that family has so increased that we find $B_{15}$ the last mentioned of the group, and most of these subdivisions are in their own right COMPLEXES too.

Eddy and Dalldorf in 1937 defined the G complex as including the flavines and the pellagra-preventive factors (the pyridoxine complex and the niacin complex). They also suggested the inclusion of the antidermatitis factor, vitamin H — later called biotin.

So much for the historical side. What we need to know today is how to identify the type of deficiency reaction we must look for to keep our health in this funny world of counterfeit foodstuffs. There are various vitamin G complexes on the market. When you feel the need for one be sure that you get one that is reputed to perform as it should, for the clinical test on human subjects is the only way to be sure that the right factors are present. Each species may need a different kind of some of the vitamin G components, so animal tests are useless in the case of this group of vitamins.[3]

**Symptoms of G Complex deficiency:**

1. Roughness, cracking and exfoliation of skin on soles of the feet.
2. Excessive oiliness of skin of face and nose.
3. Cheilosis (Cracking of skin and lesions at angles of mouth, dry, chapped and fissured lips, soreness and burning of lips, mouth and tongue)
4. Allergic tendencies, probably secondary to pancreas inhibition and reduced ability to digest proteins, permitting such proteins to enter the blood at lesions in bowel. Such lesions, leading to mucous colitis are common, first noted as burning and irritation in rectal area, or as alternations of constipation and diarrhea.
5. Fatigue. No stamina, patient tires easily, may be mentally low, pessimistic, cannot concentrate, "complains of weakness and general discomfort."
6. Sensitivity to sunburn, dermatitis in forms that show symmetrical determination, a result of spinal cord changes that alters skin reactivity in specific areas.
7. Engorged capillaries of cornea of eye. Reddened tongue, with similar engorgement.
8. Susceptibility to lesions secondary to engorged capillaries such as coronary thrombosis, blood sludging, cerebral hemorrhage or thrombosis.
9. Liver disease, cirrhosis and loss of fat metabolizing ability follows lack of the G Complex, thiamin and its synthetic form causes this condition unless accompanied by the natural G Complex factors. First symptoms may be edema (swollen ankles), unbalanced sex hormone status due to failure of the diseased liver to properly eliminate or detoxify estrone or alpha-estradiol [4]
10. Hyper-estrogenic reactions: In the female, menorrhagia, metrorrhagia, cystic mastitis, premenstrual tension, hyperadrenia. In the male, gynecomastia (common among war prisons), hyperadrenia, possible hypertension.

The general effect of G complex deficiency is fatigue, due to capillary engorgement and stagnation. This brings on the tendency to blood sludging[5] and the consequent tendency to form thrombi and the dangers of coronary thrombosis and cerebral thrombosis. It is well to recall that cancer too, has been called the disease of stagnation, it seems to never occur in tissues supplied with normal circulation, unless a local supply of toxins is present. Further, recent animal tests demonstrate that cancer is far more easily created in those animals that get a low vitamin diet than in animals getting natural unrefined foods.[6]

Psoriasis is an old and stubborn ailment that often responds well to the use of the G complex. Allergies too, often disappear in a few weeks under the use of this vitamin group. The liver produces a detoxifying hormone discovered by the Japanese that they called Yakriton[1] which seems to be a physiological anti-histamine. It is probable that this function of the liver is impaired in G complex deficiency.

Without this natural antihistamine, we are more susceptible to colds and hasten to try synthetic substances that have far less effect, and require our attention to something we would never think about if we had not been cheated of the right vitamin content in our food.

As to the synthetic enrichments supposed to take the place of the natural, never accept that smooth argument. Tests made on such synthetic "enrichments" show that their effect is to actually reduce the already low nutritional values of the impoverished product. Test animals died quicker on the "enriched" diet than on the unenriched.[8] The millions of dollars spent advertising such products do not make the claims true. Careful tests on human subjects confirmed the results.[9] One of the strange facts of modern life is how people will believe advertising propaganda at the expense of ten to twenty years off their life span.

Synthetic vitamins may have an important place as drugs. They are of no possible value as foods, according to all available tests; they act to destroy nutritional values instead. Our government should follow the example of Canada, where synthetic products of all kinds are barred from any food use.

[1] *The Vitamine Manual* Walter H. Eddy, Williams & Wilkins , 1921, P. 24
[2] *The Vitamins and Their Clinical Application*, Stepp, Kuhnau & Schroeder, 1938. English translation. Vitamin Products Co. p. 29.
[3] *Vitamin News,* p. 122 (Vitamin Products Co.)
[4] "The Biochemistry of B Vitamins" Williams, Eakin, Beerstecher, *Shive. Am. Chem. Soc*. Monograph 110. 1950. P. 382.
[5] "Sludged Blood" Knisely, Bloch, Eliot, Warner. *Science* Nov. 7, 1947.
[6] *Cancer Research,* Engel, Copeland 12:211-213, 1952
[7] *Tohoku Jol. Exper. Research*, Horiutti. Obsako. 24:505, 1934.
[8] *Science*, Morgan Agnes Fay "The Effect of Imbalance in Filtrate Fraction of B Complex in Dogs," P. 261. March 14, 1941.
[9] *J.A.M.A.,* 125:2, 175, May 13, 1944

---

**The B Vitamins (Nov. 1952)**

$B_1$ Thiamin, (1912)

$B_2$ Riboflavin, (1933)

$B_3$ Pantothenic Acid (1938)

$B_4$ Anti -paralysis factor (Adenyic Acid?) (Cocarboxylase?)

$B_5$ Niacinamide (1934)

$B_6$ Pyridoxin (1934)

$B_7$ Biotin (1935)

$B_8$ Inositol (1928)

$B_9$ Folic acid and paraminobenzoic acid (1945) (Latter acts by promoting synthesis of former).

$B_{10}$ Feathering factor for chickens (Elvehjem) (1944) Unknown composition

$B_{12}$ Organic cobalt (1948)

$B_{13}$ Growth factor. (1948) Unknown composition

$B_{14}$ An anti-anemic factor, essential to cell growth, may interchange with $B_9$. (1949)

$B_{15}$ A universally required cell oxidase (Sajous' Adrenoxidase) Pangamic Acid (1948)

THE STATEMENTS HEREIN MAY NOT AGREE WITH CURRENTLY ACCEPTED MEDICAL OPINION. NEVERTHELESS, THE PUBLISHER BELIEVES THEM SOUND.

**Edited by Royal Lee** **November 1952**

# NOTES

VITAMIN NEWS
VITAMIN PRODUCTS CO. • MILWAUKEE, WISCONSIN

VOL. 17

# VITAMINS IN DENTISTRY

Paper read before Rochester Dental Dispensary Study Club, January 10, 1940

By Royal Lee, DDS

The story of vitamin deficiency is a long one, but a few words on that subject are in order before discussing the specific reactions such deficiencies produce that are of interest to the dentist.

Alfred Hess,[1] physician in charge of the Hebrew Infant Asylum in New York, established the fact back before the World War, that vitamin deficiency definitely was the all-important cause of such conditions as heart disease of various kinds, susceptibility to pneumonia, grippe, nasal diphtheria, furunculosis, otitis, nephritis, adentis[2] as well as the more definite syndromes of deficiency such as scurvy beri-beri, or rickets. Intestinal troubles such as gastritis and constipation were invariably accompaniments of these deficient conditions.

Heart disease and pneumonia alone, the two major causes of death, are almost invariably the end result of years of deficient nutrition. White bread, other white flour products, corn syrup and glucose, white sugar, cold storage foods of all kinds, are present in all of our diets in such a percentage that it is appalling to think of the abuse to which we are subjecting our bodies.

Dr. Weston A. Price[3] was the first dentist to publish an article asserting that dental caries was primarily a result of vitamin deficiency. This was in 1927. In 1923 I had prepared a paper on the subject of "The Systemic Causes of Dental Caries" and read it to the senior class at Marquette Dental College, subscribing to the same hypothesis. I called attention to the findings of Dr. Pollina that in a survey of six thousand school children; the only ones with sound teeth were those children who had not had a history of children's diseases. That showed, I argued at that time, that the real cause for both the incidence of children's disease and the accompanying dental caries was one and the same vitamin deficiency. Dr. Price's findings were completely in accord with that hypothesis.

Dr. Price met with such opposition to his contentions that he decided to take an extended trip around the world and compile such a complete record of the damage wrought by civilized man in his commercial distribution of devitalized foods that his critics would be forever silenced. His book, entitled *Nutrition and Physical Degeneration,* shows beyond any possible doubt the real truth of the matter. He found that in all parts of the globe where the native population had changed from their natural foods to the use of commercial products, there began the infiltration of those dreaded diseases — tuberculosis, pneumonia, and influenza — together with a statistical rise in dental pathology that exactly paralleled the increase in the use of those commercial foods. Caries, pyorrhea, deformities of the dental arch, cleft palate and harelip were all now present where unknown before. It made no difference whether the change took place in a high valley in the Swiss Alps or in an island of the sea in the eastern or western hemisphere. The identically same results followed the introduction of the commercial foods of civilized man.

Vitamin deficiency conditions are not found in uncomplicated syndromes that represent conditions due to the lack of a single vitamin. They are mixtures of conditions in which there are almost invariably several deficiencies operating in conjunction. To catalog these conditions and refer each symptom to a deficiency of some one vitamin has been a difficult matter. We can deprive test animals of one vitamin at a time and observe the reductions, but two things are wrong with that procedure. One is that the different species react somewhat differently to this test, and secondly the action of a partial deficiency acting over a long period of time is unquestionably of a different nature from the effects of a complete dificiency acting over a short period of time. The reactions to deficiency I shall describe can in many instances be reproduced in test animals, but the actual facts have been determined in most cases by treatment of human patients with vitamin concentrates, and a condition observed to be consistently amenable to such treatment has been accepted as a deficiency result.

The basic reaction to vitamin A deficiency is a change in the epithelial tissues.[4] Mucous membrane become sensitive to irritation, and degenerative or metaplastic changes occur. These of course are most rapid where destructive influences require the most rapid repair.

A predisposition to infection of any kind is set up. In the mouth this may mean pyorrhea or Vincent's Infection, with a pale color of the mucous surfaces. The pyorrhea due to A deficiency differs from that in C deficiency in that the teeth remain tight, and there is not the characteristic bleeding.

The B complex[5] is necessary to mouth integrity in that an abnormal redness of the tongue and throat is present usually in pellagra with the changes ranging from simple erythema to a gangrenous necrosis such as heretofore known as "noma."

Vitamin C deficiency[6] primarily causes a degeneration of the intercellular substance of teeth and bone. The bone tissues become decalcified, and loose teeth are the result. If teeth become loose individually because of the end result of a pus pocket, that is not scurvy. But where several teeth are loose without evident infection, it is quite certain to be incipient scurvy. Gingivitis is a more early stage, except where due to infection as a consequence of the epithelial changes of A deficiency. It is obvious that the deficiency of vitamin C is favorable to rapid resorption of the alveolar ridge in edentulous mouths. It is also obvious that deficiency of A will increase the irritability of the mucous surfaces and add to the difficulty of getting a newly fitted set of dentures into satisfactory service.

Vitamin C deficiency is also responsible for a reduction in the germicidal enzymes normally present in the saliva,[7] which adds to the general tendency to infection, not only of pus germs but also of the systemic infective children's diseases. Those same germicidal enzymes protect the teeth against caries, so we have here the reason why Pollina found good teeth only in those children who had never had those children's diseases.

Vitamin D is another factor that cooperates with each of the vitamins so far mentioned, as it supplies the calcium that is essential for the metabolic changes that are regulated and controlled by those vitamins. The germicidal enzymes are inactive in the absence of calcium, and vitamin C cannot maintain the bone integrity without a calcium supply.[8)] The specific function of vitamin D is to increase the affinity of the blood serum for calcium, so that a normal assimilation of that element will take place from the alimentary supply. But another factor is required to unload that calcium again when it arrives at its destination, and that factor is termed by one group of investigators the vitamin F complex. It consists of that group of unsaturated fatty acids of which linolenic, arachidonic and clupanodonic are known to be of biological activity if present in the proper form. vitamin F is found normally associated with vitamin D in its natural sources such as butter or cod liver oil.

If vitamin F is not given with vitamin D, as when a purified concentrate is used, toxic effects can easily be produced. Those effects are purely the effect on excessively high blood calcium. In pregnancy, calcification of the placenta occurs. Nephritis and albuminuria are a common result of reckless administration of vitamin D without its accompanying synergists. I have received reports of cases like this: A nine-year-old boy, dosed heavily by fond parents with a highly concentrated proprietary form of synthetic vitamin D during the winter months, developed kidney inflammation and a severe albuminuria in the spring. The physician, on getting the history of the case, stopped the use of the D and prescribed vitamin F and warned the parents to keep the youngster out of the sun. The parents, distrusting the accuracy of the physician's diagnosis, put the young man out on the beach in a bathing suit the next day to get a "healthy tan." A half-hour of this treatment resulted in a collapse, with fatal consequences.

Cold sores and fever blisters are specific signs of low calcium in the tissue fluids. A vitamin F tablet or two with five grains of calcium lactate will produce a definite recession of the condition in two or three hours. A little vitamin D at this stage will invariably cause a prompt recurrence. It draws the calcium back into the blood stream from the pericellular fluids after the vitamin F has diffused it out. It must be kept in mind that the blood stream does not supply the cells directly. The pericellular fluids must carry the nutritive materials across the gap between the cells and the capillaries. Vitamin D is a "loader-up" of the transportation system of the body, and vitamin F is the onloader.[9] They are directly antagonistic from the viewpoint of the observer who watches only the blood calcium, but to the physiologist who sees the whole picture they are necessarily synergists that act in unison to get calcium to its ultimate designation in the body. It is significant that vitamin F has recently been found in cod liver oil and in butter.

We can see here the logic of trying to obtain a balanced intake of all the vitamins, rather than to overdo the use of any particular one. Systemic diseases, such as children's diseases, fevers, and all infectious processes exhaust the reserves of vitamin C[10] and often rapid degeneration of the dental structures follows such a case history. The requirement of many of the vitamins is subject to great variations so that an intake that is adequate at one time may be quite insufficient at another. The slow convalescence from fevers, pneumonia, etc. is mainly due to the increased requirement which is inadequately supplied at this time in the great majority of cases. If the requirement happens to be greater than the intake for any reason, the patient declines into some fatal outcome as heart involvement, or a new infection made possible by the low resistance. That is why pneumonia so often recurs several times in one winter in the same patient. It is a tragic fact that no patient is known to die until his reserves of vitamin C are completely exhausted. No vitamin C can be found in any of the tissues of a victim of an infectious disease, while it can always be shown by color tests in other cases. The conclusion is obvious. Vitamin C should be invariably used as a part of the treatment in any such case. The reduction in temperature when vitamin C is used is often amazingly rapid. The spread of infection sometimes seen after the extraction of diseased teeth calls for the immediate use of heavy doses of vitamin C. This vitamin seems to stimulate phagocytosis, and aids in the sequestration of the infected area. Hot applications aid in this result, as phagocytosis is also facilitated by heat. The high temperature in infections is, no doubt, the natural reaction of the body to stimulate phagocytosis by this means, and with the added help of the new supply of vitamin C the temperature becomes unnecessary. It is obvious that we have the first physiological remedy for fevers. Another interesting fact is that the white blood cell is higher in vitamin C than any other cell of the body, under normal conditions. The phagocyte seems to be the policeman of the body, and the vitamin C his ammunition. Without it, his digestive enzymes are ineffective against the new enemy.

Vitamin C is the most important of the vitamins, and is the most difficult to get. It is oxidized so easily, that it disappears in storage of citrus fruits and vegetables. Spinach is a good source if fresh, but loses its entire content within a week after it is cut at room temperatures. Potato is one of the good sources, and more reliable than most. In the potato, the C is combined with the protein molecule, which accounts for the statement that potato protein is a valuable nutritious principle. Baking the potato destroys the vitamin the least, boiling loses the most.

Fresh meats contain valuable amounts of vitamin C, but in cold storage it is completely oxidized. Milk is a good source unless pasteurized. Irradiation also destroys the vitamin C in milk.

A combined deficiency of vitamins C, F, and calcium in growing children can result in the condition of chalky teeth. The use of these vitamins with calcium lactate will normalize these teeth in a few weeks. Sometimes there is a phosphorus deficiency too, as characterized by nervous temperament, unruly disposition and restlessness at night while sleeping. This can be corrected by the use of phosphoric acid, glycerophosphates or lecithin.

Calcium phosphate is so insoluble as to be a poor source of that element. The lactate is quite soluble, but as it carries no phosphorus, it can aggravate a deficiency of that element.

Raw milk is, no doubt, the best source of calcium as it carries three times as much as is required by a growing child if used at a quart a day. But pasteurized milk again has lost its calcium and fails to supply enough for maintaining the growth of the infant. Certified raw milk is the only safe form of milk from a nutritional standpoint, because of its higher vitamin C content and higher calcium content.

Back in 1926, McCann wrote a chapter entitled "Iron Men" in his book, *The Science of Keeping Young*.[11] The iron men he referred to were the natives of Finland, which he said was one of the last civilized areas to resist the influx of commercial foodstuffs. He pointed out how in the Olympic games, the Finns were able to perform feats of endurance that astounded the world. They walked off with a hundred times the number of prizes that they would have won if their chances had been even in competition with such greater numbers. We are witnessing today the result of such physical superiority in their phenomenal defense of their country against the Russian invasion. What is the basic diet of the Finnish people? It is whole rye bread, high in vitamins B, E, F, and G and smoked fish, high in vitamins A, D, F and G. Plenty of fruit is available. A war correspondent writes back in January that fresh peaches are served commonly in the public restaurants, a great mystery to him, but evidently from cold storage sources.

There we have the secret of their diet. They get all the required vitamins naturally in their normal and unprocessed state. Compared to us, they are really supermen. Finns arriving in this country are noted for their perfect teeth. Here, however, they are usually unable to retain them. Our terrible food soon sends them to the dentist, who continues to find more and more repairs necessary as time passes. Dr. Price records many instances where caries became inhibited in persons who returned to their native habits, after much damage had been done by devitalized foods. The necrotic progress immediately stopped, and the cavities remained static, thenceforth without developing further, showing the evidence of the renewed production of the protective germicdal enzymes.


[1] Hess, Alfred Fabian, *Collected Writings,* 2 Volumes, Charles C. Thomas, 1928.

[2] Hess, Alfred Fabian, Infantile Scurvy. V. A Study of its Pathogenesis, *Am. Jr. Dis. Child.* November, 1917

[3] Price, Weston A., *Nutrition and Physical Degeneration.* Paul B. Hoeber, Inc. New York 1939.

[4] British Medical Research Council, *Vitamins, A Survey of Present Knowledge*, 1932

[5] Sebrell, W. H., Vitamins in Relations to the Prevention and Treatment of Pellagra. *J.A.M.A.* 110, 20:1665-1672, May 14, 1938. Sydenstricker, Geslin, Templeton and Weaver, Riboflavin Deficiency in Human Subjects, *J. A. M. A.*, 113, 19:1697-1700, November 4, 1939.

[6] Bastedo, Walter Arthur, *Materia Medica Pharmacology, Therapeutics and Prescription Writing*, Fourth Edition, Reset, W.B. Saunders Co. Philadelphia, 1938.

Daldorf, G. The Pathology of Vitamin C Deficiency. *J.A.M.A.* 111, 15:1376-1379, October 8, 1938.

[7] Editorial, Salivary Immunity, *J.A.M.A.*, 108, 15:1264-1265, April 10, 1937.

Cheyne, Virgil D., Effects of Selective Salivary Gland Extirpation Upon Experimental Dental Caries in the Rat., *Proc. Soc. Exper. Biol. Med.* 42, 2:587-590. Nov. 1939.

Pickerill, H.P., T*he Prevention of Dental Caries and Oral Sepsis*, Second Edition, Bailliere, Tindall & Cox, 1914.

[8] Aub, J.C., The Use of Calcium and the Choice of a Calcium Salt, *J. A. M. A.*, 109: 1276 October 16, 1937

[9] Mirvish, *Biochemical Journal*, 24:233-238, 1930.

[10] Abt, A.F. and Farmer C. J., Vitamin C: Pharmacology and Therapeutics, *J. A. M. A.*, 109:1276, October 16, 1937, Martin, G. J., and Heise, F. H., Vitamin C Nutrition in Pulmonary Tuberculosis, *Am J. Dig. Dis. and Nut.*, 4:368-374, 1937.

[11] McCann, Alfred W., *The Science of Keeping Young,* George H. Doran Co. New York 1926.

# NOTES

VITAMIN NEWS

VITAMIN PRODUCTS CO. • MILWAUKEE, WISCONSIN

VOL. 17

# THE SYSTEMIC CAUSES OF DENTAL CARIES

By Royal Lee, DDS

**(Reprint of paper read before the senior class at Marquette University Dental School, Dec. 1923)**

The factors governing the decay of teeth have always been the subject of much speculation by dentists. The theory accepted in recent years is that the immediate cause of the tissue destruction in this case is lactic acid, produced at the point of decay by microorganisms, which are protected in the initial stages of the process by a gelatinous plaque attached to the teeth. It has also been observed that some persons are immune to caries, and that the susceptibility in caries varies with the same individual at different times, being greatest in childhood. As it has been shown that the most careful prophylactic measures will not entirely prevent caries in susceptible persons, it is the purpose of this paper to describe the cause of the systemic conditions that are predisposing factors in the case of dental caries.

Fones says regarding the cause of tooth decay: "The only logical result of the interesting researches of Pickerill is that, in tribes and races where dental caries is the great exception and not the rule, the diet consists of unrefined and natural foods, while the peoples in whom dental caries is most prevalent are consumers of refined or civilized foods."

Howe, after extended clinical observation on children, states that caries is a result of vitamin deficiency in the food. He was able to produce, in guinea pigs, caries, bleeding gums, resorption of alveolar process, and soft tissues, and even necrosis of cranial bones by feeding a diet deficient in vitamins, in this case oatmeal and fat-free milk. He says, "The softening and carious dental effect was distinct and unmistakable." By careful feeding of proper foods Howe was able to arrest the carious processes, and again cause their recurrence by a return of the vitamin deficient diet. He states that he was unable to say which of the three vitamins was responsible for the effect, that very likely all three were of importance in this respect. He also states that it makes no difference whether these disturbances are the result of irregular calcium metabolism or the result of infection, the control (or predisposing cause) lies in the diet.

Prinz, from a long series of experimental studies, states that he has almost arrived at the conclusion that the etiology of dental caries rests with the constituents of the salivary fluids.

Howe, in later experiments on the effect of diet upon the teeth, gives the different effects of the three known vitamins which are as follows: first, known as fat soluble A, found in fish oils such as cod liver oil, in animal fats, yellow grains, bananas, green vegetables. Second, water soluble B, found in milk, germ of seeds, eggs, yeast, raw vegetables. It is destroyed by a temperature of 150 degrees Fahrenheit, so it is not present in pasteurized milk nor in cooked foods. Third, water soluble C, found in orange and lemon juice, cabbage, raw tomatoes, and green vegetables is destroyed by boiling. Howe found that as a result of these experiments upon guinea pigs and rabbits that the vitamins B and C are the most important in the production of immunity to caries. This is significant in that these vitamins are not found in cooked foods.

Pollina, after clinical observation and study of family, personal and mouth history of six thousand Boston school children, found that eleven per cent who had been totally free from infectious disease, had normal dental arches with no dental caries, well balanced in nutrition, body and mental age. He says, “Many observations have enabled me to compare, reflect and record the above data with such definiteness as to evolve the following axiom: that dental caries is the result of infectious diseases of childhood, acting on the organs' internal secretion.” Pollina claims that from clinical records he can show a history of measles, chicken pox, mumps, scarlet fever, diphtheria, etc. in every case of dental caries in children.

Here we have an apparent difference of opinion among authorities. Some believe that dental caries is the result of a vitamin deficient diet. Others think it is due to a derangement of the endocrine glands or the organs of internal secretion. Another says it is due to the composition of the salivary fluid. Again that it is due to a diet of denatured or civilized food. The above causes, however, are really one and the same. A diet of the refined civilized foods is invariably lacking in vitamins B and C. As Sajous has demonstrated that vitamin C is always present in normal saliva where it “sustains the defensive oxidation which renders bacteriolytic and antioxic enzymes effective,” we find that these scientists have been approaching the solution of the same problem from different angles, and that dental caries may be due to a vitamin deficient diet, thus starving the endocrines, or that the endocrines may be debilitated through disease, in either case the saliva is deprived of it normal bactericidal properties. Also, Howe says that lack of vitamin B causes atrophy of the parathyroids. Sajous states the parathyroids are important in the promotion of calcium and phosphorus metabolism, and as these elements form the mineral elements of the teeth, one can see that lack of vitamin B during the development of the teeth will certainly interfere with proper calcification. Thus, vitamin B is responsible for the proper development of calcification of the teeth while vitamin C promotes bactericidal properties of the saliva and is responsible for the subsequent preservation of the teeth. And as both of these vitamins are destroyed by the cooking of the food and the pasteurization of milk, one wonders how the human body is able to function at all on the minute amounts of these essential food elements found in the average diet. The deficiency of these vitamins produces many other pathological symptoms aside from the dental aspect. For instance, Howe says regarding his experiments with guinea pigs: “The nervous condition of the animals was very marked, and on handling showed signs of tetany, these are attributed to deficiency of water soluble vitamins (B and C).”

To prevent caries then, we must begin with the child as early in life as possible and see that the diet contains plenty of vitamins B and C, which means as much uncooked food as possible and non pasteurized milk. And according to the previously quoted authority Pollina, care must be taken to guard against childhood diseases, which debilitate the endocrines, and as Sajous also states, favor the necrotic dental process of caries by failing to provide nature's “germicidal oxidizing” agent to the saliva. Sajous in his celebrated treatise, *The Internal Secretions and The Practice of Medicine,* elaborates in detail upon the protective function of the endocrines, not only in respect to caries, but in regard to systemic infections such as diphtheria, measles, etc. And as he has shown that the endocrines depend upon the supply of vitamins in the diet to furnish the material for their disease fighting secretions, it is apparent that the degree of resistance to disease possessed by the individual is proportional in considerable measure to the vitamins in his diet. Therefore, the whole question resolves itself into a matter of vitamin sufficiency, and the childhood infective diseases that Pollina considers a cause of caries are really another result of vitamin starvation if Sajous is correct in his conclusions. In this way the infective disease becomes a secondary predisposing factor favoring caries, and may be many times as effective in this respect as the primary factor, the vitamin insufficiency. Pollina's viewpoint, that caries were due to exhausted endocrines, may be justified as he observed the predisposing cause that was most apparent.

Tuberculosis has been observed to predispose to caries, rapid destruction of the teeth taking place in many cases.

This is to be expected as susceptibility to tuberculosis is now known to be due to vitamin insufficiency and the disease has a particularly debilitating effect on the endocrines. We here have a vicious circle, in which the vitamin starvation produces the susceptibility to infectious disease. The overworking of the endocrines to fight the disease increases the need for vitamins, and the exhaustion of the endocrines increases the susceptibility to infection.

When we consider that the vitamins in the food are the materials from which the endocrines secrete their active principles, it is apparent that there are two ways that a glandular insufficiency may take place: (1) There may be a lack of vitamins in the diet. (2) There may be a degeneration or atrophy of the gland, sometimes being an irreparable result of the first situation. Diabetes is a good example of this, the islands of Langerhans undergoing a degeneration, possibly from overwork in attempting to secrete insulin from the blood stream that contains too little of the raw material, the essential vitamins.

It must be remembered that the metabolism of the human body, being an animal function, is a breaking down process of complex compounds that are built up by the synthetic processes of plant metabolism. The animal or human body cannot build upon organic compounds, and is wholly dependent upon the vegetable kingdom for organic foods. Vitamins are a class of organic compounds that are probably the most complex of food constituents. As before stated, all the ductless glands (the thyroid, parathyroid, thymus, pineal body, pituitary, adrenals, gonads, pancreas, islands of Langerhans, spleen), must have one or more of the three classes of vitamins in order to secrete their vital fluids, and if deprived of the vitamins will atrophy and cease to function. Such cessation of functions produces the following results:

1. Lessened resistance to all infectious diseases, including dental caries. This point could be elaborated upon to any length. For instance, Sajous has shown that the opsonin of bacteriology is a secretion of the thryo-parathyroid glands, the spleen and pancreas produce Erlich's complement while the amboceptor of Erlich is secreted by the adrenals.

2. Disturbances in metabolism, such as diabetes and rickets. Severe dental caries accompanies rickets, and teeth develop slowly or not at all in children afflicted with this disease. The cause is lack of vitamin C, which is found only in raw food, being destroyed by heat. The mysterious fact that rickets occurs oftenest in children in very poor or very wealthy families is explainable in view of these facts. The child in the poor home gets too little of all foods, while the child in the rich family gets only cooked or sterilized foods, and is not allowed in the kitchen where other children are getting raw foods, occasionally at least.

The third result of lessening or cessation of endocrine function is disturbance to organic function including mental activity. Dr. Berman of Columbia University in his book, *A Study of the Glands of Internal Secretion in Relation to the Types of Human Nature,* states, "The internal secretions constitute and determine much of the inherited powers of the individual and their development. They control physical and mental growth, and all of the metabolic processes of fundamental importance. A derangement of their functions, causing an insufficiency, an excess, or an abnormality, upsets the entire equilibrium of the body, with transforming effects upon the mind and the organs. In short, they control human nature, and whatever controls them, controls human nature." Dr. Berman shows that the temperament of an individual is determined by the relative activity of different glands of internal secretion.

To summarize them, dental caries is due to a vitamin-deficient diet, starving the endocrines, which are then unable to secrete sufficient of the germicidal ferments to prevent dental caries or other infectious disease. And the presence of a systemic infection sets up a vicious circle, as the hyperactivity of the endocrines in fighting the disease makes the vitamin starvation more acute, such starvation being the original cause of susceptibility to the infection.

*Vitamin D was just being established as another factor in rickets when this was written.

## BIBLIOGRAPHY

Howe, "Dental Caries," *Dental Cosmos*, August 1920, pages 921-929.

Editorial, *Dental Cosmos,* August, 1921, pages 836-839.

Howe, "Studies on the Effect of a Vitamin Deficient Diet on the Teeth." *Dental Cosmos,* November 1921, pages 1,086-1,092.

Pollina, "Endocrinodontis," *Dental Cosmos*, February, 1922, pages 218-223.

Sajous, "Endocrine Glands and Dental Nutrition and Caries," *Dental Cosmos,* July 1923, pages 702-713.

Sajous, *The Internal Secretions and the Practice of Medicine*, 4th edition, pages 696-699, 713-715. (Vol. 1.)

Talbot, "Late Researches on Interstitial Gingivitis," *Dental Cosmos*, August 1921, pages 795-803.

Editorial, "Endocrinology," *The Dental Digest*, March 1922, pages 183-184.

# VITAMIN NEWS

VITAMIN PRODUCTS CO. • MILWAUKEE, WISCONSIN

VOL. 17

## TOOTH DECAY

## AND ITS CAUSE

Modern teachers in dental colleges like to pretend that, "There is no scientific proof that tooth decay can result from improper diet" (A statement by Dean Noves of the Dental College of the University of Oregon at the Northwest Dental Conference, Hood River, Ore. April 15, 1952). At the same conference a Department of Agriculture official stated, "There is no scientific proof that a poor soil can cause poor health." These are samples of the bending of scientific facts to suit the despots who rule a totalitarian state.

The truth about dental caries was well expressed by Bicknell & Prescott in *The Vitamins in Medicine,* (1942, Grune & Stratton, p. 688) under the caption of "Refined Foods." They point out the fact that in the Pacific Islands a number of occasions are matters of history where tooth decay was practically non-existent until refined foods were introduced, when in only five years time the incidence of caries in children became common and in adults between forty and fifty years of age had increased fifty percent. These authors state that when human teeth are incubated with white flour or white sugar and saliva the enamel is destroyed, while with raw sugar or whole grain flour they are "hardly affected, especially with the unrefined sugar."

They quote the findings of Osburne & Noriski (*J. Dental Res*. 1937. 16:431), who found that unrefined cereals and sugars have a protective action on tooth enamel. Children eating raw sugar cane, having teeth that were covered with sticky sugar most of the time, were relatively immune to decay. These authors also state that raw milk has a similar protective action on the teeth. They quote Sprawson who found a sudden startling fall in dental caries in a children's institution after a schedule of one pint per day of raw milk was instituted. Other instances of caries differences due to the raw vs. pasteurized milk were cited.

These are final tests on human subjects. These results show how caries can be prevented properly without mass poisoning of water supplies through fluorine. (If you think this term of "poisoning" is too strong, recall that one fifteenth part per million of sodium fluoride in water will cut the activity of lipase, a vital cell enzyme, 50%) (Reported in a *Bulletin of the State of New Mexico*, 1939.

This book, *The Vitamins in Medicine,* by Bicknell and Prescott here quoted has disappeared from the book marts. You cannot buy a single copy. The modern racketeers know that they can only carry on their criminal adulterations of food by suppression of the truth. That seems the only explanation of why this important reference work that every physician needs, has been made to disappear without a trace.

The extent to which employees of medical and dental organizations cooperate in this criminal racket is shown by the fact that there is an almost universal acceptance of pasteurized milk, acceptance of the fluoridation program, acceptance of criminally adulterated foods like white bread, refined and synthetic sugars, synthetic fats, and imitations of butter as glaringly crooked as the green shavings that the fabled Scotchman tried to feed his horse. Even butter today is artificially flavored (perfumed) and colored with coal tar dyes to cheat the buyer. The Scotsman had not thought to flavor his green shavings with new-mown-hay perfume. The modern sneak thieves of our life and health have been a little more subtle. No wonder the *Drug Trade News* of July 16, 1945 editorially commented "We Need More Guts." That we need "professional men" with "the guts to say in the open, in court and on the witness stand the truth that they say behind closed doors, but which they fear to say publicly." The editor points out the fact that men who know the facts fear to express their opinions before Congressional committees, because they know that they will be subjected to retaliation. He says that many experts refuse to defend the facts because "it will get them in bad" with their "scientific" society or with organized medicine.

By this system of maintaining their "poison cult" the drug and adulterated food industries are directly responsible for your dental disease, and your ill health, your heart disease and arthritis — by so confusing scientific thought that the truth cannot be recognized. As the above editor winds up: "Well, what do you think of it? Can we expect Congress or anyone else to fight our battles when we don't dare to do so ourselves?"

When the Shute Brothers in Canada showed the merits of vitamin E in heart disease and other common ailments, they were viciously attacked by those wolves of organized medicine. This vitamin, only present in fresh cereal products, never found in chemically aged and oxidized, criminally adulterated flour, must not be permitted recognition. Even after fractions of this complex are shown to affect the heart so favorably in some acute diseased states of that organ that the change can be shown in a few minutes on cardiographic recordings, the value to the human is denied. How crooked can man become, how stupid can their vitamins get? For a complete review of the value of this vitamin, get a copy of the *Annals of the New York Academy of Sciences,* 1949, Volume 52, Art. 3 pages 62-428. (New York, American Museum of Natural History).

Our pureblind authorities prate, "There is no scientific proof that vitamin E has any value to the human economy." While at the very same time they accept pasteurized milk without a scintilla of evidence that it will support life as well as raw milk, with volumes of evidence to the direct contrary. In one test at an orphan asylum over a period of years, where the food was identical for two groups except for milk pasteurization for one, there were 14 times as many new cases of tuberculosis among those using pasteurized milk as among those on raw milk.

If you want to know what happens to a medical man who slips up and publishes such a fact as a new test that shows heart degeneration from the use of refined foods in time to halt the consequences of sudden death, read the item in the *New York Times,* Tuesday July 12, 1949 where "Heart Test Report Stirs Medical Row," and "Physician Loses Hospital Post after Appearance of Unauthorized Article." A new test for coronary disease and suggesting a dietary approach for diagnosis and possible prevention caused Dr. Ernest Klein to be summarily dismissed from his position with University Hospital. His findings were the result of his study for over three years of the blood of 200 to 250 persons per day at the Hospital Blood Bank.

He had been told by his superior, "You have no right to do any research work here any more than the maid who cleans the place." Certainly, all research must be done under such auspices as will insure no publication of results that will hurt and business racket than may have its control set up to keep the truth from their victims.

Personally, I tire of calling attention to these morbid facts. I prefer to go further into the interesting exploration of the vitamin complexes that can save life. But what is the use of finding a vitamin that relieves most prostate gland victims, a vitamin that restores missing pulsations of the heart, vitamins that perform naturally and physiologically what nitroglycerin does as a poison, vitamins that bring down the temperature in infections as quick as any antibiotic or wonder drug without any possible repercussions, vitamins that restore oxygen to the tissues of heart victims that are gasping for breath, vitamins that wipe out allergic reactions, when most professional followers of the healing arts are so gullible as to blindly fall for the wiles of the Pied Piper of the Wonder Drug advertising industry — so gullible that they cannot see the vast difference between physiological methods of therapeutics, and the monkey-wrench into the machinery methods of the poison cult and the razor-happy surgeon?

Yes, research is the most pleasant, even if it has to be done with one hand — the other being busy fending off the attacks of slimy creatures ensconced in the editorial staffs of national dental magazines, ensconced in the Food & Drug Administration (where they spout the dictum "no disease can result from any deficiency") ensconced in the Federal Trade Commission (where they spot the dictum "a natural product is not superior to a synthetic imitation"), the OPA where vicious attempts are made to use the law to wipe out competition of products that support life against criminally adulterated products that cannot, ensconced in the Post Office where fraud orders are actually issued against book publishers who sell literature that fails to agree with "consensus of medical opinion" (God help out freedom of speech today). Just to list a few of the diversions that will automatically follow any attempt to bust even a little segment of that vast empire of deception that feeds on the unsuspecting American public. As Alios Senefelder said 125 years ago after establishing the science of lithography: "one spends 98% of his time trying to convince people that a new discovery is true, and 2% of his time on the research necessary to making the discoveries."

We have even gone to the lengths of developing special microphones to pick up heart sounds that are below the normal limits of audibility and special amplifiers and special recording devices to prove that these changes so readily created by some of the vitamins are really actual physiological responses instead of a temporary reaction to clever salesmanship. This instrument is the Endocardiograph (U.S. Patents #2,305,626,2,392,487-2,479,072) available at a nominal rental fee to any physician who would like to see for himself what vast improvements may occur in the cardiovascular reactions of the average patient to the use of scientifically prepared vitamin concentrates from natural sources.

If you want to know what honest cereals can do as a health builder get a copy of *Reader's Digest* for September 1952, and read about "Sweden's Supergrandpa" (page 23) the old gentleman of 66 years whose mainstay of diet was rye bread and water, who beat 50 young athletes in a 1,000 mile bicycle race. Such stamina in our country is unthinkable and certainly unheard of. If you look back a few pages in *Vitamin News* you will note that scientific studies some years ago established rye as the cereal that was by far the best as a muscle builder, wheat in animal tests in comparison being a fat builder.

But do not forget that rye only reflects the mineral quality of the soil it was grown on. Those silt-filled rocky valleys in the Scandinavian peninsula are full of real minerals. The Finns you will recall take home ten times their share of long-distance running trophies from the Olympic Games. Now maybe you see a light? "There is no scientific proof that a poor soil can cause poor health." So says the propaganda of the Death-food Flour Industry. "Eat White Bread and Reduce" say full-page ads in the *AMA Journal.* As we see it, the only thing you could possibly reduce thereby, would be your health.

## A FEW COMMENTS ON THE RELATION OF ABNORMAL HEART SOUNDS TO MALNUTRTION

Extra systoles, heart block, fibrillation: These phenomena are due to the loss of conductivity of the heart tissues for the impulses that otherwise maintain synchronism of the contractile rhythm of the heart muscle.

Heart block first starts as a skipping, then finally becomes a "pulsus alternans" situation, the heart muscle has become so insensitive that it responds only to a "second call" from the control apparatus that normally regulates pulse rate.

The cause is a deficiency of the cereal germ vitamins, $B_4$ in particular. This fraction of the B complex is essential to normal function of motor nerves. It has also been called the "anti-paralysis vitamin." It is inseparable from natural thiamin: never found in synthetic thiamin.

It is, further, the physiological remedy for enlarged heart, for it is this factor in the B complex that maintains vascular and muscle tone.

A continued deficiency of $B_4$, of course, results in more or less degrees of nerve and muscle degeneration, but all the above effects of its deficiency usually respond quickly in some degree to its administration.

An enlarged heart, with its distorted and leaking valves, as shown by murmurs, usually becomes almost normal in its performance except for a prolong first sound — the indication of tired muscle, within a few minutes after ingestion of the natural B complex carrying the wheat germ concentrate. Fibrillation responds as quickly if the degenerative changes have not progressed too far.

Heart block requires more time. Its presence indicates a relatively extended degree of degeneration.

Muscular fatigue and hypertrophy usually is treated with digitalis. A new extract of heart muscle, known as Cardiotrophin, seems to be better for the purpose. Its action is quicker than digitalis when tested on the patient with a weakened and flabby heart, as shown by the weak and extended first sound.

The second sound of the pulse is commonly supposed to be made by the closing of the valves at the end of the heart contraction, in fact later than this, at the end of the outflow of blood, the blood reversal tending to close these valves. If the second sound at the aortic microphone position is accentuated, the general conclusion may be made that the systemic blood pressure will be found above normal. (It is important to distinguish an accentuated second sound from a diminished first sound).

If the pulmonary system happens to be engorged and hypertensive, the accentuated second sound of the pulmonary position will be definite.

This is common with patients having hypoadrena, and they will complain of distress in the chest on exertion due to this congestion. Vitamins to support the adrenals are indicated. Remember cortisone and probably the other adrenal hormones require vitamıns C and B complexes for their formation. These patients usually do very well if they get proper natural vitamin supplements. They are incipient asthmatics, and need adrenaline. Their systemic blood pressure is usually low.

Sometimes the second sound is absent or barely perceptible in the mitral valve position of the microphone. One or two Vitamin F tablets usually restore the second sound here within a few minutes.

Since we know that this vitamin increases the supply of ionized calcium required in muscular activity, it is probable that the absence of the second sound here is because of consequent muscular incompetence — the contraction losing its vigor at the end of the effort, permitting a more gradual slowing of the blood output than normal, thereby eliminating the second sound at this valve.

It is important to note the rest period duration — the time between the end of the second sound and the next first sound. If it is shortened to where it is no longer than the contraction period that follows the first sound, a so-called "tic-tac" rhythm is produced.

This is a serious state of damaged heart muscle — usually an indication of coronary insufficiency. It responds slowly to the use of the vitamin G complex and the $E_2$ fraction. Both these vitamin products are vasodilators — the $E_2$ as rapid as nitroglycerin and useful for the same purpose, but far more constructively. (Certainly, it is unsound to use a poison as a substitute for a food.)

In the angina pectoris case, $E_2$ is often effective after nitroglycerin has failed.

Vitamins $E_2$ and the G complex are vasodilators, essential for the coronary and angina patient. The B complex is bad for these patients until they have had their deficiency of the vasodilators taken care of — otherwise their acute symptoms may be aggravated.

There is a little confusion regarding the vasoconstrictor and vasodilator effect of the vitamins, hormones and drugs because the dilation of the vessels or capillaries that are in the walls of the arterioles will promote constriction of their muscular fibers by supplying fresh blood. Therefore a vasodilating factor may be a vasoconstrictor for certain areas, and vice versa.

Adrenaline is a vasoconstrictor for most of the body, but is a vasodilator for the coronary and lung vessels. The vagus nerve acts to decrease the blood supply to some tissues, increase it for others. Therefore, it is essential to follow the empirical rules for the use of many of these principles.

Another note: wherever adrenaline is used, be sure to use Park-Davis' natural adrenaline. It has a much better action than the synthetic imitation, will not cause toxic side effects and after-pains due to pyrogenic impurities in the synthetic.

Eye specialists have found the synthetic product entirely too irritating for use in eye preparation.

Paroxysmal Tachycardia: This is an apparent loss of pulse rate control normally exercised by the sympathetic nervous system. Potassium deficiency seems to be the most frequent cause — the use of organic potassium as available in Minaplex tablets is usually effective in bringing the control back into normal rates within 15 or 20 minutes. (In two to three tablet dosage.)

Otherwise, the load on the heart is mainly regulated by the oxygen demand of the tissues. This demand has been found to increase as much as 250% by reason of vitamin E deficiency, which normally inhibits unnecessary tissue oxidation. The vitamin C complex is necessary to maintain the red cell oxygen carrying capacity; a deficiency may cause a loss of half the capacity of the blood to carry oxygen. It is very obvious that these two vitamin complexes can be a matter of life or death, and tells us why test animals put on E deficient feed die from heart failure before any other symptoms are observable that might arise from the deficiency.

That is, no doubt, why we have so much heart disease in this country, while it is almost unknown in China where refined foods are also unknown.

The patient who presents himself with a marked shortness of breath is usually relieved within fifteen minutes after taking three or four tablets of vitamin C complex.

The patient who is kept awake with a "pounding heart" after eating too much is usually relieved in the same period after taking two or three "Minaplex" (1) tablets, the organic mineral complex taken from Alfalfa and Sea Lettuce. The potassium content is the active principle. The same dosage usually relieves paroxysmal tachycardia in the same time.

Nervous tension also may affect the heart in this manner; the basic disorder may be mainly the potassium deficiency that incapacitates the sympathetic nervous controls.

The use of unrefined sugar and whole grains in place of white flour products and refined sugar is an important part of the advice needed by this type of patient, unless he prefers to pay the higher price of the minerals in the tablet form for the rest of his life.

Hypertension can be aggravated, too, by potassium deficiency, but there are usually other contributing factors. The most common one is liver damage, and this will be shown by a high sedimentation rate. The remedy then is the fat-metabolizing complex that is needed for liver regeneration, available as a beet-molasses extract sold as Brtslco (2) tablets.

The active factors are betaine, choline and the alcohol-soluble minerals.

Where cholesterol accumulations are involved, the use of the buckwheat juice tablet Rutaplex (3) will be found indispensable. It releases the cholesterol from the tissues. If the liver can take it out, the blood cholesterol will not rise, may even drop: but if the liver cannot do its job, the blood pressure will drop and the blood cholesterol will rise at the same time.

To promote the disposal of the cholesterol through the gall bladder and keep it in solution meanwhile, the beet leaf extract "Betaris" (4) tablets will be found very helpful. They are indicated in all gall bladder troubles, such as gall stone formation simply a state of bile in which cholesterol is precipitated out instead of remaining normally in solution. The use of beet greens in the diet will accomplish the same thing.

*Similar products are available from the Therapeutic Foods Company:
1. Organic Minerals 2. Betacol 3. Cyruta 4. Betafood

THE STATEMENTS HEREIN MAY NOT AGREE WITH CURRENTLY ACCEPTED MEDICAL OPINION. NEVERTHELESS, THE PUBLISHER BELIEVES THEM SOUND.

Edited by Royal Lee March 1953

// VITAMIN NEWS

VITAMIN PRODUCTS CO. • MILWAUKEE, WISCONSIN

VOL. 18

# VITAMINS AND HEART DISEASE

It is truly remarkable how government experts and medical authorities can officially keep their collective heads buried in the sands of referred ignorance. Below we offer the latest example of how the "consensus of opinion" leads on the innocent and trusting layman to his slaughter just as the Judas goat leads the sheep to the abattoir axeman.

Seven hundred thousand people a year die of preventable and curable heart disease — the disease caused by vitamin deficiency, directly consequent to the illegal sale of criminally adulterated flour and cereal products that should deliver vitamins to the consumer, instead of cheating him of essential nutrients while delivering unessentials. The makers of bleached flour admitted 47 years ago the criminal nature of their practice of bleaching with oxidizing agents that destroy vitamins and other nutritional values of fresh wheat.[1] It is strange that at the same time the medical authorities are so obtuse to the benefits of the lost vitamins that we are cheated out of in wheat flour, they fall so easily for the arguments in favor of water fluoridation, which at best is trying to correct nutritional deficiency reactions with a vicious poison. (A poison proven dangerous in one-fifteenth the concentration recommended for water medication, according to unquestioned tests.)[2] Dr. Harold Hawkins proved years ago that unless malnutrition is present, immunity to dental caries is inevitable.[3]

The vitamin fractions that are needed to protect the heart are $B_4$, the C complex, the G complex, and the E complex. The latter contains one factor that has the identical effect of nitroglycerin ($E_2$), and another (vitamin F) that relieves the muscular weakness of deficiency, shown by the absence of the second sound when the stethoscope is placed over the heart apex.

Whether or not these reactions occur is simple to determine by making phonocardiographic recordings of the heart sounds on any human subject, or on horses, dogs, or monkeys. In most cases where arrhythmias, fibrillation, extra systoles or heart block are present in any degree the use of natural concentrates of wheat germ will improve the sound pattern in a few minutes. If the apical second sound is weak or absent, in the vast majority of cases a little of the F fraction of the E complex will eliminate the aberration inside of five minutes.

Where the patient has seizures of angina pectoris the $E_2$ fraction of the E complex (the phosphlipid component) will promote relief more satisfactorily than the drug substitute for this food, nitroglycerin.

These matters are not subject to any argument whatever. Tests can be made in any group of people and 9 out of 10 will be found to be radically deficient, typical victims of bleached flour.

The Vitamin Products Company will supply both the Endocardiograph and the vitamins for such tests on a moment's notice.

The funny part of this picture is the fact that the same people, who for fifty years or so have encouraged for their own private profit, the criminal adulteration of flour by bleaching, are now promoting the wide use of fluorine in drinking water

— no less criminal adulteration to offset the terrific accumulated tendency to tooth decay that flour refining and bleaching has unquestionably brought about. (If you question this statement, read pp. 688 and 689 in *The Vitamins in Medicine* by Bicknell and Prescott.

It is still funnier to see the august American Dental Association and the American Medical Association using all the combined political influence to force these criminal practices into general acceptance with complete disregard of all moral principles and constitutional rights of the unsuspecting victims. We see such remarkable spectacles as the dean of a large dental college publicly spouting off at a convention of dentists: "There is no scientific proof that dental caries can result from malnutrition."[4]

Only a moron needs proof that something can be made out of nothing. If food minerals are deficient, as Hawkins long ago demonstrated, the teeth will be deficient. Not even the lactogenic germ is necessary, for simple erosion will rob the teeth of minerals to build bone.

It is interesting to see how all unprincipled and incompetent (mentally and morally) politicians leap to the assistance of racketeers who seem so powerful in their wire pulling. Most of these political opportunists fail to realize how an aroused public can react once they find out how they have been duped, robbed, poisoned and starved by crooks who admit their criminal intent — admitted almost fifty years ago. Crooks that in the flush of their success in pulling the wool over the eyes of the public, professions, and law enforcement officers, have the frightful gall to say that their opponents, like skunks, are not to be argued with but exterminated. Anyone who criticizes white flour products as a source of disease is a 'predatory quack' to be exposed. (*Food, Drug and Cosmetic Journal,* Oct. 1951 p. 788) Crooks that can only continue their criminal destruction of public health by corrupting the Federal Food and Drug Administration and the Federal Trade Commission, who are paid to protect the public, but are now, according to Dr. Harvey W. Wiley, protecting the adulteration of foods and drugs.[5]

The Federal Trade Commission says that the synthetic vitamins put into flour to facilitate its sale after the natural ones are destroyed are exactly equal to the original natural ones taken out in processing or destroyed by bleach, and they will prosecute anyone who ventures to call attention to the inferiority of the synthetic imitations in sales literature for natural foods. But in the U.S. Army, in its official *Nutrition Manual* for 1949, says this:

"Wherever possible, the nutrients required should be obtained from natural foods, rather than synthetic preparations. This is particularly true of the vitamins. Synthetic concentrates, tablets and pills may not contain all of the known nutrients, either as such or in optimal proportion. Furthermore they obviously may not contain lesser known or unknown nutrients which are, however, provided by natural foods."

This manual also properly appraises the commonly encountered deficiency states as follows:

"The fact that vitamin deficiency diseases do occur in this country, however, indicates that dietaries are not always adequate. These deficiencies occur as a result of poor food habits, improper selection of foods, lack of proper funds, or disturbed metabolism due to other causes. More widespread and therefore of the greatest importance are the subclinical deficiencies resulting from a sub-optimal intake of vitamins. Here the symptoms are vague and ill defined, and it requires considerable skill to recognize and diagnose such conditions. Whereas, a severe vitamin deficiency is incapacitating, the subclinical deficiencies may result only in fatigue, inefficiency, malaise and discontentment."

This Army Manual might have gone on further and told us how these 'subclinical deficiencies' may not attract any attention until so much damage has been done as to cause sudden death by heart failure. We often call attention to the 28 test animals put on a diet lacking the same important vitamin for the heart, the E complex where the effect of one year of the equivalent of white bread feeding caused the sudden death from heart seizures of 13 of these animals. Death before any warning illness, loss of weight or other signs were apparent.[6]

A similar investigation on the nutritional value of skimmed milk, plus vegetable oil is in progress. The animals live only a few months. Such a diet cannot support life.

Now look at the latest thing in baby foods. You will find skimmed condensed milk plus cheap vegetable oil. Why take out the butter and replace with Oleo? To cut the wholesale price, my dear Sir. To take the business away from the maker of an honest food.

The consumer pays the same price until some retailer decides to get go and try to get more business by 'cut-throating.'

Even the baby food made by our largest dairy combine is so adulterated. Why? Because they must meet the competitive price, or lose the business. What is wrong here? Simply that the Food and Drug Administration is asleep at the switch. In any game, the rules must be enforced by an impartial umpire, or crookedness springs up. So they take out the butter fat and sell it to the government at a high price, and cheat the baby of its rightful vitamins. As good butter is our most important source of vitamin E, the little fellow begins to develop heart and muscle degeneration on the bottle.

The National Dairy Council says good butter has 1/10 as much vitamin E as wheat germ oil. It is our best source of vitamin E, also an important heart vitamin. The A.M.A and the Food and Drug Administration try to tell you that there is no such vitamin as F, but again that is a deliberate misrepresentation, a bald faced lie in plain language, to keep you in ignorance of its importance. Look up the section in the 1949 *Annual Review of Biochemistry* on this subject. There it is stated that a deficiency of F is suspected to predispose to cancer. Or look at the latest issues of the *International Review of Vitamin Research* (Berne, Switzerland), Vol. XXV. No. 1 and see the two articles on vitamin F, pp. 62 and 86. Both of these publications are officially using the term vitamin F, and anyone who says it does not exist is deliberately keeping his head in a sand pile. By denying its existence, these foul crooks are putting off the day of reckoning when its widespread deficiency can be recognized and corrected. Heart disease and arthritis in particular. Go back to Dr. Weston Price's book, *Nutrition and Physical Degeneration,* page 273, and read how the crippled and pain-wracked little boy who was told his fate was death by ignorant doctors, and who recovered perfect health on butter containing vitamin F that Dr. Price obtained from Deaf Smith County, Texas. (Dr. Price called vitamin F at that time the 'X' factor of butter, since identified as a member of the F complex).

Modern politics has put half our production of butter, this finest of food fats, into storage where it rots until sold for soap grease, while full-page advertisements in our home papers sell us fool's counterfeit butter at three times what it is worth as soap stock.

A basic principle often forgotten:

"There is well-controlled experimental evidence that of vitamins A and C increased liberality of intake continues to yield increased nutritional well-being up to at least four times the amount demonstrably needed; and there are clinical indications that something similar may be true in the case of vitamin C." Page 521 of *Chemistry of Food and Nutrition,* 5th Edition. H.C. Sherman. Macmillan 1937.

"Increased food calories without regard to increased vitamin intake results in shortening of the life period of test animals. Increasing the calories with attendant increase of vitamins and minerals by the use of natural foods resulted in increased life span." H.C. Sherman, *Food and Health*, page 200. Macmillan 1936.

By this reasoning, we should never eat white bread, candy or soft drinks, because they add to our calories without supplying a quota of vitamins.

Let us beware of propaganda. Let us beware of mass medication to cure our deficiency diseases. Let us beware of crooks on the public payrolls who conspire to destroy our health for their own selfish ends.

The man who tells the truth can prove it. The man who is trying to mislead you cannot cite the facts. He must refer to opinions. Have you noticed how only opinions are cited to support water fluoridation? How its opposers, who have nothing to gain (and a lot to lose) are so viciously vilified?

**REFERENCES:**

[1] Reprint No. 1. Lee Foundation for Nutritional Research - North Dakota Agricultural College — Experimental Station — *Bleaching of Flour* — 1906.

[2] *University of Arizona Bulletin* by M.C. Smith and E. M. Lantx.

[3] *Applied Nutrition* by H.F. Hawkins, DDS.

[4] Northwest Dental Conference. Hood River, Ore. April, 1952.

[5] *Special Reprint 11-50*. 'The History of a Crime Against the Food Law' by Harvey W. Wiley, MD.

[6] Gullickson and Kalberly — Anals of New York Academy of Science, 1949.

**Edited by Royal Lee** **February 15, 1954**

# SOME TYPICAL HEART ABNORMALITIES AND THE FUNCTION OF SPECIFIC NUTRITIONAL FACTORS IN EACH TYPE.

Cataplex B, which contains $B_4$ (anti-paralysis factor) as one of its natural components, seems to be extremely effective in certain heart conditions such as: heart block, bundle branch block, auricular fibrillations, auricular flutter, arrhythmia, enlargement, and the type of Bradycardia which is caused by impaired nerve conductivity, all of which no doubt are due to the lack of the $B_4$ factor, removed in cereal processing. One of the amazing things about the activity of Cataplex B is its immediate response in cases of deficiency. As a rule any of the above conditions will show noticeable improvement in 5 minutes, as indicated by any sensitive heart-recording device. Below is a typical case with a graph taken before Cataplex B administration and another graph 5 minutes later.

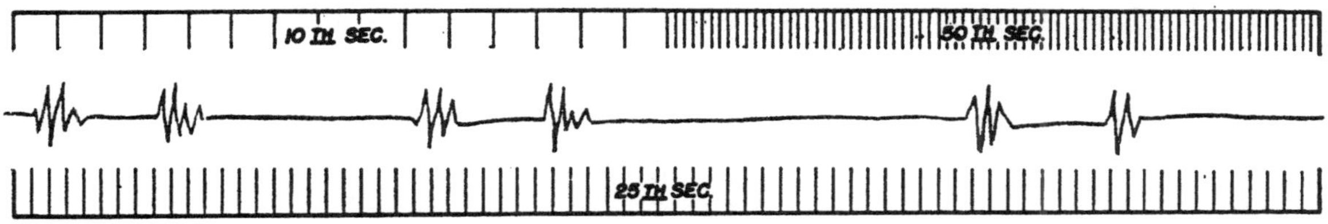


After the administration of Cataplex B.

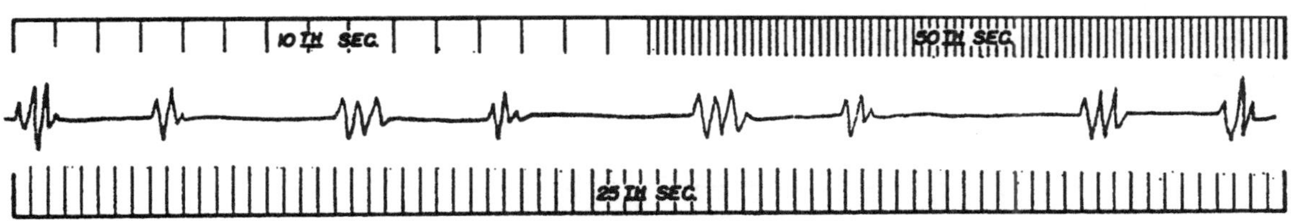


Cataplex G contains nerve relaxing factors and is usually indicated for the high strung, hypertensive, jumpy patient who has the exact opposite heart picture of the one shown above (i.e. he will have a shorter than normal rest period instead of the abnormally long one of a heart block patient — above). The G complex relaxes the B complex contracts or creates muscle tone. "Cataplex $E_2$" which is noted for its nitroglycerin action, is usually used in combination with "Cataplex G" because of their joint action in the same type of heart picture. Both Cataplex G and Cataplex $E_2$ are vasodilators and are the nutritional factors indicated in Coronary Thrombosis, Coronary Insufficiency, Angina Pectoris or any other vascular constriction. All of these conditions will show a shorter than normal rest period on a heart graph. Alleviation of pain etc. is usually experienced in 5 to 10 minutes. The graph will not return to normal for about two weeks and upwards of continuous nutritional treatment. Below is a typical graph of this type.

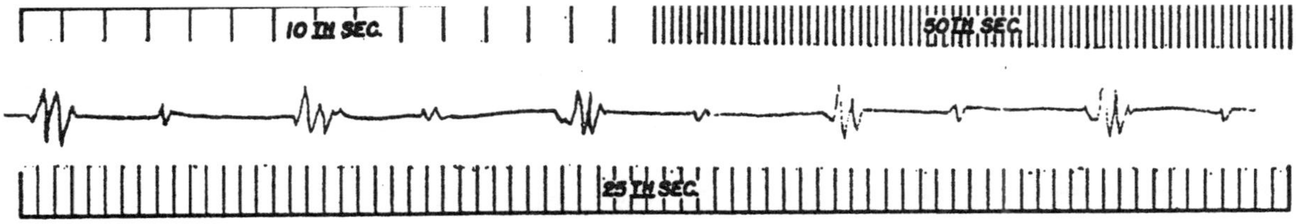

After the administration of Cataplex G.

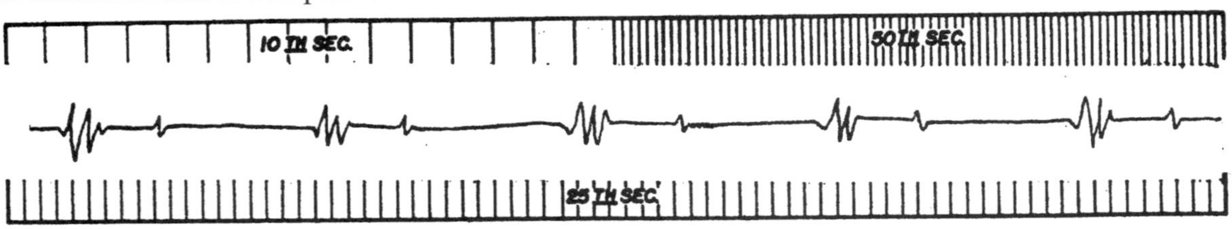

Cataplex C is indicated where there is a relatively higher second sound in the pulmonary area than in the other valvular areas. When the pulmonary circulation becomes engorged and hypertensive, a heart graph will show an accentuated second sound and will usually be associated with a distressed or heavy feeling in the chest on exertions. This condition is associated with a hypoadrenia and "Cataplex C" is known to support adrenal activity. A graph of the type mentioned appears below before and after Cataplex C administration.

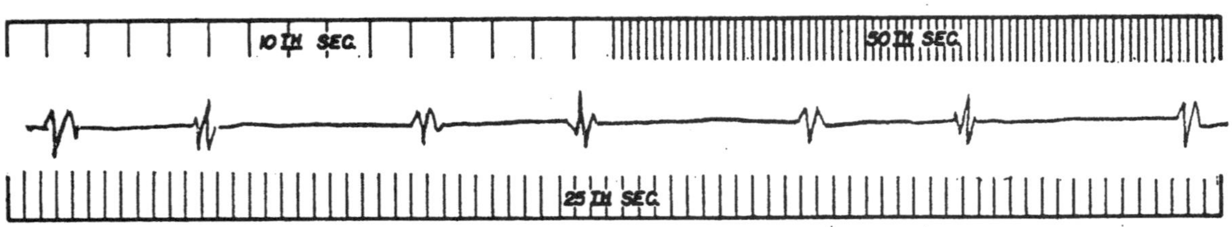

After the administration of Cataplex C.

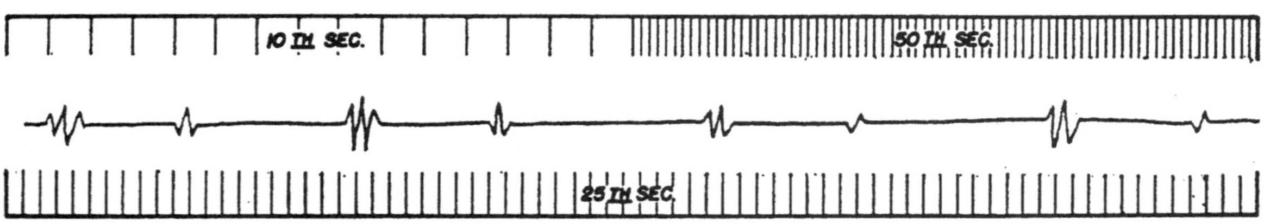

Minaplex is indicated in paroxysmal tachycardia in which condition there is an apparent loss of pulse rate control, which is normally exercised by the sympathetic nervous system. Minaplex will stimulate the sympathetic nervous system and is usually effective in bringing the control back to normal within 15 to 20 minutes after the administration of 2 or 3 tablets. A graph of this type follows.

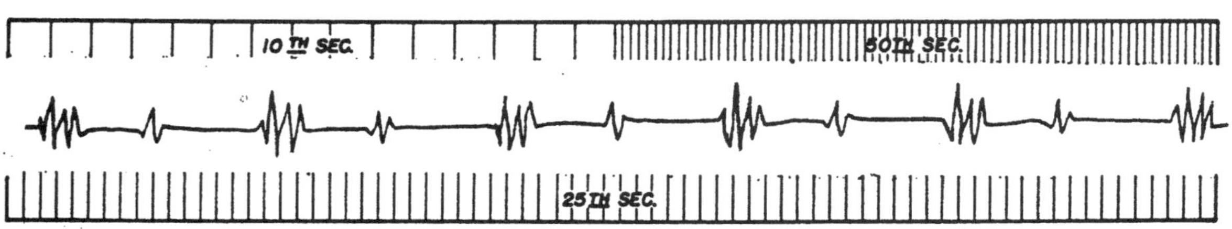

After the administration of Minaplex.

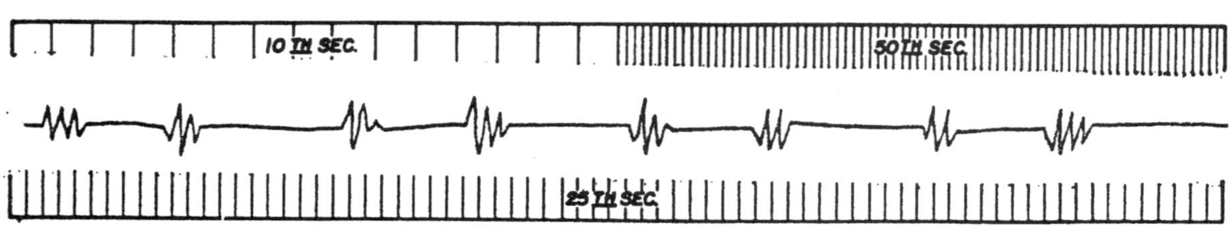

Cardiotrophin is a new heart muscle extract that acts as a heart muscle tonic, as indicated by cardiograph tests. Its action is usually immediate on the patient with a weakened and flabby heart. As indicated by the graphs below of a typical patinet at 5-minute intervals. It is indicated where the patient's heart has poor muscle tone, muscular fatigue, or hypertrophy. These conditions usually show up on a heart graph as a weak first sound of low amplitude together with an abnormally high second sound.

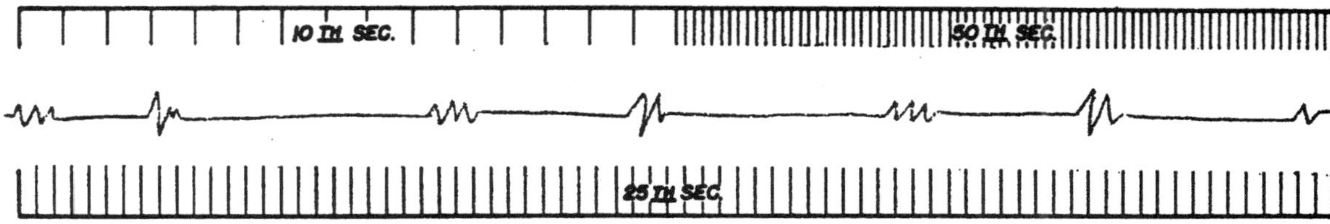


After the administration of Cardiotrophin.

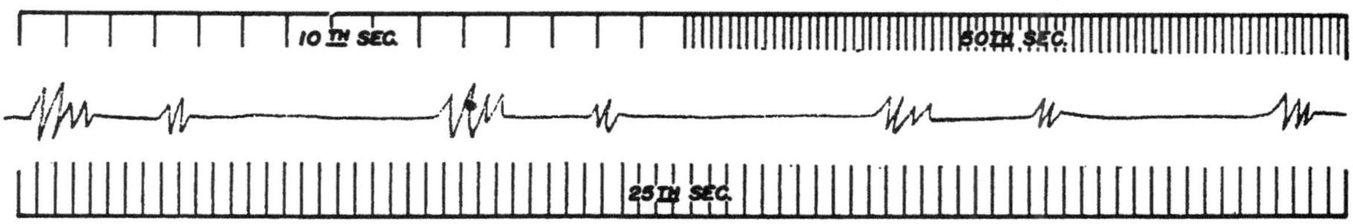


Cataplex F increases the supply of ionized calcium, which is required in muscular activity. Where the second sound is absent or barely perceptible in the mitral or tricuspid area, there is apparently a weakness of the muscular layer of the large arteries and hence a lack of snap in the reaction of the supply of blood that is pumped into them at each heart cycle. This lack of reaction shows up as an extremely low second sound and indicates the need of Cataplex F and the ionized calcium that it makes available.

Note the typical graph below together with one taken 5 minutes later showing the expected improvement.

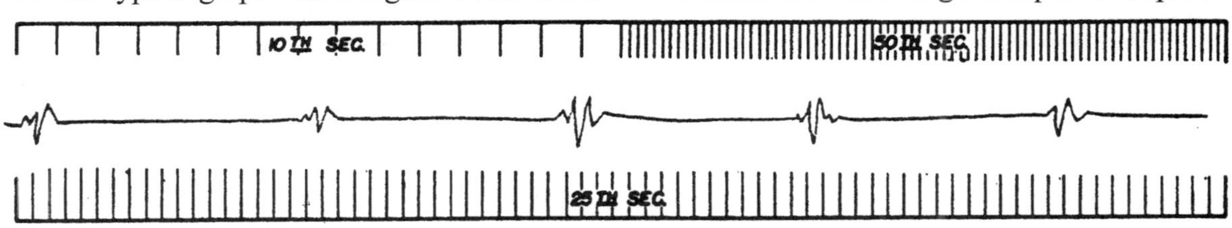


After the administration of Cataplex F.

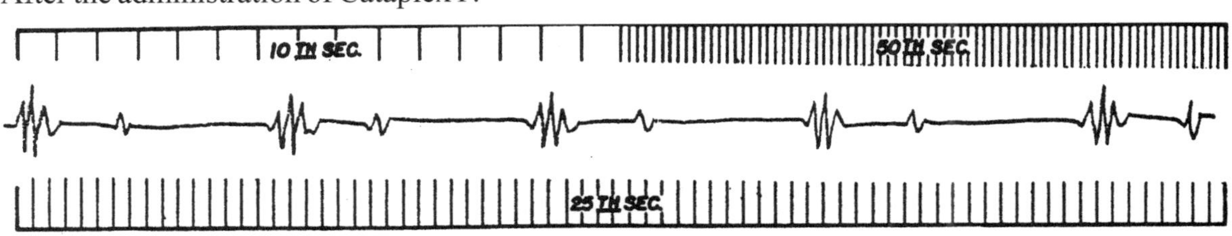

# NOTES

VITAMIN NEWS

VITAMIN PRODUCTS CO. • MILWAUKEE, WISCONSIN

VOL. 18

# THE ETIOLOGY OF DIABETES MELLITUS

The statistically rapid rise in diabetes mellitus in this country is alarming. One cause has been reported in these pages before. The action of synthetic sugar, glucose (dextrose, corn sugar) is unique among sugars, no other sugar being capable of causing diabetes even when fed in large amounts to test animals.

When incurably diabetic test animals are desired for experimental use, it has been found that small doses of alloxan will quickly destroy the islets of Langerhans in the pancreas without disturbing any other body tissues. The animal is thereby rendered permanently diabetic.

Is there any possibility that we are getting alloxan in our foods that act similarly.

Yes, with definite certainty. Alloxan is formed by the action of oxidizing agents such as chlorine, chlorine oxides, etc. or xanthine, a normal constituent of tissues (muscle, liver, pancreas, thymus, spleen) and of urine, which carries 0 to 1 percent, and of common foods like cereals, malt and yeast, and of meat foods, as mentioned.

And where might we get chlorine and chlorine oxides in our food?

We all know that much of our water supply is doped with chlorine to poison the bacteria in the sewage it may carry. Not all cities are as well equipped as Milwaukee, where the water after chlorination is filtered through activated carbon to eliminate the chlorine in a 15 million-dollar treating plant. (Maybe the fact that Milwaukee breweries are the city's best water customers is the real reason — you cannot successfully make beer with chlorinated water; it poisons the yeast.)

We all know that the latest patented flour bleach is chlorine dioxide, succeeding the nitrogen trichloride — agene — which after its patents ran out was conveniently found to cause epileptic reactions of a fatal nature in dogs, and was eliminated from all use in foods by the Federal Food and Drug Authorities. It, too, functioned as a bleach and bug killer by releasing free chlorine, so the quite probable action of flour bleaches as diabetogenic factors has been adversely reacting on the public health for some time.

Since these poison chemicals destroy both the xanthine and the vitamin E of the cereal germ, it is of interest to learn that xanthine can reduce the need for vitamin E in animal feeding tests. (Reported in *Nutrition Review,* Jan. 1948, p. 118). In fact, we might legitimately consider xanthine as a member of the vitamin E complex. A xanthine compound — theophylline — is used in medicine to relieve heart symptoms of vitamin E and G deficiency. And xanthine is found associated with E and G vitamins in wheat germ.

Xanthine seems to be a synergist of vitamin E in protecting from oxidation and enzyme damage the genes of the chromosome of the cell. It seems also to be a part of the liver mechanism that delivers excess cholesterol to the bile route of elimination. (See *Protomorphology*, p. 208-209 for details.)

Truly, as Herbert Spencer so long ago said, the neophytes in any field are likely to be so absorbed in observing the actions of their new schemes as to neglect to note the reactions.

In dealing with foods, the Food and Drug long ago set up the principle that any added poison in any food was too much. It is regrettable that principle cannot be the guiding force in government instead of commercial expediency — and political expediency.

There is only one way to judge a food. That is by its effect as a food.

Here is how honey stacks up in feeding diabetics. Dr. Kilian of the University of Frankfurt has just published the results of his tests. He found that the administration of equivalent amounts of honey and sugar to diabetic patients, the honey gave a remarkably lower blood sugar curve. And the addition of 10 to 20 grams of honey to the usual diet of diabetics did not disturb the sugar balance. Summer honey was slightly superior to winter. (*Chemical Abstracts*, July 10, 1953; p. 6527g).

No product that has not stood the test of time as such should be permitted to enter any schedule of nutrition. Mineral oil once was commonly used in reducing diets as salad oil.. It was even commercially much used in doughnut frying.

Here is the present status of mineral oil as an alimentary component:

1. It promotes ano-rectal infection of crypts.
2. As much as 60% may be absorbed and be deposited in the liver. (from which it is impossible to remove)
3. It interferes with the assimilation of calcium, phosphates, vitamins A, D, E and K.
4. Tends to reduce prothrombin levels.
5. Interferes with estrogen metabolism.
6. Indirectly causes pruritis ani, may contain carcinogens, may cause lipid pneumonia. (See *Jol, AMA,* Feb. 7, 1953)

This reviewer comments that mineral oil should be discussed from the standpoint of toxicology, not from that of pharmacology. But remember the vast sums spent to assure the public that it was harmless, a perfect laxative? Today the doctor is being bombarded with new propaganda, no less reckless, about a constant array of new wonder drugs, mainly for the purpose of treating victims of starvation, who are ill because their cereals were bleached, their sugar refined, their syrup of synthetic glucose, their doughnuts cooked in petroleum, their drinking water chlorinated and fluoridated. All promoted by gentry who are "too absorbed in observing the action of their schemes to be aware of the reaction."

Please review the following. It may afford you a better perspective, and help immunize you against unsound commercial propaganda.

## SIDELIGHTS ON THE PHYSIOLGOY OF FOOD ASSIMILATION

The permeability of the intestinal wall is regulated by the posterior pituitary hormone.

Hoskins says that posterior pituitary secretion is necessary to the health of the intestine, that it prevents constipation, prevents atony and paralysis of the muscular layer, promotes deposition of fat in the liver where it is burned to supply energy.

Gordon estimated that 86% of the obesity in children was attributable to posterior pituitary weakness. (*Jour. Pediat.* 10, 204-220, 1937).

It is evidently not the vasopressor factor (pitressin) that does these things, as victims of basophil pituitary cell have hypertension, ecchymoses simulating scurvy, brittle bones, obesity, hirsutism, and hypogonaidsm but no gastrointestinal aberrations. (Cushing, *Harvey Lectures,* 1932-33 pp. 90-158.) Such as severe hyperchlorhydria, as produced by pituitrophin.) (Dodds et al, *Lancet,* 1-1099, 1935.)

The normal hormone seems to have been split into three separate fractions by previous investigators — pitressin, oxytocin and the anti-dieresis factor — for recent discoveries show these are all combined into one principle in the living gland. (Pat. #2, 342, 172.)

Alkaline phosphatase and ribonucleic acid (from yeast) are known to contribute to normal production of this hormone. (opposing basophilism.) Freckles and "liver spots" are known to be indications of basophil overbalance. (Cushing, *Harvey Lectures* 1932-33, pp. 90-158.)

This is of interest in view of occasional reports of the successful use of vitamin F for "liver spots" since we now know that this vitamin favors alkaline phosphatase activity by supporting prostate function — the prostate being the normal source of this enzyme.

That is why prostate tumors cause heavier bone growth, and Cushing reported bone weakness and fractures common among his basophil pituitary patients. The effect of such posterior pituitary activity in causing arteriosclerosis and angina pectoris as well as the hypertension reported by Cushing has been previously referred to in these pages as well as its action in promoting fatty degeneration of the liver.

These effects are quite likely due to a secretion of an incomplete hormone complex, where the gland is capable of only elaborating a part of the normal balanced complex as described in Pat. #2, 342, 172.

Since the use of natural vitamin G complex immediately relieves such adverse reactions of the posterior pituitary principles essential to those normal physiological reactions, it is to be suspected that where its incompetence is observed, the real situation may be a recession of activity because the secretions have become toxic in the state of the victim's deficiencies, just as thyroxin becomes toxic in patients deficient in vitamins C and F.

## VITAMIN C — THE ORGANIC COPPER VITAMIN

*Vitamin News*, Sept. 1933, carried the comment that the elaboration of hormones was suspected to be dependent upon vitamin availability. Today it is known that cortisone cannot be produced unless vitamin C is present. In scurvy the administration of the adrenotrophic pituitary factor is not followed as it normally is, by a stimulus to cortisone output.

Our comment at that time was to point out that the endocrine functions were, in the main, concerned with toxin removal. Today we find cortisone being used to aid in the elimination of the tissue toxins produced by burns. (And the title of that 1933 issue was "Vitamins for Pain and Shock.") This statement and quote was prophetically made:

"The use of gland extracts and hormone preparations has not been as successful as would be expected for treating these conditions for the reason that it is far more difficult to supply a full complement of the hormones that are elaborated from the vitamins than it is to supply the relatively few vitamins. By that we mean that it is far more difficult to maintain a balanced endocrine function by giving the gland extracts, and success is possible in far fewer cases, than when the proper supply of all the vitamins is made available.

"We might add that in the latter case, Nature is permitted to choose the remedy, while in the former the Physician makes the choice.

"It is becoming increasingly apparent that most, if not all, maladies heretofore attributed to the presence of toxins are, in reality, caused by a deficiency of vitamins."

— Dr. D. T. Quigley, M.D., F.A.C.S.

We know a lot more today about vitamin C complex than we did at that time. But we did know at that time that the best vitamin C complex came from potato and mushroom. Now we know why.

Naturally citamin C complex contains traces of copper. When this is separated out, it is found to be tyroainase. Just as when the $B_{12}$ fraction of the B complex was finally isolated, it was found to be organically combined cobalt.

---

## *THE NATION'S LARDER AND THE HOUSEWIFE'S PART THEREIN*

By: Sir Robert McCarrison, Dr. L.H. Lampitt, Prof. V.H. Mottram, Dr. Franklin Kidd
(G. Bell and Sons, Ltd., London)

Page 27...

... Here I am constrained to repeat, with some modification, what I said of vitamins twenty years ago, when as yet their numbers had not gone beyond the letter C: "Whether there be three or legion, they will be found to exist — and this is the important point — in natural food stuffs, in quantities and in combinations adequate for the needs of the body." Perplexed as we sometimes may be by the mounting numbers of the vitamins, it is well to remember this and to rely upon fresh, natural foodstuffs for their supply.

Page 44...

... So from infancy and childhood through adolescence to adult life, dietetic malnutrition, aided often by infection, leaves its trail of morbidity, and this although the food fault or faults may not be extreme. So long as they are sufficient in degree to impair the function of nutrition, they will, sooner or later, directly or indirectly, give rise to disease. The constant drop will wear away a stone; the constant imperfection of nutrition, though this be relatively slight, will wear away the body.

VITAMIN NEWS

VITAMIN PRODUCTS CO. • MILWAUKEE, WISCONSIN

VOL. 18

Reprint No. 25A Supplement to "Are Vitamins Drugs?"
Lee Foundation for Nutritional Research
Milwaukee 3, Wisconsin

# CLINICAL NUTRITION (— FOODS VS. DRUGS —)

**by Royal Lee**

The literature in English on clinical nutrition is very limited, both in volume and quality. Probably the conservatism of official medical opinion has served to discourage publication of new ideas, further, there is a well established program in organized medicine to block progress in the dissemination of facts that relate to health building foods or therapeutic use of natural foods, vitamin and mineral supplements. This pernicious and corrupt misuse of the facilities of medical education has been so effective in creating the idea that nutritional therapy is futile and leans toward quackery that we feel it imperative to clear the slate on this matter by offering in a special booklet the proof of this state of affairs: *Why Organized Medicine Has Been Fighting Vitamins.*

The intent and purpose of this organization to steer interest away from nutritional deficiency as a cause of disease is shown by frequent periodic news releases similar to the one published through Associated Press just as this is being written (Nov. 6, 1948) "Doctor Warns of Cold Remedies ... As for vitamins 'only one tenth of one per cent of the people who take them without medical advice get any good from them. Most people get enough of the vitamins in their food.'"

(Comment by Dr. Austin Smith, Director of the division of therapy and research of the American Medical Association.)

This is obviously a misstatement; as everyone knows who has had a kindergarten grounding in vitamin knowledge. Just compare it with the comment of Dr. Thomas Parran, Surgeon General of the U.S. Public Health Service, who at the Hot Springs Food Conference expressed the opinion that improved nutrition would add ten years to the "Virile life span of the average human being."

Official editorial comment of organized medicine takes pains to say the opposite; "All substances required by normal adult human beings can be supplied under ordinary conditions by a balanced diet." And "Foods common to the American Dietary properly selected will contribute everything that foods can give to the maintenance of good health"[2] and a well known medical writer Dr. Clendenning tells us "there is no general deficiency — the public is getting its vitamins."[3]

This trend began many years ago, when the definition of a drug became involved in the theory of specific effects as opposed to empirical therapeutics, in the effort to make drug therapy "scientific."

A discussion of any subject may best begin by a definition of terms. For a definition of Therapeutics let us quote Potter: "Therapeutics comprises all the science and art of healing and includes the use of medicines and all other agents and measures which are known to alleviate or cure disease. The operations of nature herself are properly embraced in the general term "therapeutics," which may be subdivided as follows:

"Natural therapeutics, includes the operation of the healing power of nature, those modes and processes of healing which occur independently of art and tend to spontaneous decline and care of disease. There is no scientific dogma better established than this, that the living organism is in itself adequate to the cure of all its curable disorders ... This part of the subject is taught only casually in the schools, but it deserves a special chair and more systemic treatment than it receives.

"Applied therapeutics embraces the application by art of agents foreign to the living organism for the purpose of aiding nature to restore the body to a healthy condition.

"Empirical therapeutics is a term applied to the use of ... therapeutic agents for the sole reason that they have been tried previously with successful results in cases apparently identical with the one under treatment ... It was necessarily the original method in therapeutics, has conferred many rich gifts upon medical science, and has been advocated by many able physicians...

(Author's note: We might interpose here the comment that Potter in this definition did not differentiate between natural therapeutic agents that are common to the living organism and agents foreign to the organism to which he confined applied therapeutics: apparently empirical therapemics may include both types of agent.)

"Rational therapeutics means the use of remedies based on the knowledge of the pathological conditions present in the subject and the physiological action of the agent employed ... The illustrious Albrecht von Haller, the father of physiology and the author of the doctrine of irritability, was the real originator of modern physiological therapeutics. In the preface to his *Swiss Pharmacopoeia* (circa AD 1755), occur the following remarkable directions — the first recorded of their kind:

"'In the first place the remedy is to be tried on the healthy body, without any foreign substance mixed with it: having been examined as to its odor and taste, a small dose is to be taken, and the attention directed to all effects which thereupon occur: such as upon the pulse, the temperature, the perspiration, the excretions. Having thereby adduced their obvious phenomena in health, you may pass on to experiment upon the sick body.'

" ... Medical colleges have recognized physiological drug experimentation as a part of their regular curricula: laboratories are fitted up in many of the schools with costly instruments of precision, for the more exact prosecution of this study ... The medical press of every civilized country is filled with the results of these labors, and no medical student is permitted to pass the graduating ordeal until he has mastered the essential characteristics of the physiological action of the important medicaments so far established .... What has hitherto been the conviction of but a few, is daily growing into a fixed canon of professional belief ... that all real advance towards the establishment of therapeutics as a science must be made upon the lines laid down by Haller, namely drug-proving upon the healthy human organism."

We have quoted Potter at length to illustrate the way in which modern medical science was led into a blind alley from which it has not as yet been able to extricate itself.Note our question marks after each use of the word "physiological." How could a "foreign agent" be accepted without question as a physiological influence?

And how could a nutritional deficiency or a vitamin ever be discovered by men experimenting with "agents foreign to the organism" tried on "the healthy body?"

And since a drug must be an agent having a demonstrable effect on "the healthy human organism," all nutritional factors — vitamins, enzymes, minerals, proteins, amino acids — were excluded from the drug category. They were, in fact, rendered absolutely invisible to the investigator conditioned by this viewpoint. Only drugs can remain in his view.

Only the discredited adherents of empirical therapeutics would be competent to detect a natural nutritional therapeutic agent. These in late years were represented by the homeopathic school, which has been practically eliminated through the passing of the control of medical education into the hands of its enemies.

Theoretically, the rationalists were right. But if we are still too ignorant to understand the human machine, is it not ridiculous, to turn over to those who possess only theories, the exclusive privilege of experimenting upon the machine?

And is it not still more ridiculous for those experimenters to confine their activities in principle to tests of agents "foreign to the organism" really all known poisonous substances, and to turn their backs and close their minds to suggestions of possible merit in nutritional factors?

It will at once become evident that no nutritional substance will ever become identified for its value in treating deficiency disease by this method of investigation, simply because it can have no effect whatever upon the healthy body.

Forty years ago the materia media literature of this country began to adopt this principle to the exclusion of empirically determined facts, and all food products and concentrates became "quackery."

Cod liver oil was condemned as being far less useful than butter, linseed oil with its vitamin F was thrown out to admit cotton seed oil (as "sweet oil") in its place in prescriptions, rye and buckwheat with their reputation for curing capillary disease, such as crysipelas were dropped, scurvy grass was forgotten (once a specific among mariners as a cure for scurvy), barley water with its wonderful vitamin B pattern that had such a reputation for babies and invalids was immediately ignored by the teachers and textbook writers, and such mineral tonics as the phosphates and manganese were relegated to the patent medicine trade (cf. Horsford's Acid Phosphate and Gude's Pepto-Mangan) where they would be sniped at as "unorthodox" and unscientific.

The drug companies of course had to fall in line and eliminate anything in their catalogs that did not conform to "scientific" thought. Eli Lilly had a highly effective syphilis remedy, a botanical product that no doubt owed its effectiveness to vitamin C content, the formula of which they had actually and in fact "obtained from the Indians" known as "Succus Alterans" in their 1898 drug list. Cheaper synthetic arsenicals soon pushed this product into the background.

Today we use sulfa drugs, antipyrin and aminopyrine, not knowing that they probably act wholly by mobilizing into the blood stream the tissue reserves of vitamin C where the vitamin can promote phagocytic action and thereby cure the disease at the same time leaving the patient with an "overdrawn bank account" of the essential vitamin which may be more serious than the original infection.

The *Journal of the American Medical Association* printed not so long ago[4] a full page condemnation of

Upjohn's "Citrocarbonate" as a fraud because it claimed nutritional value for its mineral content which happens to be ideal to replace the blood serum salts depleted by kidney and sweat gland activity. These actions officially closed the doors of orthodox medicine to nutritional therapy.

When Jacques Cartier, exploring the St. Lawrence Valley, followed the advice of the Indians in treating the scurvy of his men with pine needle tea 400 years ago, he was practicing "empirical" medicine.

Fluid extract of common thornapple, known to be one of the best sources of vitamin C was once a highly respected remedy. Ellingwood[5] states that this product was as "near specific" in cardiac disease including "angina prectoris, valvular deficiency, endo-myo and pericarditis, trachycardia, rheumatic heart, cardiac neuralgias, palpitation, vertigo, apoplexy, dropsy and functional derangements." The value of thornapple extract in angina pectoris is confirmed by Dr. W.N. Macartney.[6] Now that we know that the vitamin C complex deficiency reduces the oxygen-carrying capacity of the red cell so the heart is called upon to do much less work if given more of this food factor, we can understand why thornapple extract can be good in so many affections of the heart. Further, the "rheumatic heart" is today being suspected to be purely a result of vitamin C complex deficiency, the vitamin P of the C Complex being found a valuable remedy,[7] and the only known physiological treatment.

It is such a definition of "drug" (something used to treat disease which "is foreign to the body and with a specific action on healthy subjects") that has caused the establishment of the drugless healing professions, the osteopaths, naturopaths, etc. These are practitioners who felt that disease usually was a departure from nature's normal state, and that health would be restored if the offending conditions were corrected, and that the administration of drugs was no rational procedure if the objective were the removal of causes.

It is obvious that any substance that has any effect on a healthy subject must be foreign to the body, unless used in other than normal amounts, in which case its use would be thta of a drug. For instance, common salt is an emetic if used in drug dosages, but if a food if used in nutritional dosage.

Unquestionably, here is the dividing line between the practice of medicine and the practice of drugless therapy.

Nutritional factors can only become drugs by their use in such amounts as to produce effects other than nutritional effects.

Cushny, in his *Textbook of Pharmacology*[3] agrees with this. He says, "Pharmacology is the study of the changes induced in living organisms by the administration in a state of minute division of such organized substances as do not act merely as foods ... These substances are known as 'drugs.'"

He adds, "It is quite impossible to distinguish between drugs and poisons. Almost all remedies given in excess cause dangerous or fatal symptoms ... (it is certainly possible to distinguish between foods and poisons.)"

Of late, there has been an attempt on the part of many law administrative bodies to so define foods as to put them into the drug category in a legal sense, so as to bring into the realms of medical practice, the drugless practice of food therapy. This permits the prosecution of the drugless practitioner on a charge of "practicing medicine."

As a matter of fact , the ability to select such foods as will prevent deficiency disease or starvation is incumbent upon every living being. There should be no interference with any sources of either foodstuffs or information. The only reasonable laws are already in effect, those that punish fraud. And the biggest fraud in connection with foods is going unpunished — the sale of devitalized cereals that in all probability causes the United States to lead the world in deaths from heart disease, and aggravates every degenerative disease.

## REFERENCES

[1]. Potter, S.O.L., "Therapeutics, Materica and Pharmacy," *Blakistons*, 12th Ed., 1913, page 3.
[2] *Jol. A.M.A*, October 25, 1941. Editorial, page 1447.
[3] Ibid. September 20, 1941, page 1035.
[4] Ibid. May 20, 1933, page 1597.
[5] Ellingwood, F. (MD). *Materia Medica and Therapeutics,* Chicago Medical Press Company, 1898, page 264.
[6] Macartney, W.N. (MD) *Fifty Years a Country Doctor,* E. P. Dutton & Company, 1938
[7] *Am. Jol. Rheum. Dis.* (1), 11, 1945

# NOTES

VITAMIN NEWS
VITAMIN PRODUCTS CO. • MILWAUKEE, WISCONSIN
VOL. 18

# THE CONTROL OF GROWTH, HEALTH AND VITALITY BY PROTOMORPHOGENS

A protomorphogen is a cell secretion given off by all living cells at all times in minute amounts that promotes the synthesis of protein for cell repair and cell maintenance on the outside of the cell wall, after which it is absorbed by the cell. Protomorphogens are chromosome end products, made in the cell nucleus, probably the agents by which the basic functions of the chromosome are exercised. All living proteins carry a protomorphogen component by which the protein is made specific in nature, specific in causing organic reactions, specific in function, specific in its ability to act as an antigen in provoking immune reactions. All antigens may be antigenic by reason of accompanying protomorphogens — in some cases instead of being attached to a protein molecule the protomorphogen may be attached to a lipoid or polysaccharide aggregate. When a protein has been separated from a protomorphogen, it is said to be denatured, and is no longer fully capable of antigenic action; that is, it cannot create an antibody specific to it in the circumstance of its injection into an anilal blood stream.

Since no cell can grow or maintain itself unless protomorphogens as secreted by itself are available in the percellular fluids, it is obvious that here we have the possible biological growth regulator. Suppose that the immune-body producing mechanism of an animal, heretofore looked upon only as a defense against invading organisms (cells) from the outside, were to be found to exert the same controlling action on every organ and cell of the body, we would have the answer to the long-sought question of why animal organs and living creatures in general were able to regulate their growth exactly according to a well-ordered plan.

We find, on investigation, that there is just such a reaction of the immune body producing mechanism (the reticulo-endothelial system) and it has been described under the general designation of "natural tissue antibody" (NTA).

There is a specific NTA for every different kind of organ in the human body. Suppose a patient with a history of tuberculosis or chronic bronchitis shows evidence that his lung tissue has a very low vitality, refuses to heal after damage or irritation. It certainly will not be far-fetched in reasoning to assume that there is present in the blood stream an excessive amount of the lung-specific NTA that is acting to inhibit unduly the vital repair activities of the lung cells. The more protomorphogen released into the blood stream by lung lesions, the more NTA will be created, it is reasonable to assume. The reactions of a tubercular patient are exactly such as one might assume from this hypothesis. They seem to have lost much of their healing vitality; their incentive for tissue repair is no longer up to normal. The same is true of heart patients who have had extensive heart damage. The same may be true for many other organs and tissues. Pernicious anemia seems to be just this, as well as the dystrophies of muscle and atrophy of nerve tissue in the wasting and paralytic diseases. The patient simply has become allergic to some of his own tissues. Philosophically speaking, such a mechanism of this kind has, of necessity, to exist. The body must have as much ability to tear down and discard as to build and repair. Normally, both operations properly balance to create health.

Now for the clinical side of this new philosophy. Protomorphogens have been made by extraction of chromosome material from heart, lung, liver and other organs. The lung protomorphogens in tests on various patients with tuberculosis, bronchitis, smoke-burned lungs (of firemen) has almost invariably proven useful in speeding recovery. More, it often seemed to turn the tide where the patient was making no favorable progress.

The heart protomorphogen was really spectacular. With the cardiograph to record the performance, immediate improvements in heart action can be observed. A few minutes are enough for the change in the heart's reaction to the new blood stream with its lowered content of NTA to be apparent. It seems that as soon as the heart protomorphogen is absorbed into the blood stream by the alimentary route, it combines with NTA in the blood, and such blood is more friendly to the heart cells.

The effect is much like that of digitalis. The heart becomes stronger and the pulse rate slows; the rest period becomes longer in proportion to the contraction and systolic time. The dosage must be small at the start, as the combination of heart protomorphogen with the NTA is a poison, normally produced in relatively small amounts, but usually put into the category of "fatigue toxin." Too much may make the patient feel slightly toxic, like the onset of a cold — which may be accompanied by the same type of reaction between an antigen and an antibody — here the antibody that protects us against the "cold virus." After this first dose, the protomorphogen (any of which seem to be capable of this primary upset in patients with a long history of disease) is perfectly well tolerated.

Protomorphogens never can be administered by injection, as in that case they will aggravate the target organ instead of helping it. This is because injected protomorphogens are immediately picked up by phagocytes and carried off to lymphoid tissue where they instigate the production of more, instead of less, NTA. Alimentary administration, on the other hand, simply promotes the reduction of the NTA blood levels, no doubt by direct combination with the NTA as fast as the protomorphogen is absorbed into the blood stream. The different effect may entirely be due to the concentration on arrival in the blood, the alimentary absorption being so diluted that phagocytic pickup cannot be accomplished.

I may divert here to say that it appears that cortisone does its work by flocculating blood antigens so that they can be picked up by phagocytosis. Cortisone, therefore, promotes an immediate reduction in blood antigens, most of which are toxic, and creates a temporary feeling of well being. But, by reason of the phagocytic route of disposal it creates, the latter effect is an excess of antibody productions of all kinds, and if it happens to be muscle antibody that is overproduced (as would happen if the cortisone injection took place after a day of hard muscular effort which had loaded the blood with muscle protomorphogens) the effect 14 days later would be an obvious attack of asthenia, that might mean the beginning of a serious muscular dystrophy for which no cure might be found (other than muscle protomorphogen).

Heart protomorphogen, being heart muscle extract, may act favorably on all muscular tissue.

The protomorphogen of bone tissue has been found of great value to the dentist, bone regeneration around loose teeth has been readily accomplished where the decalcification has not been accompanied by too much necrosis. Its biggest field in dentistry may be in its highly beneficial effect in improving the toughness of the mucous membranes under dentures and eliminating the common complaint of sore spots under the false teeth, which are no more successful than the natural teeth without a healthy bone support. The effects of the bone protomorphogen are very prompt, the denture patient reports improvement within a few days. X-ray pictures may show recalcification of bone within two weeks.

This short review of this new field in promoting specific nutritive activity of any specialized body tissue is intended as an introduction only to the subject. We suggest your further study of the book *Protomorphology,* if you desire to know more about the theories invovled.*

Meanwhile, protomorphogen extracts are now available as follows:

Bone– BIOST tablets
Heart — CARDIOTROPHIN tablets
Lung — PNEUMOTROPHIN tablets
Liver — BETALCO and BETACOL tablets (combined with lipotrophic factors)

OTHERS SOON TO BE AVAILABLE

* "Protomorphology" is published by Lee Foundation for Nutritional Research, Milwaukee 3, Wisconsin and is available through the International Foundation for Nutrition and Health: 858-488-8932 or online at: www.ifnh.org.

THE STATEMENTS HEREIN MAY NOT AGREE WITH CURRENTLY ACCEPTED MEDICAL OPINION. NEVERTHELESS, THE PUBLISHER BELIEVES THEM SOUND.

**Edited by Royal Lee** **May 1954**

# NOTES

VITAMIN NEWS

VITAMIN PRODUCTS CO. • MILWAUKEE, WISCONSIN

VOL. 18

# POLITICS

# AND BABY FOOD

The effects of the acts of unthinking politicians have unlimited ramifications. When Congress started to buy the votes of the farmers by purchasing butter and allowing it to rot in warehouses, they did not realize that they were buying those votes with the health of the American people, and most particularly with the health of the future babies of the country. For not only was oleomargarine substituted in many a diet for butter, but in most baby foods of today, you will find butter has been removed from the condensed milk and cheaper "vegetable fats" put in its place.

Why this change? Simply because the counterfeit can be sold for less than the genuine. Look at the labels on any of the proprietary baby foods. Cheap glucose instead of milk sugar, oleo instead of butter fat.

As discussed before in *Vitamin News*, glucose has no place in any food because it favors the incidence of cancer and diabetes, and blocks the assimilation of calcium. Lactose (milk sugar) is the only sugar suitable for baby food, as it promotes the assimilation of calcium.[1] (We refer here to the synthetic glucose [dextrose] made from corn and potato starch, in Germany from sawdust, by cooking with sulfuric or hydrochloric acids.)

It was noticed that babies on these new formulas were too often afflicted with attacks of convulsions, tetany from a lack of diffusible calcium, no doubt.[2] It was found that the addition of vitamin $B_6$ (pyridoxine) would prevent these convulsions. It has long been known that vitamin $B_6$ would relieve symptoms of deficiency of vitamin F, the important vitamin of butter,[3] apparently assisting the bacterial flora of the intestinal tract to produce forms of vitamin F.

It was also found that the autoclaving of the baby food at too high a temperature had destroyed the natural $B_6$.[2] It is a good example of what Dr. F. M. Pottenger, Jr. had demonstrated in his tests on animals of the futility of depending on pasteurized milk as a food — it caused loss of teeth, constipation, liver diseases, heart disease, homosexualism and finally death from arthritis.[4] Dr. Pottenger reports that autoclaving (high temperature cooking) greatly speeds up the degenerative changes produced by pasteurization. Condensed milk was far more potent than pasteurized milk in creating disease.

It is a proven fact that cooking protein and sugar together destroys nutritional values.[5] Essential amino acids are lost, amino acids essential to bone and tooth formation.

SPECIAL NOTE: Clinical tests show that honey (10% solution) was much better utilized than synthetic dextrose when intravenously administered to either healthy subjects or patients with liver disease. Just another example of how real foods are superior to imitations. (Abstract p. 52, *Jol. Clinical Nutrition, vol. 2,* #1)

## REFERENCES

1 *The Vitamins in Medicine,* by Bicknell, A. Prescott, 2nd ed., p. 641.

2 *Jol. Clinical Nutrition,* Vol. 2, No. 1, p.44.

[3] *Jol. Biol. Chem.*, Schneider, Steenbock, and Platz, 132:539, 1940.
[4] *Reprint No. 27*, Lee Foundation for Nutritional Research — Milwaukee 3, Wisc.
[5] *Jol. Nutrition,* Vol. 40, No. 2 (Friedman and Kline).

## THE BIOCHEMISTRY OF GOUT

Gout, once quite prevalent, is today less well-known than a hundred years ago, but the disease is not by any means extinct. Many cases are associated with or concurrent with arthritis. It is characterized by deposits of sodium urate in the cartilage and ligaments of the joints, first appearing often as an inflammatory state of a toe or finger that is extremely painful and sensitive.

A single dose of sodium phosphate as a laxative is known to bring on such a joint flareup in patients having no previous experience with the condition. It seems that sodium phosphate readily reacts with the blood uric acid and forms this insoluble sodium urate. A high sodium content of the body fluids is considered a predisposing cause.[1]

The origin of most uric acid is probably by the oxidation of guanine, adenine or xanthine. (Guanine by the influence of guanase becomes xanthine. Adenine is likewise converted to hypoxathine by adenase. Hypoxanthine oxidase converts hypoxanthine in the presence of oxygen into xanthine. The xanthine is oxidized to uric acid by xanthine oxidase.)

These precursors are metabolic waste products of the cell nucleus. They are available in greater amounts when active leucocytosis is increasing the availability of such toxic waste products. That means in case of chronic or acute infectious disease, excessive use of certain high protein and highly cooked foods. (See Kouchakoff's work on poisons produced by cooking that increase leucocytosis, in which even cooked water is found toxic because of bacterial residues always present, "pyrogens.")[2]

Xanthine being the source of uric acid, let us look into the function of this substance, a relatively unsoluble waxy material. It appears to be a protector against toxic substances, as injections of suspensions of xanthine prevent liver damage following chloroform poisoning.[3] How does chloroform cause such damage? By releasing the components of chromosome structures that are ordinarily essential as determinants, such release being due to the solvent effect of chloroform on the wrapping films of the chromosome.[4] (Recall that the chromosome is a lamellar structure of alternate monomolecular films of fatty wrappers and layers of lipoproteins high in nuclein — the blueprints of the cell that guide repair and growth, without which *deformed structures replace the normal.*)

Vitamin E is a part of this wrapper film substance (the tocopherols promote monomolecular films, are used in industrial lubrication to increase film strength of oils, and to reduce their tendency to oxidative destruction). Xanthine is found to reduce the amount of vitamin E to be required in the food scheduled, so must be a partner in this protective progress.[5]

Normally, the administration of exogenous guanine and xanthine does not result in increased excretion of uric acid.[6] Probably only in deficient or diseased states this occurs.

Vitamin P complex (the flavonoid group) inhibits xanthine oxidase, therefore blocks the loss of xanthine and the production of uric acid.[7]

And vitamin E is an oxidation inhibitor; in its deficiency the tissues may require up to 250% more oxygen, other factors being the same.[8] (No wonder the heart breaks down in E deficiency, with its load possibly increased 250% trying to get this oxygen to its destination.) The production of uric acid conceivably might be, too, increased 250% if this oxidation excess is all related to xanthine destruction.

We do not have to go much further to list a few habits to avoid if we wish to give gout a wide berth:

1. Eat no foods that have lost their content of vitamin E. (All commercial cereals are devoid of this vitamin. It is lost by oxidation promptly after nature's seal of the seed germ is broken.)

2. Rancid fats destroy vitamin E on contact. (Stale meats are likely to have rancid fats, if the animal was in need of this vitamin, his fats may have been rancid before he was butchered. Sausage, etc. — very bad.)

3. Stale vegetables likewise may have lost their vitamin E content by oxidation, also their vitamin P of the C complex.

4. Foods high in potassium are protective against gout. Black molasses, raw sugar, vegetable leaf & juice in general carry potassium. Cereals do not, root vegetables do.

5. Sodium intake in any form except table salt (chlorides) being very bad. No laxatives containing sodium, no bicarbonate (potassium bicarbonate is preferable to soda in cooking).

6. Our best common source of vitamin E is good butter. (The best butter carries one-tenth as much of this vitamin as wheat germ oil. It is one-tenth the price. You get the fat free — oleo cannot meet this competition.)[9]

Our best common source for vitamin P is deep freeze grape juice concentrate. (Do not confuse this with grapefruit juice, which carries so much citric acid that it may disturb calcium transport in the tissues unless used in very small amounts.)

The homeopathic school recommended formic acid for gout. Now we find that formic acid reduces uric acid to xanthine and thereby may render it harmless as a gout excitant.[10] One to three drops of the 25% solution in a glass of water is about the flavor of citric acid and was reputed to relieve gout in a hurry.[11] Now that we know why, it may become more popular. But the basic cause still is the malnutrition that deprived the victim of his true body-building health food, the food that was "made worse so it could be sold for less," thereby driving all honest competition to the wall, bringing us to the point where people are starving to death on all sides (dropping dead from heart disease) and we accept it as "acts of God" when in fact it is simply the end result of criminal adulteration of our staple foods.

[1] Waugh & Abbot: *Text Book of Alkaloidal Therapeutics,* p. 307.
[2] Kouchakoff, P,: *Proc. 1st Int. Cong. Of Microbiol.*, Paris, 1930.
[3] Ravdin et al: J. *Clin. Invest. XVIII* (6): 633-639, November, 1939.
[4] Turck, F. B.: *The Action of the Living Cell,* page 264, MacMillan, 1933.
[5] Hove & Harris: *J. Nutrition,* 34:571-579, 1947.
[6] Plimmer et al: *J. Physiol.*, 39:98-117.
[7] Beller & Martin: *J. Biol. Chem.*, October, 1951.

[8] Houchin & Mattil: *J. Biol. Chem.,* 148:301, 1942.
[9] *Dairy Council Digests*, 21:6, July, 1950.
[10] Thorpe: *Dictionary of Applied Chemistry,* vol. 5, p. 791, 1917.
[11] *New, Old & Forgotten Remedies,* Anshutz (Boericke & Tafel, Philadelphia), page 231, 1917.



**Edited by Royal Lee** **September 1954**

VITAMIN NEWS

VITAMIN PRODUCTS CO. • MILWAUKEE, WISCONSIN

VOL. 19

# VITAMIN E COMPLEX

The vitamin E complex is now known to embrace the tocopherol group, the xanthine group, the phospholipid group, the lipositols, and the sex hormone precursors.

The tocopherols were the first to be recognized and, as usual, have stolen the show, just as thiamine did in the case of the B complex. The tocopherols appear to act purely as anti-oxidants, and to be the protective agent for more complex parts of the vitamin E assemblage. As such, it conserves and extends the effect of any one of the other members of the vitamin complex, and therefore its wide scope of action is explainable.

Two books on the subject of vitamin E deserve a place in the library of every physician interested in the effects of malnutrition. One is the *Annals of the New York Academy of Sciences*, Vol. 52, Art. 2, pages 63-428. It contains contributions from over one hundred authorities, and discusses the role of vitamin E deficiency in causing the following diseases:

*Acute and subacute vascular obstructions, angina pectoris, diabetes mellitus, Dupuytren's contracture, fibrositis, leg ulcers, multiple sclerosis, myocardial degeneration, Peyronie's disease, rheumatic diseases, stasis dermatitis, stasis ulcer, Sydenham's chorea, urethral stricture.*

It also contains the report of Dr. Gullickson of the Minnesota Agricultural College on his feeding test on 28 cattle where 13 dropped dead from the effects of a one year's deprivation of vitamin E complex.

The other book is *Alpha Tocopherol in Cardiovascular Disease* by W. E. and E. V. Shute and six other contributors. (Shute Foundation for Medical Research, London, Ontario, Canada, 1952.) It lists, among others, the following diseases as amenable to tocopherol therapy:

*Acute glomerulonephritis, arteriosclerosis, coronary occlusion, coronary thrombosis, diabetic ulcers, exfoliative dermatitis, indolent ulcer, leukoplakia, peripheral thrombosis, phlebitis, pruritis, purpura, thromboangitis obliterans, thrombocytopaenia, thrombophlebitis.*

In this book, Dr. E. V. Shute says (page 188): "Many people have advanced the proposition that a natural vitamin is superior to a synthetic. The evidence adduced for this is very tenuous and unsatisfactory and we are not convinced of it."

Dr. Shute makes a very common mistake in assuming that one fraction of a natural complex is the vitamin itself. If that fraction only is under consideration, it is possible for the synthetic to be equivalent to the natural if the natural could be completely purified, and provided that the molecular structure of the synthetic were identical to the natural, isomerically speaking, and were not contaminated with identical but isomerically unlike and biologically inactive (and often not only inactive but biologically toxic) molecules. (See Lee Foundation Report No. 6 for elucidation on this.) (It is known that only laevo-pantothenic acid is useful biologically, the dextro form is toxic, for example. Synthetic pantothenic is normally half of each form.)

We admit the evidence is "tenuous," but nature made it that way. It is up to us to be "tenuous" enough to follow the facts.

The other reason for natural to be superior to synthetic is the presence of essential synergists in natural crude extract. Dr. Shute needs unnaturally high dosages of alpha-tocopherol because he lacks these partners, he depends on the antioxidant effect of the tocopherol to preserve the real vitamin factors present in the patient's tissues rather than to depend on administering more of the sadly deficient complex in toto.

Dr. Shute's method is again to use pharmacologically high doses of one fraction of a complex, rather than to use a complete complex. He is not to be blamed — he is reporting clinical results.

He is treating angina pectoris, for instance, with tocopherol and getting results that actually are due to the protective action of the tocopherol on the tissue reserve of the vitamin $E_2$. We prefer to supply the $E_2$ itself (of natural source) where indicated, for it is as specific in its effect for this purpose as nitroglycerine.

Dr. W. E. Shute reports frequent reversal of effect, the patient is made worse if overdosed, and the right effective dose may vary for each patient (page 103). It is obvious that if the alpha tocopherol is the protective agent for a real factor that is available to each patient in varying amounts, depending on his own dietary vagaries, the protective agent must be given in an adjusted dose to match the real factor. We have discussed this reversal of action where missing synergists were involved before in these pages. It is common effect with synthetic "vitamins" and almost never seen in natural complexes.

In coronary thrombosis, the G complex is far more important than the tocopherol, the effect is immediate, almost as spectacular as the $E_2$ in the angina syndrome. Since the G complex, the $E_2$ and the tocopherols are all found in wheat germ, the part of the wheat discarded in white flour making, it is reasonable that all may be required by the cardiac patient who owes his predicament to his attempt to live on white flour.

The effect of the G Complex is to promote better coronary circulation; in fact, vasodilation in general, cooperating with the vitamin fraction $E_2$ in this effect, and opposing the action of thiamin which tends to aggravate the coronary patient by its vasoconstrictive effect.

And where the general effect of the E complex is desired, we refer to the reports of clinical use in *The Vitamins in Medicine* by Bicknell and Prescott (Grune & Stratton, 1953). They are emphatic in expressing their preference for natural forms of vitamin E as a complete complex, even saying that the entire wheat germ is preferable, so as to include the whole missing link of the B and G, as well as the E and A complexes removed from our cereal foods. (These authors fail, however, to recognize the fact that commercial wheat germ has lost its E potency by oxidation, its oils go rancid in a few days after milling and the only vitamin values are the B complex remaining.)

Bicknell and Prescott condemn high dosages of tocopherols because of their tendency to cause bone and tooth decalcification. We also can report a case where a patient lost all his otherwise sound teeth within a month after an intramuscular shot of alpha-tocopherol, given as a remedy for arthritis. His dentist reported that his teeth were so decalcified that they had lost 90% of their strength, the tooth crowns could be broken off by thumb pressure.

There is only one way to get natural vitamin E. Fresh butter contains 1/10 as much vitamin E as wheat germ oil, costing ten times as much, and whole wheat bread made from flour ground from the wheat at the time the bread is baked. Commercial "whole wheat" flour is devoid of vitamin E, the oil content is rancid and will destroy tocopherols on contact. "Wholeness" here can only be true of fresh made flour. The same is true for any other processed cereal food. White flour is less toxic than stale whole wheat flour, as it has lost its oil.

Dr. Shute makes the interesting point that the human body stores up vitamin E to the extent of a three years' supply in the fatty tissues, and that if we reduce by fasting, we release a lot of this vitamin for use in the other tissues. (We are told, too, by toxicologists that we can accumulate DDT in fat reserves to the extent that we can be poisoned by a fast, or in case of illness where weight loss can be rapid. The DDT is one of those insidious poisons that waits to "kick us when we are down.")

A rat has a life span of less than three years, and it is known that a rat can receive enough vitamin E from his mother to last him all his life. That does not mean that we can live all our life without it.

The chromosomes disintegrate and liquify when the protective vitamin E has disappeared. (*The Vitamins* by the A. M. A., 1935, page 585.)

That is why ulcers fail to heal, and any overworked organ cannot repair itself in case of E deficiency. The chromosomes must be intact for tissue growth or repair. They supply the blueprints for the job. This function of vitamin E complex was described in *Vitamin News* back in 1936 with reference to "petroleum dermatitis" where the hands of screw-machine operators and others who are excessively exposed to oils contract a skin condition that refuses to heal. The cause as then stated was loss of vitamin E (and A) from the skin cells, blocking repair. The internal ingestion of our E complex tablets often healed up these victims inside of a few days. Surgeons, dentists, and housewives who wash their hands frequently or have them in contact with detergents too much have a similar trouble, and a similar cause. (*The Vitamins*, A. M. A., 1935, p. 594.)

Dr. Shute reports an opposing effect between tocopherol and estrogens. That is because the estrogens promote the release from the chromosome of the "blueprint" factors, and the tocopherols protect the chromosome from agents that tend to break it down, or release its components. The tocopherols act favorably in peptic ulcer, and estrogens are also useful in treating such ulcers.

How does it happen that tocopherol and estrogen oppose each other in one case and in another act parallel? No doubt the reason for the tocopherol acting to assist estrogen in peptic ulcer is that the "blueprint" factors, once released, are enabled to better resist enzymatic digestion in the stomach by the added protection of the tocopherol, and thereby speed up the healing rate. The adverse effects of estrogen that normally are observed are the effects of the toxic residues of enzymatically split "blueprint materials," the histamine, necrosin and pyrexin known to follow local tissue damage, and which are systematically released in case of too much estrogen and too little tocopherol. (The placental production of estrogen is for the purpose of making available to the growing embryo ample supplies of "blueprint" material, and without protective vitamin E, the toxic residues can create eclamptic seizures by chain reaction effects, once the blood levels rise to critical degrees.) The normal effect of estrogen, otherwise, is to make available "blueprint material" for the fabrication of the chromosomes of the germ cells in the gonad.

Dr. Shute's success in treating indolent ulcers with tocopherol ointment is understandable in view of this theory. The long-known value of poultices of bruised plant tissues to such wounds is also understandable, for green leaves are one of our best sources of the vitamin E Complex. The healing effect of chlorophyll may be due to tocopherol or other synergist factors, for it is usually impossible to purify such natural materials completely.

The presence in the natural vitamin E complex of the estrogen precursor (as reported by Levin et al) appears to be unknown to the Shute group, for Dr. E. V. Shute on page 187 discusses wheat germ oil as if its only value were in its tocopherol content. The other known synergists of the E complex are no less important, the xanthine (which can spare up to 50% of the tocopherol requirement) (*Jol. Nutrition,* 34:571-79, 1947), the lipositols, which appear to be important in the cholesterol-metabolizing effect of vitamin E (as stressed by the Shutes on pages 131-157) the sex hormone precursors, and the phospholipid group (vitamin $E_2$, the nitroglycerine-like factor and vitamin $F_2$, the "blueprint" protector that restores appetite to children and adults who fail to assimilate their blood reserves of fats and proteins) and vitamin $F_1$, the active form of unsaturated fatty acid factor described in the *Annual Review of Biochemistry*, 1949, where it was hypothesized as a cancer preventive, and which restores calcium to the tissue fluids so fast that a phonocardiogram shows improved heart action within five minutes where the second sound has been suppressed by reason of such deficiency (previously discussed in *Vitamin News*). (This vitamin was first discovered in wheat germ oil by Burr in 1932.)

This makes six separate complexes within the E complex, each of which is of a multiple nature, the members being still un-numbered and new relatives popping up periodically.

The Shute group have accomplished a wonderful job in demonstrating the extent of our refined cereal-induced diseases, and we must not be too critical of their failure to accept the facts that have been so successfully ignored by the medical profession in general.

According to *Thorpe's Dictionary of Chemistry,* xanthine is converted into alloxan by the action of flour bleach chemicals, or chlorine (as in drinking water). Alloxan is a specific poison for the Islets of Langerhans (causing diabetes) and Dr. Ugo Butturini has contributed a chapter on diabetes in the Shute book where he goes into much detail on the damage that can be done by alloxan, and he speculates on how it may be produced in the human body, but apparently he was not aware of this source. Since diabetes is known to be one of our most rapidly increasing diseases, and tends to become hereditary, we need to know the real cause as soon as possible.

Dr. E. V. Shute (page XV) notes that coronary disease was first recognized at autopsy in 1896 and now kills half the men dying over 50 years of age. Since the tocopherols are destroyed by flour bleaches (or any other oxidizing agent including chlorine in drinking water) it may be more than a coincidence that it appeared just as flour bleach was introduced, and its increase parallels the extent of the use of such poison. It is interesting to recall the efforts of Dr. Harvey W. Wiley, the first head of the Federal Food and Drug Administration, to stop the use of bleach poison, and that the U.S. Supreme Court concurred in a decision in 1918 that the use of any such poison in whatever small amount was illegal (But never enforced).

Here is a horrible price we are paying for a lack of integrity on the part of our law enforcement personnel. No wonder there are political pressures to block the acceptance of the hypothesis that vitamin E is needed in the metabolism of the human machine. No wonder that the Shutes were "unable to get their work published in any medical journal."

How long will it take for people in general — and the medical profession to realize that:

1. The human body cannot make something out of nothing?

2. The use of refined and demineralized foods causes our body to disintegrate. First, we lose our teeth, then may follow the common forms of gastric ulcer, arthritis, and heart disease (plus those listed previously).

3. Any poison added to food or drink is too much — we are being submitted to illegal mass experimentation when this rule is violated.

## SLANTED SCIENCE

It is quite interesting to watch the planted propaganda in our journals of "science" that diverts public opinion from the facts of life.

Recently (in *Agricultural and Food Chemistry,* Sept. 15, 1954, page 978) there appeared a report that purported to show that pasteurization had no effects on the nutritive properties of milk. If this report is right, Dr. F. M. Pottenger, Jr. was wrong when he observed that cats lost their teeth, became decalcified in bone structures, incurred liver disease, heart disease, constipation and stomach ulcers when fed pasteurized milk.

How did Bixby, Bosch, Elvehjem and Swanson succeed in getting opposite results?

Simply by rushing through short term experiments on short-lived animals like rats. It takes time for vitamin deficiency to do its dirty work. A rat can live all its life on the vitamin E it received from its mother. It the intake is cut in half, it no doubt could run several generations before it showed definite reactions. Chinchillas had to accumulate fluorine for several generations before they began to die spontaneously from the lethal accumulations.[1]

Are such gimmicked experiments common? Yes, quite. Aluminum was declared quite safe as a contaminant in food by careful tests in which the antidote was added to the ration along with the aluminum.[2]

In another case, vitamin E was declared ineffective where iron chloride was added to the ration to destroy the E.

And oleo has often been tested to show that it was a perfect food, but milk solids were used to afford the phospholipids otherwise essential and only available from honest natural fats, milk solids or butter. (Even purified casein carries enough of natural lipoprotein to avoid the deficiency reactions due to use of refined or synthetic hydrogenated counterfeit imitation fat.)

Elvehjem is known as a scientific Judas, the goat leading the sheep to slaughter. Once, he declared no trace element needed to be in an organic form to be useful in nutrition.[3] Only a few months later, it was found that cobalt could not be assimilated by the human unless in the organic form of vitamin $B_{12}$, and that we cannot live without it. Why believe him now?

There are simple clinical proofs of the evils of pasteurization. Rat tests are pure propaganda.

[1] *Chinchillas, Test Animals — or You and Your Grandchildren?* W. R. Cox — Lee Foundation

[2] *Lee Foundation Report No 5.*

[3] *A Critical Discussion of Trace Elements and Biodynamic Agriculture* (reprint free from Vitamin Products Company).

[5] *A Practical Way to Avoid Malnutrition* (reprint free from Vitamin Products Company).

THE STATEMENTS HEREIN MAY NOT AGREE WITH CURRENTLY ACCEPTED MEDICAL OPINION. NEVERTHELESS, THE PUBLISHER BELIEVES THEM SOUND.

**Edited by Royal Lee** **March 1955**

VITAMIN NEWS

VITAMIN PRODUCTS CO. • MILWAUKEE, WISCONSIN

VOL. 20

## MORE ABOUT

## "UNFITTING THE UNBORN"

Ex-President Herbert Hoover, in a radio interview on November 6, 1955, stated that the effects of starvation on a population created such mass damage that such people became a continuing liability to the world; that to save them, you had to get them young before irrevocable changes in their bodies had occurred, and that otherwise they "became the parents of the world's bandits and gangsters."

I know of no one who has had a better opportunity to see malnutrition in action. Children can be born with warped minds, as well as with warped bodies, as a result of the mother's ignorance of what honest food might be, and who has tried to live by eating counterfeits and imitations.

A good example is the retrolental fibroplasia that today is the main cause of infant blindness. The cause is unquestionably bleached flour. Bleach destroys vitamin E, so essential to prevent waste of oxygen in the tissues and prevent oxidation where it is not wanted. Exposing the baby to oxygen, such as is common with premature infants, precipitates the condition. It can be prevented by a better intake of vitamin E in test animals (p. 478, *Annual Review of Biochemistry,* 1955.).

A recent article in the *Journal of Clinical Nutrition* (July-August 1955) concludes with the comment, "The pathological states observed in vitamin E deficiencies have been suggested to result from the action of lipid peroxides on sulfhydryl-sensitive enzyme systems." It is significant that the best remedy to save eye tissue from developing opacities after injury is sulfhydryl, known to all eye doctors. The author of this article calls attention to the fact that lipid peroxides have also been found present in human venous diseases. (Edwin L. Hove, *Anti-Vitamin E Stress Factors as Related to Lipid Peroxides*, page 328.)

Whether or not you lost the sight of an eye after an accidental injury might depend on how much you had been cheated by counterfeit food makers, it appears. And the eyesight of your baby might be just as much a similar matter of how much the mother had been cheated in buying her food.

The tragic circumstance is accentuated by the fact that these defects, due to malnutrition, tend to be hereditary and require a number of well-fed succeeding generations to eliminate the tendency. This was well demonstrated in my paper "Malnutrition and Heredity — Unfitting the Unborn."

More evidence is available today. In *Science* (November 9, 1951, p. 479) you will find an article showing how the deficiency of only one of the B Complex vitamins can cause the following congenital abnormalities:

Facial, cranial and eye deformities, umbilical hernias, hydrochephalus, exencephalus, anencephalus, abdominal herniations, harelip, polydactylism, syndactylism, retardation in growth, misshapen bones, cleft palate, absence of ossification centers, and other deformities. *Drug Trade News* of May 25, 1952, reports cleft palate and skeletal deformities from riboflavin deficiency (page 36). Also note comment on page 308, *Annual Review of Biochemis-*

*try,* 1935.

These are a few of the penalties Mother Nature exacts for your departure from her plan and pattern of living, and the use of counterfeits of natural foodstuffs. These consequences are biological time bombs that we fix for ourselves. No sudden death from heart disease occurs unless there is a great contribution by accumulated food deficiencies. We let the counterfeit food promoter tell us that "There is no proof that there is any need for vitamin E complex," or whatever other vitamin is under discussion. Certainly, there never can be any such proof, until we put a few hundred human guinea pigs into cages and destroy them by an artificial deficiency. That dastardly liar who makes such a statement should be shipped to the Siberian salt mines. I know of no more acute punishment. He deserves the worst, for he is selling us down the river for his own measly welfare.

We can put you or any other subject into a chair and record your heart sounds on a tape and read off the various serious deficiencies, just as easy as we can record the sound of a ball-bearing in a machine and tell the operator just how many more months of service he is going to get. The same machine will do both jobs.

If one fraction of the E complex is seriously lacking, the second sound of the heart (in some microphone positions) may be entirely lacking. Supplying the victim with a tablet or two of this vitamin will bring back the sound in a few minutes.

Another fraction of the E complex has exactly the effect of nitroglycerin on the vascular system and relieves angina pains as quickly as the drug. But it is the physiological remedy, for which nitroglycerin is a poor substitute.

Another fraction of the B complex will correct skips, extra systoles and fibrillation, often effective in minutes. Another may stop valve leakages by restoring normal tone to the heart muscle, and again the change may take only a few minutes. There can be no argument as to these results. They correct the damages of starvation, and unless corrected, the patient is in danger and is dying by inches. All so totally unnecessary.

Everybody today is becoming cholesterol conscious; cholesterol in excess in the blood is so commonly a contributory cause to cardiovascular disease. Again, it is now discovered that a high blood cholesterol can be caused by one thing — by the use of synthetic fats in the diet. Feeding hydrogenated fat to rabbits, chickens or humans — the result was the same, a doubling of blood cholesterol.

How to reduce blood cholesterol? Simply use unrefined vegetable oils instead of the synthetic counterfeit, and the blood cholesterol may drop *below* normal.[1]

It has been said that it is the vitamin F content of the natural oil that is effective. We believe that is true, but do not confuse vitamin F with "unsaturated fatty acids." Such fatty acids may not have any vitamin activity. Only fresh extracts with no taint of rancidity can be expected to be of value. They must be made from sources of known clinical effectiveness. If you really want a good vegetable oil with natural vitamin content, you will have to liquify sesame seed in a liquefier and extract the oil in a small press or centrifugal juicer. (The juicer bowl will have to be lined with filter paper.)

All oils in the stores (except an unrefined oil in a health food store) have been refined and heat-treated to the point again of such diminishing nutritional value as to be pathetic. Olive oils may be the exception. Gallstones are cholesterol and olive oil dosage has been a remedy of long repute, but much maligned as a "quack remedy" by the surgeon. There is also something in beet leaf juice that helps to eliminate gall stones, at least to eliminate any symptoms of trouble. Two ounces twice a day (best in tomato juice) of beet leaf juice — cooked or raw — has immediate effects.

Natural fats with a high protective action against cholesterol are found in avocado, in all raw nuts, olives however prepared, raw peanut butter (made by liquefying raw peanuts in a liquefier with a little mustard and thousand island dressing or grating in a nut flaker and mixing separately), liquefied sesame seed (available as "tahini" in food stores, a staple Armenian and Turkish food), as the oil in all fresh ground cereals, whether whole wheat, rye or rice. (Beware of rice unless you know the source. We find all store rice, except that in some health food stores, is treated with methyl bromide, a poison that will remain absorbed in some degree if once exposed. We suggest you get organic rice direct from growers advertising in *Prevention* or *Natural Food and Farming*.)

[1] *Federation Proc.*, June 1955, p. 661, Kinsell and Michaels. *Food and Nutrition News,* October 1955, F. A. Kummerow, p. 1.

> "Knowing that vitamins act as components of enzymes in the body, we may visualize a vitamin deficiency and a defective gene having identical effects and leading to the same congenital abnormality." Page 131, *Bulletin of the National Research Council,* No. 123, Nov. 1950. "Maternal Nutrition and Child Health."

THE STATEMENTS HEREIN MAY NOT AGREE WITH CURRENTLY ACCEPTED MEDICAL OPINION. NEVERTHELESS, THE PUBLISHER BELIEVES THEM SOUND.

**Edited by Royal Lee** **January 1956**

# NOTES

VITAMIN NEWS

VITAMIN PRODUCTS CO. • MILWAUKEE, WISCONSIN

VOL. 20

## COUNTERFEIT FOODS

## AND THE MEN WHO FRONT FOR THEM

In the April issue of the *Journal of the Southern California Dental Association* you will find two articles by Dr. Lucien A. Bavetti ("Sugar — Natural or Refined" and "Food Faddism") with an editorial on them entitled "Debunk and 'D' Truth" by Dr. J. C. A. Harding.

Both of these worthy gentlemen seem to be ignorant of the basic principles of nutritional science. To get all the cards on the table, let me set up a few principles that I defy any authority to twist, to use as a measuring stick to see how far these fellows have departed from the established facts and principles.

1. All animal life, including man, must depend upon organic foods elaborated by the plant kingdom. The plant and its symbionts build up inorganic materials, minerals, air and carbon dioxide by the aid of the Sun's energy into the tremendously complex foods all animal and human life absolutely depend on for its existence; animal and human life being the opposite of plant life in that instead of building up inorganic materials into organic, it reverses this process and breaks down the organic compounds into simpler ones and releases the energy they contain for their support and activity. All this was designed and consummated long before man was aware of the process, and who is just now becoming somewhat aware of the complex patterns of its operation.

These organic foods are like charged electric batteries; the energy they contain can be released by the animal cell and the energy put to work. When a horse draws a plow, he is using this energy. When we use our muscles, we are releasing the energy of the Sun put into the food we eat by the Sun's rays. When we think, we are using the same energy in another way.

2. All foods are complexes of almost infinite variety and form. They are living mechanisms, not inert chemicals.

Proteins are the living fractions of plant or animal cells, incapable of supporting human or animal life if destroyed by heat or otherwise.

Fats are complex assemblies that contain not only fuel, but also vital vitamins and phospholipids, many of which are incomprehensible to the chemist because they are again, complex mechanisms, not chemicals, just as a watch is a mechanism, not a piece of brass, but to the chemist would be crudely categorized as "organized brass." Yes, organized to do a job, that of keeping time. Organic foods are organized to keep our brains functioning as well as to keep us warm. A chemist might as well try to make a synthetic watch out of brass without the assistance of a watchmaker, as for him to try to make a synthetic food without the assistance of the plant kingdom.

Carbohydrates are just as complex, in fact no natural carbohydrate is found without accompanying natural fats, vitamins, and phospholipids, essential to its use by man.

Vitamins and minerals are in plant tissues, parts of enzyme systems, and enzymes are the living mechanisms of the cell. To remove one single component — say ascorbic acid — and call it a vitamin is asinine in its concept, for every vitamin is again a complex of partners and synergists.

No victim of malnutrition is ever deficient in one such chemical. He will be deficient in a whole array of factors, for if he has used refined foods, he will be deficient in dozens of single factors that might be described by a chemist who has investigated food composition. But only a nutritionist who has studied food reactions in the human subject could act intelligently in setting up a remedial diets, and synthetic chemicals would have no place in his recommendations, for chemicals are not food. As before, only a watchmaker can correct malfunctions in a watch, not the chemist who might know all about its composition, and who might not even know what the actual function of the watch might be.

Foods only become chemicals after they have been taken apart, each component carefully purified, any impurities still left carefully assayed and put on the label. A chemical must be of known composition. To assay every food before use to convert it into a chemical would destroy its usefulness as a food, just as a watch after the chemist has taken it apart is no longer a watch, but still the same material chemically.

Drs. Harding and Bavetti would have us believe:

There is nothing wrong with synthetic foods.

Natural sweets are just as bad as refined sweets in causing dental caries.

Natural and refined foods are of equivalent value, nutritionally.

As to the first statement — if synthetic food is capable of supporting life, we no longer need the plant kingdom in all its complexity to support us. Synthetic "foods" are in general, vicious and insulting counterfeits. What are a few? Hydrogenated fats, oleo, phony "vegetable" shortening, all hydrogenated oils that should be called "death foods" by law because they cannot possibly act as natural fat does. In careful tests on rabbits, chickens and human subjects, these hydrogenated "death food" fats caused a great rise in blood cholesterol, where honest unrefined vegetable oils reduced the blood cholesterol. What is the significance of a high blood cholesterol? Simply that it helps to bring on heart disease and sudden death.

Another synthetic food used to dilute and adulterate many real foods is glucose (corn sugar, dextrose). It, like hydrogenated fats, has no food value, unless you consider calories alone food, which I do not. Who ever needs calories alone? You cannot eat calories alone without cheating yourself of the minerals and vitamins that normally should accompany those calories, and furthermore, you no doubt are trying to get nutrition without calories alone; for the universal disease, if there is one, is overweight, the doctors tell us caused by too many calories.

And about natural sweets — Dr. Weston A. Price once related in a letter to me how an island colony had no tooth decay, though they almost lived on sugar cane. But after a sugar refinery was set up, they developed the same universal tendency to tooth decay we see here. The tests reported by Dr. Bavetti were not honest tests; refined foods were a part of the food pattern of the persons involved. Sugar cane juice cannot stop tooth decay if the victim is still eating white bread. Dr. Pottenger in his famous cat tests found pasteurized milk still caused arthritis, loss of teeth, gastric ulcers, etc., regardless of raw meat feeding. Crooked tests like this are a part and parcel of the counterfeit food racket. I could write a book about the gimmicks used to create false results. "Figures don't lie, but liars figure."

Now, about natural vs. refined foods, in general. Our worst offenders are refined cereals, white flour, etc. Flour has had its germ removed. Why? Because the oil in the germ goes rancid in a few days, destroys the flavor, and in fact, renders stale whole wheat flour with its rancid oil, a poison instead of a food. Rancid oils act to cause muscular dystrophies, heart disease and various kinds of nerve paralysis. Cereal oils go rancid in a very short time after the grain is crushed or ground. That is why no bread can be wholesome unless made from fresh flour. That is why animals will not eat the stale cereal foods we use, unless starved into the necessity. On top of this, we eat flour and bread bleached with a vicious chemical, an oxidizing agent that hastens rancidity and that converts part of the vitamin fraction of the cereal into a poison that specifically causes diabetes. (All bleaches convert xanthine into alloxan.)

It is a first principle of all pure food laws that the addition of any poison, regardless of the smallness of the amount, to any food or drink is a criminal violation of law. The U.S. Supreme Court has concurred in this. Still, we are forced to eat such foods. Why? Simply because such creatures as Dr. Harding and Dr. Bavetta spout off with such weasel words as you will find in the articles in question, as the mouthpieces for their professional society.

For forty years, we were fed in our butter tons and tons of the vicious carcinogenic agent "butter yellow." No doubt that is an important reason why cancer is more prevalent in countries where the most of this, "butter yellow," carcinogenic butter and yellow cheeses were eaten. As far as I have been able to discover, butter yellow was never made for any other important purpose by the coal tar industry. Every ounce of the butter so colored with cancer-causing coal tar dye was colored for the purpose of deceiving the buyer of the butter as to its quality. Every ounce was a criminal fraud, intended to get money by false pretenses. Even if the most harmless of dyes were used, it would still be a criminal fraud. The buyer is entitled to get what he pays for. The highly-colored spring butter from cows getting new grass always commanded a higher price, so the butter industry decided it would make all butter look as "nice." They didn't know the gun was loaded. But the victims were just as dead as if killed by a robber's gun. In this case, it was a "robber's gun.".

The apologizers for the counterfeit food makers always deny that we have any deaths in this country from food deficiencies. They refuse to admit that our 700,000 deaths from heart disease can be due to white flour and refined sugar and synthetic fats, even though countries that do not get these foods do not have these diseases. Along with poliomyelitis, only in countries eating death foods do we have these deaths.

I cannot believe that the executive management of the American Dental Association and the American Medical Association is unaware of these basic facts.

The truth is evident to any doctor who takes the trouble to record the heart sounds of almost any person. Evidences of degenerative changes in the way of valve leakage, muscular in-coordination, muscular degeneration, fibrillation, skipping beats, split sounds, disappearance of the second sound and many other aberrations are common, which usually improve or disappear on the administration of a few tablets of natural vitamin concentrates of the cereal germ vitamins. There can be no argument about the whole matter. If the 700,000 people who die each year could have been reached by these tests, there is no question that 90% could have been saved.

It is this counter-publicity by such stooges as Drs. Harding and Bavetti that stops the doctors and their patients from knowing that they are suffering from a simple form of starvation, and that their condition is easily treated by better food.

Dr. Bavetti remarks that patients become victims of "quacks and food faddists" after their doctor has told them that they have an incurable disease, and that "I am sorry, there is nothing that we can do about it."

The real quack here is the medical man who is not permitted to tell his patient that he is starving to death. Medical treatment anyway is the cult that is obsessed with the idea that most disease can be treated with poisons — do not forget that the official definition of a medicine is that it first must be a poison. (See Foundation Report 26A.) That is a part of the whole essential principle of the control exercised over the medical and dental professions by the food industry racketeers, and for whom Drs. Harding and Bavetti are mouthpieces.

As I write this, I note in the *St. Louis Globe-Democrat* (Oct. 10, 1955) that Dr. W. S. Priest, President of the American College of Cardiology, at the meeting of the St. Louis Academy of General Practitioners, announced that the cause of heart disease is the building up of fat molecules into large sizes that causes blocking and clotting in blood vessels. He said: "When we find out how to homogenize these fat molecules of the human blood, we will have the answer."

And in the *Kansas City Star* of October 18, Dr. William Dock tells us too much fat in the diet is the cause of the "arteriosclerosis that accounts for so many heart attacks, brain strokes, and kidney failures."

These men have not heard that it is the phospholipids in natural vegetable oils that absolutely prevent any such building up of large fat molecules. All phospholipids are emulsifying agents, "homogenizers," that promote the transport of cholesterol and other fatty materials in the body fluids. Without a proper supply of these phospholipids, cholesterol and fats cannot remain in suspension, cause gall-stones as well as the heart disease etc. here listed by the best medical authorities, who are so abysmally ignorant in nutritional science, and who never would admit that the synthetic shortenings and oleo we are criminally swindled with are the basic cause of the appalling incidence of heart disease, so peculiar to America.

A most remarkable piece of dishonesty is Dr. Bavetti's claim that soil deficiencies do not matter — crops and milk from cows fed poor feed may have no less nutritional value than those produced on the most fertile soil. This idea is also being promoted by other men who certainly should know better — Dr. Maynard at Cornell, for one. They get away with this lie by citing tests on milk showing the same chemical content regardless of the feed given to the cow. But they say nothing about the fact that the cow robs her body to maintain milk quality. Cows in Florida, where the soil is worst, live only one-fourth as long as if fed better feed. It requires carefully planned crookedness to weasel these facts, I would say. Then, Dr. Bavetti cites all the government authorities to show where "reliable" information can be obtained. Sure! Write to the Food & Drug Administration. Who is the executive director? The vice president of a leading death food flour milling company in Minneapolis. Certainly, he will see that you are properly informed to shorten your life by adding to his volume of businesses. He will warn you against "food faddists" who do not believe in counterfeit foods, being in the counterfeit business himself. He will not tell you that in Germany a few years ago, when it was found that flour bleaches destroyed vitamin E, the practice was quickly stopped. He will not tell you that our own U.S. Supreme Court in 1918 said that flour bleaching was a criminal act, a violation of the Federal Pure Food Law, and that his job is to see that the law is not enforced. I imagine about thirty million deaths can be directly charged against these careful planners of propaganda against "health food quacks." The Southern California Dental Association should be a little less than proud of these Judas front-men for the counterfeit food industry. Dr. Pikerill in 1911 said that all dental disease was a result of the use of counterfeit foodstuffs. Are they underwriting more business for themselves by supporting these food crooks?

Drs. Harding and Bavetti may not like these plain words, but when they call believers in honest natural foods "quacks and faddists," the quacks and faddists are entitled to a public hearing to find out exactly who is a quack and what makes him tick. The billions of dollars invested in counterfeit food rackets seem to be quite well in control of both the AMA and its aping sister the ADA. The AMA has quite a history of criminal activity. Do not forget it was fined for trying to set up a monopoly of medicine and surgery in Washington D.C. a few years back, and was later again convicted at the state level for the same offense in the State of Washington.

## HOW COUNTERFEIT FOODS PRODUCE DEFECTIVE OFFSPRING — THE PRICE WE PAY FOR OUR COMPLACENT ACCEPTANCE OF THE PROPAGANDA PUT OUT BY FOOD RACKETEERS

Test animals subjected to deficient diets give birth to offspring having deformities "similar to those that occur in humans:" cleft palate, harelip, clubfoot, missing bones or fingers, or excess numbers of fingers or toes, as well as "deformities of heart, blood vessels, bones, brains, eyes, kidneys and sex organs."
(*Science News Letter*, Jan. 28, 1956.)

This article goes on to say that there is no evidence that humans encounter such severe deficiencies as these test animals were subjected to. This I emphatically differ with. The fact that human mothers do give birth to offspring having these exact deformities seems reason enough to suspect the same cause. Plus the fact that many mothers actually live on refined foods and soft drinks entirely, while pregnant, not knowing the penalty for their indifference to the facts of life. They are sublimely indifferent to the obvious axiom that you cannot make something out of nothing.

The above article winds up with this statement: "The mother test animals did not suffer despite the effect on the young. They gained in weight and remained in good health throughout the experiments."

"Nature will never let you down — if you are intelligent enough to be faithful.."
—— Edward Yoemans

THE STATEMENTS HEREIN MAY NOT AGREE WITH CURRENTLY ACCEPTED MEDICAL OPINION. NEVERTHELESS, THE PUBLISHER BELIEVES THEM SOUND.

**Edited by Royal Lee** **April 1956**

# NOTES

# VITAMIN NEWS

VITAMIN PRODUCTS CO. • MILWAUKEE, WISCONSIN

VOL. 20


## POLIOMYELITIS AS A DEFICIENCY DISEASE

The resemblance of poliomyelitis to beriberi has been recently remarked by McCormick.[1] He suggests that the paralysis of polio may be directly due to vitamin $B_1$ deficiency, and that a virus infection of the nervous tissue involved should be suspected.

As far back as July 9, 1916, the possible deficiency background of poliomyelitis was suspected by Professor Simon Baruch, who may be quoted: "There is a striking similarity in some of the causes predisposing to infantile paralysis and beriberi. Both occur chiefly in overcrowded localities, in hot weather, and more among males than females. Both are accompanied by fever and paralysis, and both are extremely fatal. Both have prevailed as epidemics, and their fatality has caused terror and despair.

"Beriberi was formerly regarded as an infectious disease from undiscoverable sources, but is now known to be due chiefly, if not solely, to absence of vitamins in the diet.

"May not infantile paralysis, which has eluded thus far the most searching investigations, be likewise traceable to some defect in diet that may be discovered?

"It is not a new idea that beriberi, as well as polio, may develop from an infective agent. In fact, many early experimenters isolated various bacilli from the tissues of beriberi patients and reproduced definite symptoms of beriberi by injecting the cultures into test animals."[2] If a virus were present and acted as the real causative agent as a contaminant of invisible nature in each case, it would account for the wrangle among the different early investigators, each of whom were sure that their own variety of bacteria was the cause of the disease, and which disagreement resulted in the abandonment entirely of the whole idea on an infectious cause, and the establishment of the deficiency theory.

Tuberculosis today is accepted as an infectious disease, which has a primary cause, lowered resistance secondary to malnutrition. Originally, when the bacterial nature of the immediate cause was first discovered, it was assumed that the immediate cause was the primary cause.

In beriberi, it is quite possible that the infective cause has still to be identified, as our knowledge of virus diseases is in its infancy.

But in the case of polio, it is pretty well established today that it is actually a virus disease. Burnet tells us that carriers are known (usually children) who are apparently healthy, but continually excrete polio virus by the faecal route.[3] This virus then acts to infect susceptible individuals.

The next question is, "Why does the victim become susceptible?" We may find clues in the behavior of other virus diseases, for example, herpes simplex, also discussed by Burnet. This virus is known to continually exist in the patient's body throughout life, once the subject is inoculated, and the antibody is found in the blood of a constantly higher percentage of patients tested in increasing age levels.

Now it is definitely known that the symptoms of herpes simplex are never exhibited unless the patient has a lowered content of calcium in his tissue fluids. Factors that increase blood calcium at the expense of tissue fluid calcium aggravate herpes simplex, and factors that accomplish the opposite quickly eliminate herpes simplex. (Vitamers D and F, respectively, accomplish this — D increases blood calcium content and F vitamin reduces it by diffusion into the tissues. These effects are supplementary, rather than antagonistic, and natural sources of vitamer D, such as fish oils, are known to carry definitely active components of the F vitamer. The normal action is for the vitamer D to accelerate intestinal calcium absorption by the blood stream, and for the vitamer F to unload the cargo at the destination.[4] The effect of the D without the F is usually an aggravation of herpes.

Doctors Reese and Frisch (of Madison, Wisconsin) have promoted a theory that polio virus often enters the subject through tooth cavities, offering as evidence the fact that in a survey of 272 polio victims, cavities were present in 2.6 times the number of a comparable group of non-infected persons. Further, that in communities having fluoride enough in the water to reduce tooth decay to 75% of normal, polio incidence was 22 to 34% less than usual.

This evidence, however, may also be adduced to mean that where more calcium was metabolized, there was not only less tooth disease, but less polio, for natural fluoridated water contains calcium fluoride.

Dr. McCormick points out that the demineralization of flour by the roller mill was to be suspected as a major cause of polio. In fact, he points out that the first roller mill to manufacture white de-germinated flour was set up in Vienna in 1839, and the first case of polio reported was found there in 1840.

The effect of muscular exercise in precipitating an attack of polio is also explainable, in that the muscle sugar reserves burned up thereby are held as phosphagen and loss of the sugar component releases phosphorus ions, which, in turn, can combine with the diffusible calcium bicarbonate moiety, and lower the diffusible calcium of the tissue fluids below the critical point. This form of calcium seems essential to the control of virus activity.

At this moment, it is important that we grasp the full significance of the concept of tissue reaction to malnutrition, by which the receptivity to specific agents is produced. Crotti, in his lifetime study of goiter and thyroid disease, looked for and seems to have unquestionably found, a specific micro-organism that exists in all goiters, and which causes goiter, if injected into healthy thyroids. But the presence of this organism does not preclude the accuracy of the conclusion that all goiter is a consequence of deficiency. Crotti found that he could cure goiter with bichloride of mercury about as easily as with iodine.[5] That certainly does not justify the treatment of goiter with this drug; in similar fashion, malnutrition consequences in general may be successfully treated by various substitutes for the physiological remedy, and medical science has not fully awakened yet to its obligation to see that such mistakes are not too common. A good example of such a mistake is the treatment of infective diseases with sulfa drugs, which accomplish their effects solely by drawing into the blood stream vitamin C, which thereby stimulates the phagocytic elimination of the micro-organisms. It is obvious that the use of sulfa drugs is made necessary only by a deficiency of the vitamin, and a too great deficiency in a patient will cause a failure of the drug, and instead of recovery, death will follow. The vitamin could never cause harm, and should be given first, and the sulfa only used as a last resort.[6]

[1] McCormick, W. J., M.D., *Medical Record*, February 4, 1942.
[2] McCarrison, *Studies in Deficiency Disease*, Oxford Press, 1921.
[3] Burnet, F. M., *Virus as Organism*, Harvard University Press, 1945, p. 60.
[4] *Calcium Metabolism*, Lee Foundation for Nutritional Research, Milwaukee, Wisconsin, Report #3.

[5] Crotti, Andre, M.D., *Diseases of the Thyroid, Parathyroids and Thymus*, Lea & Febiger, 1938.
[6] *Vitamin News*, Vitamin Products Company, Milwaukee, p. 154.

THE STATEMENTS HEREIN MAY NOT AGREE WITH CURRENTLY ACCEPTED MEDICAL OPINION. NEVERTHELESS, THE PUBLISHER BELIEVES THEM SOUND.

**Edited by Royal Lee** **May 1956**

# NOTES

# VITAMIN NEWS

CATALYN — NATURES SOURCE OF VITALITY — MADE IN U.S.A.

VITAMIN PRODUCTS CO. • MILWAUKEE, WISCONSIN

VOL. 20

## THE ENDOCARDIOGRAPH AS AN INDICATOR OF NUTRITIONAL DEFICIENCIES

As many types of nutritional deficiency affect the heart, it is evident that any instrument that affords an exact indication of the heart performance should be valuable as a "deficiency indicator."

Outstanding amount these deficiency reactions are:

1. Vitamin F. As a calcium ionizing agent, it provides diffusible calcium for the use of muscular tissue, without which the muscle contractions become reduced in range, (total deficiency causing tetany) so that in the heart, the power to complete the contraction cycle is limited, and the cycle is not completed, the second sound on the cardiographic being weak or totally absent. The administration of vitamin F and calcium lactate brings back the normal cycle within ten minutes. (See Fig. 1) It is understandable why calcium lactate and vitamin F are the first thoughts in "That tired feeling." (The C complex is the next to think of.)

FIG. 1 MRS. W. B. - AGE 23

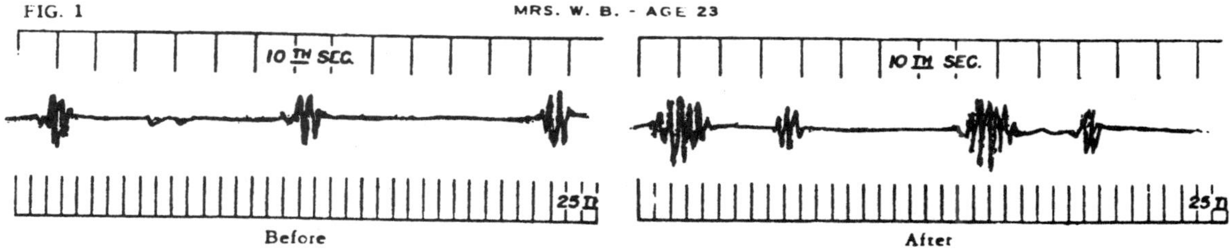


2. Vitamin C. The most important part of the C complex is tyrosinase, (organic copper) (just as $B_{12}$ is organic cobalt) which is essential to all muscle, and the heart muscle in particular, which undergoes "atrophy with replacement fibrosis" in case of a lack of enough of this element.[1] Where the heart shows a greatly increased contraction time, indicating an overworked (incompetent) muscle, natural vitamin C complex (containing tyrosinase) affords a spectacular change, both in the cardiogram as well as in the sate of the patient, who usually remarks about the disappearance of the "shortness of breath" sensation (Fig.2).

FIG. 2 A. P. - AGE 19

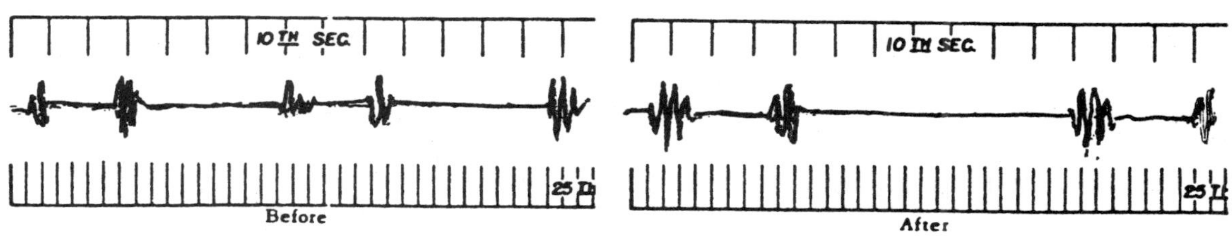


3. B Complex deficiency. Here we stressed the $B_4$ factor, the one that prevents nerve paralysis, or loss of conduction power. In the heart, this shows up as a loss of coordination between the various muscular areas so that a split first sound is the first sign, due to delay in part of the heart muscle to respond to the contraction impulse. Fibrillation is the final result of this deficiency. Fig. 3 shows the improvement in a few minutes of a patient with fibrillation after taking a few tablets

of natural B complex. (No synthetic product we have seen has favorably affected a cardiogram.) Fig. 4 shows the change in a split sound in ten minutes.

By its essential influence in maintaining nerve conduction, $B_4$ is a key factor in preventing heart dilatation or enlargement. This distorts the heart valves, and causes leakage (regurgitation) as exhibited by murmurs. As soon as the heart contracts to normal, the leakage stops. We have seen congenital causes of heart leakage permanently repaired by the B complex, after being kept under treatment for some years by the use of this vitamin.

FIG. 3

MRS. H. E. - AGE 65

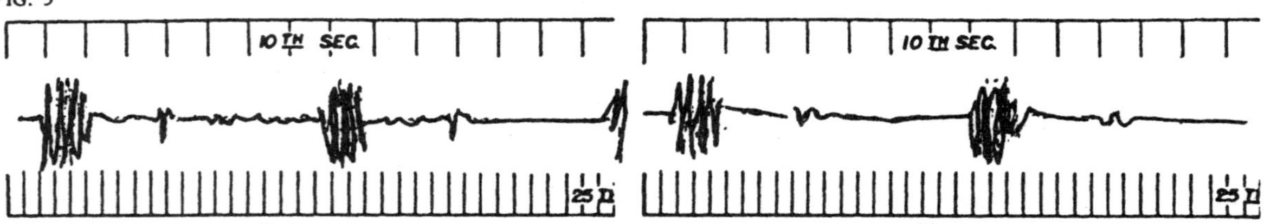


Before After

FIG. 4

B. B. - AGE 27

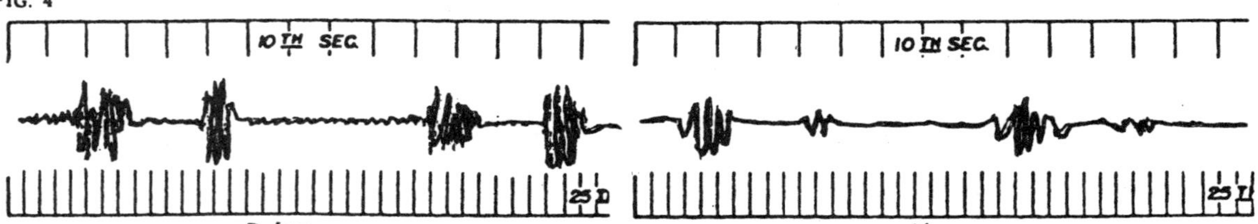


Before After

4. Vitamin $E_2$ complex. Since in vitamin E deficiency the tissue demand for oxygen may rise 250%,[2] it is important to prevent such a load from being imposed on any heart, much less a weakened and diseased one. Plus the fact that vitamin E deficiency specifically causes necrosis of heart muscle fibers.[3]

It is easy to see how vitamin E deficiency results in sudden death, the heart muscle is undermined and the load is increased at the same time. A special fraction of the E complex ($E_2$) has an effect quite similar to nitroglycerin, long used as a drug to relieve the pains of angina pectoris, a cramp-like attack that may be fatal. Angina pectoris is in all probability as specific a deficiency disease as scurvy.

5. Vitamin G complex. This is the protein-linked group of the B vitamin family. It has the opposite effect of thiamin and its synergists in that it relaxes muscular tissue, with particular effect on the coronary arteries, probably by its activation of the adrenal functions. (The pantothenic acid phase.) (Adrenalin tones up most arteries, but relaxes the coronary.) The patient with a "coronary thrombosis" is the victim we believe of this specific deficiency. At least the "coronary" patient gets remarkable relief in a short time (characterized by a disappearance or reduction in the "arm pains" and heart pains, if any with other symptomatic improvement) after getting started on a schedule of vitamin G complex. Fig. 5 shows the changes obvious in the Endocardiograph recording. Possibly the commonest of the heart reaction might be called "bleached flour disease." It is no doubt preceded by years of an enhanced pulmonary second sound, which suggests pulmonary hypertension and coronary spasticity — the syndrome of weakened adrenal function. The victim reports a "tight feeling in the chest" on exertion. (See Fig. 5 for normal pulmonary position sound, and this accentuated second sound.)

FIG. 5 J. B. - AGE 24

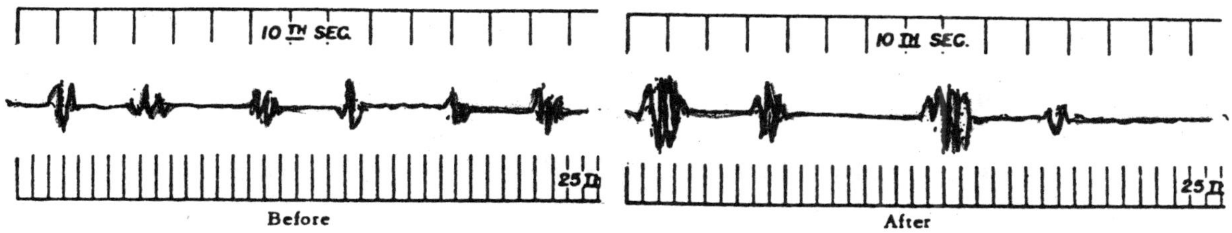


6. Potassium deficiency. Characterized by tachycardia, paroxysmal tachycardia in acute form. Potassium is absorbed from the blood by the stowing away of sugar after heavy carbohydrate meals and this can bring on heart laboring and tachycardia. Victims of this reaction should eliminate from their diet, especially the evening meal, all sugar and sugar products. The overloaded heart may be pushed beyond its limit, many a death called "acute indigestion" is in part at least due to this set of circumstances. Without blood potassium, the normal autonomic control of the heart is lost. It is an "engine without a generator" and may race to destruction.

This heart racing has been attributed to hyperinsulinism, but is purely potassium deficiency. Sugar is stored as phosphagen (instead of glycogen). Phosphagen is "di-potassium creatine hexose phosphate," a compound that is as loaded with energy as gunpowder for those who do little work and do not use up their stores of calories regularly. Too much phosphagen seems to make the human body as combustible as guncotton. Cases are on record of rapid combustion of living victims.

Normal metabolism releases the potassium into the blood again as the sugar is consumed, ready for the next mealtime load of sugar, but if the potassium intake is limited, the shortage can result in the serous state above described.

The remedy is tablets of organic minerals having the usual preponderance of potassium, or some "potassium broth," potato juice and alfalfa tea being high in this element.

## REFERENCES

[1] Bennets, H. W.. A. B., and Harley R., On the Pathogenesis of "Falling Disease," *Australian Vet. Jol.*, 24:237, 1948.
[2] Houchin, O. B., and Matrill, H. A., *Proc. Soc. Exper. Biol. Med.*, 50:216-18, 1942.
[3] Mason, K. E., and Emmel, A. F., *Vitamin E and Muscle Pigment in the Rat, Anat.* Rec., 92:33, 1945.

## FOOD SOURCES OF THE VITAMIN FACTORS LISTED

Vitamin F: All seed and cereal oils, but only if fresh and unprocessed. Wheat germ oil, soy bean oil, peanut oil, sesame oil. If stale, the rancidity destroys both the vitamin E and F content. The rancid oils in commercial cereal products, bread etc., seem to be the main cause of F and E deficiency. The oil in whole wheat flour becomes rancid inside of two weeks after milling. That is why flour is de-germinated and refined, the rancid oils otherwise cause the consumer to dislike the product automatically.

Vitamin C and tyrosinase: Potatoes and mushrooms are the best sources.

Vitamin B complex: Fresh whole wheat flour, the $B_4$ so important is available only from fresh seed germs.

Vitamin E complex: Same as F. In fact, F is a fraction of the natural E complex.

Vitamin G complex: Fresh whole wheat and other cereal and seed germs. Meat sources include the liver, kidney and sweetbreads, calf brain.

## COMMERCIAL SOURCES OF CONCENTRATES OF THE VITAMINS LISTED

Vitamin B available as CATAPLEX B (V-P 712)* or as VITAMIN B COMPLEX (C-Y 1712)**

Vitamin C available as CATAPLEX C (V-P 713)* or as VITAMIN C COMPLEX (C-Y 1713)**

Vitamin $E_2$ available as CATAPLEX $E_2$ (V-P 732)* or as VITAMIN $E_2$ (C-Y) 1732)**

Vitamin F available as CATAPLEX F (V-P 716)* or as VITAMIN F COMPLEX (C-Y 1716)**

Vitamin G available as CATAPLEX G (V-P 717)* or as VITAMIN G COMPLEX (C-Y 1717)**

Organic potassium available as MINAPLEX (V-P 721)* or as ORGANIC MINERALS (C-Y 1721)**

* *Vitamin Products Company, Milwaukee 1, Wisconsin*
** *Therapeutic Foods Company, Milwaukee 2, Wisconsin*

THE STATEMENTS HEREIN MAY NOT AGREE WITH CURRENTLY ACCEPTED MEDICAL OPINION. NEVERTHELESS, THE PUBLISHER BELIEVES THEM SOUND.

**Edited by Royal Lee** **October 26, 1956**

# Index

# C



# D

# S



# T

# X



# Y

# IFNH Recommended Clinical Reading List

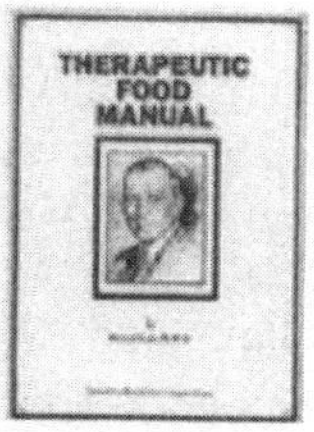


**Therapeutic Food Manual – Royal Lee, DDS**

A reprint of Dr. Lee's "finalized" treatment protocols. After some introductory material, it presents an alphabetical list of most illness classifications. Included under each listing are: a general description, a treatment protocol, physiological considerations, synergistic products and coordination suggestions. A highly recommended "source" for the practitioner developed by the "nutritional genius" himself. [#1101 $39.95]

**The Product Bulletins – Royal Lee, DDS**

The original guideline articles for the Standard Process products developed by Dr. Lee. It gives an in-depth presentation on each of the "early" products. A useful work to understand the background of Dr. Lee's approach to treatment with nutrition. [#1102 $34.95]

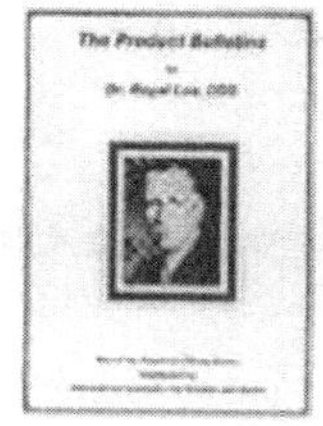

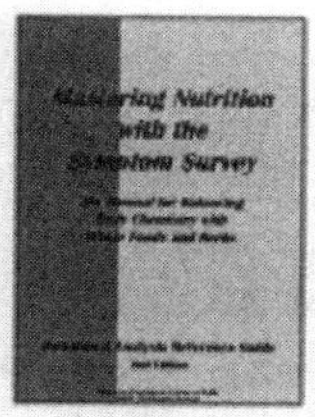

**Mastering Nutrition with the Symptom Survey – IFNH**

The manual for balancing body chemistry using the Symptom Survey is a must for any healthcare practitioner learning nutrition. This complete workbook consists of several sections including a full description and commentary regarding symptoms, biochemistry and balancing nutrition. Contemporary research and commentary for this manual are due largely to the contributions of Jeremy Kaslow, MD, Michael Dobbins, DC, Bruce Pacetti, DDS, Leo Roy, MD, ND, Bruce West, DC, and Robert Peshek, DDS. [#2701 $35.00]

**Health vs Disease – Melvin E. Page, DDS and H. Leon Abrams, Jr.**

A clear general presentation of the variables affecting health. Although an older manuscript, it still provides a thorough background to the basics of body chemistry. Almost all of the information provided is still applicable and practical. Like all classic works, it stands out despite the passage of time and further knowledge gained with modern research. [#1201 $16.95]

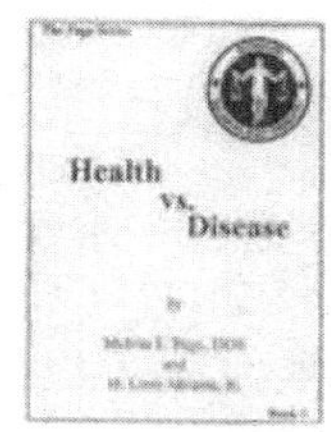


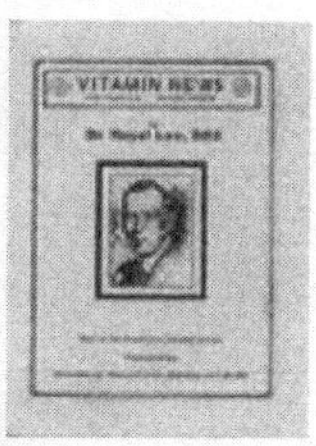


**Vitamin News – Royal Lee, DDS**

A compilation of all the newsletters published by the Vitamin Products Co. Milwaukee, Wisconsin. These monthly newsletters provide useful information to support the practitioner. They offered a wide range of topics Dr. Lee thought were necessary to understand nutrition therapy during the 1930s, 40s, and 50s. [#1106 $39.95]

**Clinical Reference Guide**

An updated guide to the Standard Process product line. It has a section for each product that provides the following information: formulation, indications for use, synergists, and a descriptive sketch by long-time Standard Process biochemist, John Courtney. Mr. Courtney worked with Dr. Lee and directed research and development after Dr. Lee's death. The final section covers additional topics that support the practitioner in using the individual products, including a treatment protocol guide, best known as "the gray pages", and tests from Foundations of Nutritional Therapy course. [#2501 $19.00]

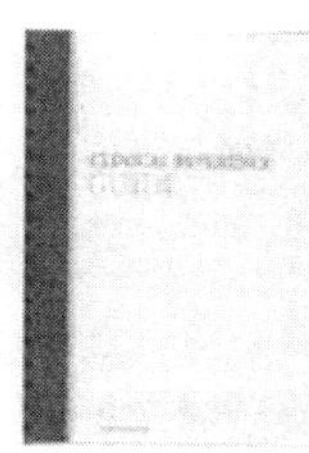

**International Foundation for Nutrition and Health**
3963 Mission Blvd.
San Diego, CA 92109
Tel (858) 488-8932
Fax (858) 488-2566

A Tax-Exempt Non-Profit Organization



E-mail: ifnh@ifnh.org
Website: www.ifnh.org

# Announcing the IFNH Professional Membership Program

***Time To Act***

Patients need the right answers to stay healthy. On a daily basis, they're bombarded with so much confusing and contradictory information about their food choices, their lifestyles, and medications that they often don't know what to do. As a result, the health statistics are worsening. According to recent headlines, we have more children in our school systems than ever before that are suffering from childhood diabetes, ADD, and ADHD. To top it off, childhood obesity is approaching epidemic proportions. The newest adult statistics on heart disease and cancer are that 37% of us can look forward to dying of heart disease and 25% of us can look forward to dying of cancer. If that isn't sobering enough, another 4% of us can look forward to dying from complications from prescription drugs that we are told will make us better.

Another recent headline showed a study by Georgetown University stating that most patient testing was useless and uncalled for. These tests frequently produce "false positives", leading to more testing and anxiety, costing taxpayers billions of dollars a year. No wonder our healthcare system is collapsing.

How can your practice help pull people out of this vicious cycle and give them the right answers to stay healthy?

***New Professional Program***

In response to your requests, the Foundation is launching a New Professional Membership Program that will focus on practice management and patient support, with a special emphasis on the Foundation of Nutritional Therapies (FNT) seminar series.

When we were lecturing around the country with the FNT course, some of you might remember an example I used of two successful practitioners. One saw over 100 patients a day and the other saw between 20-25 a day. They both did well over a quarter of a million dollars a year and this was back in the late 1980's. They had two very different practices. One practitioner sold a little bit of nutrition to a lot of people but didn't manage to keep patients long term. The other practitioner created patients who ordered product from him on their maintenance program for years and his patient list continued to grow.

Was one right, and the other wrong? I think not. But today, what you keep asking for is, "How do I get my practice running smoother and create long-term patients?" That doesn't happen by just giving them a protocol. It only happens when you have educated your patients to be better patients. This requires creating a system for you and your staff that works! With that you can have the long-term success you've been looking for!

***THE BENEFITS OF PROFESSIONAL MEMBERSHIP:***

- Special access to the fast-track certification program in whole food nutrition
- Free subscription to *The Perfect Crime* Health Report.
- Access to referrals of like-minded healthcare professionals from around the country
- Access to the newly formed IFNH team of Practice Management and Clinical Consultants
- Access to the twice-monthly discussion groups on practice management and patient education.
- Discounts on selected seminars, lectures and workshops.
- Access to liability insurance
- Certified Professional Member Certificate
- Patient referrals. Additional discounts on selected catalog items (over regular membership)
- For only $360, you will have access to thousands of dollars worth of tools and consulting.

Help support IFNH, the only independent nutrition foundation in the world that is dedicated to the healthcare practitioner and whole food nutrition.

***Make the professional membership work for you!*** Join IFNH's fall lineup right in your own office with speakers like Jeremy Kaslow MD., Jay Robbins DC., Ernie Caldwell DC., Holly Carling OMD, Lac, Phd, Art Capperauld DC., Ray Bisesi DC., and Kim Schuette CN. This faculty will oversee the FNT seminar series, as well as new modules especially designed for patient education and practice management. As a member who has taken or is in the process of taking the FNT series you are on the fast track to a certification in whole food nutrition CCWFN. (Check web site ***ifnh.org*** more information)

***The Perfect Crime Health Report.*** Most of you have read or heard of Mary Frost's book, *Going Back to the Basics of Human Health.* For those of you who haven't tried using it as a patient support tool, I highly recommend it. In fact, we have one doctor who says he got 52 referrals from one book (don't give it away!). Mary's newest offering, The Perfect Crime Health Reports will educate you and your patients on issues that are threatening your health that most people don't really understand the scope of. ***(Get your free sample report on our web site www.ifnh.org).***

***Join Us Today and Watch Your Practice Grow***

The Foundation is reaching out to you, our members to be on the ground floor of our *New Professional Membership Program.* For only $360, you will have access to the tools and consulting to really help you build the practice of your dreams. The first 250 to sign up for the Professional Membership will be Charter members and will receive 3 free original "Applied Trophology" articles from the original series (These are not reprints). For more information go to our web site at www.ifnh.org to download your application today or call 858 488-8932.

As the stewards of the Lee Foundation IFNH is only able to carry on its mission through your generous financial support and donations. It's only through your contribution that we can continue our work. Join us in keep the spirit of the ***Lee Foundation Alive!!***

Yours Naturally,

John R..Brady, III
Director